LEARNING DISABILITIES

Learning Disabilities

From Identification to Intervention

JACK M. FLETCHER
G. REID LYON
LYNN S. FUCHS
MARCIA A. BARNES

THE GUILFORD PRESS
New York   London

To our spouses—Patricia McEnery, Diane Lyon,
Doug Fuchs, and Mark Drummond—
for many years of love and support

©2007 The Guilford Press
A Division of Guilford Publications, Inc.
72 Spring Street, New York, NY 10012
www.guilford.com

Printed in the United States of America

This book is printed on acid-free paper.

Last digit is print number: 9 8 7 6 5 4 3 2

Library of Congress Cataloging-in-Publication Data

Learning disabilities : from identification to intervention / Jack M. Fletcher . . . [et al.].
  p. cm.
 Includes bibliographical references and index.
 ISBN-13: 978-1-59385-370-9 (hardcover : alk. paper)
 ISBN-10: 1-59385-370-X (hardcover : alk. paper)
 1. Learning disabilities. 2. Learning disabilities—Research. I. Fletcher, Jack M.
(Jack McFarlin)
  LC4704.L386 2007
  371.9—dc22

                                        2006029984

About the Authors

Jack M. Fletcher, PhD, is a Distinguished University Professor of Psychology at the University of Houston. For the past 30 years, Dr. Fletcher, a child neuropsychologist, has completed research on many issues related to learning disabilities, including definition and classification, neurobiological correlates, and intervention, and has written over 200 articles in peer-reviewed journals. He is Principal Investigator of a Learning Disability Research Center grant funded by the National Institute of Child Health and Human Development (NICHD), as well as an NICHD program project grant on math disabilities. Dr. Fletcher has served on and chaired the NICHD Mental Retardation/Developmental Disabilities study section and is a former member of the NICHD National Advisory Council. He was the 2003 recipient of the Samuel T. Orton Award from the International Dyslexia Association and a corecipient of the 2006 Albert J. Harris Award from the International Reading Association.

G. Reid Lyon, PhD, is the Executive Vice President for Research and Evaluation at Best Associates and Whitney International University, headquartered in Dallas, Texas. Prior to joining Best Associates, Dr. Lyon served as a research psychologist and the Chief of the Child Development and Behavior Branch within the NICHD at the National Institutes of Health, where he was responsible for the direction of research programs in developmental psychology, cognitive neuroscience, behavioral pediatrics, reading, and learning disorders. In addition, he has taught children with learning disabilities and was a third-grade classroom teacher as well as a school psychologist in the public schools in New Mexico, North Carolina, and Vermont. Dr. Lyon has authored, coauthored, and edited more than 120 journal articles, books, and book chapters addressing evidence-based education and learning differences and disabilities in children.

Lynn S. Fuchs, PhD, is Nicholas Hobbs Professor of Special Education and Human Development at Vanderbilt University, where she also codirects the Kennedy Center Reading Clinic. She has published more than 200 articles in peer-reviewed journals and sits on the editorial boards of several journals, including the *Journal of Educational Psychology, Scientific Studies of Reading, Elementary School Journal, Journal of Learning Disabilities,* and *Exceptional Children.* Her research focuses on classroom-based assessment as well as instructional methods for students with reading disabilities and math disabilities. In addition, Dr. Fuchs has conducted programmatic research on assessment methods for enhancing instructional planning and on instructional methods for improving reading and math outcomes for students with learning disabilities.

Marcia A. Barnes, PhD, is an Associate Professor of Psychology and University Research Chair at the University of Guelph and Associate Professor of Pediatrics at the University of Toronto. She is also an adjunct scientist at the Toronto Hospital for Sick Children. Dr. Barnes's research focuses on math and reading comprehension disabilities in children with and without brain injuries. She also studies the typical development of reading comprehension skills, and has written over 60 papers. She is a member of the editorial board of the *Journal of the International Neuropsychology Society* and on national grant review panels in the United States and Canada. Dr. Barnes recently served as a member of the Expert Panel on Literacy and Numeracy Instruction for Students with Special Education Needs for the Ontario Ministry of Education.

Preface

In an era of increased focus on the evidence base that supports different educational practices, this book integrates different domains of scientific inquiry, practice, and policy involving learning disabilities (LDs). Representing several disciplines in psychology and education, the book is an exposition and analysis of the scientific research base that has accumulated over the past 30 years on LDs, ranging from identification and assessment, to cognitive and neurobiological factors, to intervention. The heart of the book is its focus on research on different domains of LDs involving reading (word recognition, fluency, and comprehension); mathematics (computations and problem solving); and written language (handwriting, spelling, and composition). A clear link is made between what is known about the typical development of these skills and how to teach them, reflecting evidence that the academic difficulties of LDs are not qualitatively discrete entities but the lower end of a continuum of academic ability.

We argue that an understanding of LDs must stem from a classification model that leads to definitions of and methods for identifying LDs that epitomize the historically central construct of unexpected underachievement. Also based on the classification, specific LDs can be identified according to their core academic deficits, providing the capacity for systematically studying the neurobiological and environmental factors that interact to produce an LD. Although the book has a research focus, it extends into practice, with considerable attention to assessment and intervention methods that have demonstrable efficacy in each domain of LDs.

Our interest in writing the book was stimulated in part by recognition of the major changes in U.S. public policy involving education, beginning with the focus on scientifically based instruction in the reauthoriza-

tion of the Elementary and Secondary Education Act, through the No
Child Left Behind Act of 2001, and continuing with the 2004 Reauthorization of the Individuals with Disabilities Education Act (IDEA 2004).
For the first time since the initial legislation supporting IDEA in 1975,
IDEA 2004 allows the U.S. public education system to examine new
approaches to identifying and treating LDs under the general rubric of
response to intervention (RTI) models and specific expectations for appropriate instruction in general education as a prerequisite to identifying
LDs.

Although RTI models can be used to help identify LDs, a major purpose of these models is to enhance education outcomes for all children
through closer integration of general and special education. A frequently
asked question about these models is whether the necessary assessment
and intervention methods needed for implementation are sufficiently developed. We review much of this research, identify gaps in the knowledge base, and conclude that, although some issues require additional
scientific inquiry, a substantial research base does exist and many of the
issues regarding RTI models represent not an absence of assessment and
intervention tools, but rather the need to scale them.

We hope this book facilitates the capacity of educators and schools
to identify sound tools for assessment and instruction and to implement
them in the service of better outcomes for students at risk for or identified with LDs. We believe that the research incorporated in this book
shows that LDs are real, that the field does have a strong scientific basis,
and that the development of the field continues in a positive direction
and will continue to flourish. Most important, robust instructional
methods for each of the specific LDs are identified in the book, reflecting
the accumulation of substantial scientific information on LDs that can
be used to inform practice and policy.

This volume evolved from a series of chapters on LDs that appeared in
several recent books published by The Guilford Press (Fletcher, Morris,
Francis, & Lyon, 2003; Lyon, Fletcher, & Barnes, 2003; Lyon, Fletcher,
Fuchs, & Chhabra, 2006). For part of this book, we reorganized these
chapters into five specific domains of LDs and directly linked the intervention components with the components involving identification, cognitive
correlates, and neurobiological factors. New chapters were written on
classification and definition and assessment of LDs. The research has been
thoroughly updated, and an overarching model is proposed to integrate
the different sources of scientific evidence reviewed in the book. The result
is a single volume that integrates research on classification and definition,
cognitive processing, neurobiological factors, and instruction.

We thank Rochelle Serwator, our editor at Guilford, who proposed
the idea for this book, and Eric J. Mash, Leif G. Terdal, and Russell A.

Barkley, who edited two of the volumes in which parts of some of the chapters were originally composed. We also thank Rita Taylor, Michelle Hoffman, and Susan Ciancio for many hours of support in completing the book.

Grants from the National Institute of Child Health and Human Development (NICHD) to Jack M. Fletcher helped support some of the research in the book, including P50 HD052117, Texas Center for Learning Disabilities, and P01 HD46261, Cognitive, Instructional, and Neuroimaging Factors in Math (which also supported research by Lynn S. Fuchs and Marcia A. Barnes). Additional support for Dr. Fletcher was obtained from NSF9979968, Early Development of Reading Skills: A Cognitive Neuroscience Approach (funded under the Interagency Educational Research Initiative by the National Science Foundation, NICHD, and the Institute for Educational Sciences (J. M. Fletcher, Principal Investigator); P50 HD25802, Center for Learning and Attention Disorders (S. E. Shaywitz and B. A. Shaywitz, Principal Investigators); and R01 HD38346, Brain Activation Profiles in Dyslexia (A. C. Papanicolaou, Principal Investigator). Dr. Fuchs's work was also supported by NICHD Grant R01 HD46154-01, Understanding/Preventing Math Problem-Solving Disability; H324V980001, Center on Accelerating Student Learning, and 324U010004, National Research Center on Learning Disabilities, Office of Special Education Programs in the U.S. Department of Education. Dr. Barnes's work was also supported by funding from the Canadian Language and Literacy Research Network and NICHD Grant P01 HD048497, Preschool Curricula: Outcomes and Developmental Processes. The contents are solely the responsibility of the authors and do not necessarily represent the official views of any of the sources of grant support.

Contents

CHAPTER 1

Introduction

Since learning disabilities (LDs) were federally designated in the United States as "handicapping conditions" in 1968, the proportion of children identified with LDs has increased steadily, with such students now representing approximately one-half of all children receiving special education services (U.S. Department of Education, 1999). Although there was relatively little research on LDs at the time that the original federal disabilities legislation was enacted, significant progress has been made in understanding and treating LDs involving reading, mathematics, and written expression. With the area of word reading leading the way, major advances have been made in classification and definition issues (Fletcher, Morris, & Lyon, 2003; Lyon et al., 2001), cognitive processes (Siegel, 2003), neurobiological correlates involving the brain (Eden & Zeffiro, 1998; S. E. Shaywitz & B. A. Shaywitz, 2005) and genetics (Grigorenko, 2005; Plomin & Kovas, 2005), assessment practices (Fuchs & Fuchs, 1998; Speece & Case, 2001), and intervention (Swanson, Harris, & Graham, 2003). The advances in intervention are especially promising in the reading area, as the research shows that reading disabilities are preventable in many children, and that intensive interventions can be effective with older children who have severe reading difficulties. Moreover, in the reading area, research is converging on a comprehensive model of the most common LD—dyslexia—that is grounded in reading development theory and accounts for neurobiological and environmental factors as well as for the effects of intervention (Lyon et al., 2001; Plomin & Kovas, 2005; Rayner, Foorman, Perfetti, Pesetsky, & Seidenberg, 2002; Vellutino, Fletcher, Scanlon, & Snowling, 2004). Indeed, the same theory that explains how children develop reading skills explains why some fail, unifying the research on LDs in reading and the normative development of reading ability.

Given these advances for dyslexia, similar advances for other LDs cannot be far behind. Presently the construct of LDs and the many definitions that serve as conceptual frameworks for their identification and treatment continue to be frequently misunderstood. The field is beset by pervasive disagreements about the definition of LDs, diagnostic criteria, assessment practices, treatment procedures, and educational policies (Lyon et al., 2001). In writing this book, our goal is to help integrate the disparate sources of information into a more coherent account of LDs, beginning with an evidence-based approach to definition and classification and the implications of this approach for assessment and identification. With an adequate classification, it becomes possible to comprehensively discuss research on the nature, types, causes, and treatment of LDs, thus beginning to integrate science and practice. This book is about the horizontal integration of knowledge on LDs, providing less depth within different domains of knowledge in favor of the connections across these domains and the boundaries across disciplines. It is less about new ideas on LDs and more about a comprehensive accounting of the evidence base and its implications for enhancing outcomes for LDs.

AN OVERARCHING MODEL

Figure 1.1 presents a framework for understanding the different sources of variability that influence outcomes in children with LDs. We used this framework to organize our reviews of the major types of LDs in reading, mathematics, and written expression. The framework is anchored in a hypothetical classification of LDs based on strengths and weaknesses in academic skills. For each LD, the primary manifestation of the disability represents specific academic skill deficits (e.g., in word recognition, reading comprehension, reading fluency, mathematics computations/problem solving, and written expression). We believe that a classification of LDs can be validated that has its origins in these academic skill deficits, representing a set of achievement markers that are the basis for the classification.

The second level of analysis involves child characteristics, including core cognitive processes (e.g., phonological awareness and rapid letter naming) that directly determine the academic skill deficits (e.g., word recognition skills and reading fluency) as well as academic strengths. The performance or operation of academic strengths and weaknesses is also influenced by a second set of characteristics that are in the psychosocial domain, such as the child's motivation, social skills, or behavioral problems involving anxiety, depression, and/or attention that interfere with performance in academic domains. The arrow between

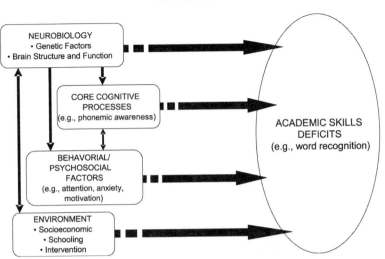

FIGURE 1.1. Framework representing different sources of variability that influence academic outcomes, the primary manifestations of the disability, in children with LDs.

core cognitive processes and behavioral/psychosocial factors is bidirectional, as cognitive difficulties can also lead to problems with, for example, attention and social skills.

The third level of analysis represents the influence of neurobiological and environmental factors. The neurobiological factors include neural and genetic sources of variability that impact academic skill deficits either through their influence on child characteristics or directly on the academic skills themselves. Environmental factors include the social and economic circumstances that attend the child, as well as schooling influences, such as the quality of the school and different interventions. The arrow linking neurobiological and environmental factors is bidirectional, indicating an interaction of these domains. In an integrated account of LDs, all of these levels of analysis must be considered. In this book we focus on the relation of academic skills and core cognitive processes, neurobiological factors, and intervention. We used different empirical and conceptual syntheses of a particular domain whenever possible as opposed to detailed reviews of individual studies.

ORGANIZATION OF THE BOOK

To understand advances involving LDs, and the material in Chapters 3–9, one must understand the field's struggle for a scientific foundation.

We believe that these efforts are tied to progress in classification and definition, and we present a hypothetical classification of LDs based on variation in achievement markers. In Chapter 2, we review the historical events that have molded the field of LDs into its present form, with a focus on the origins of current policy-based definitions of LDs through the 2004 reauthorization of the Individuals with Disabilities Education Act (IDEA, 2004). A review of the history shows that LDs have been difficult to define, partly because they do not constitute a homogeneous disorder. In fact, LDs by definition refer to deficits in one or more of several domains of academic achievement, including reading disabilities, mathematics disabilities, and disabilities in written expression. Each type of LD is characterized by distinct definitional and diagnostic issues, as well as issues associated with heterogeneity. However, the heterogeneity is best accounted for by variations in academic skills, so that a classification that explicitly incorporates this variation permits strong linkages with normative research on the development of different academic domains and a coherent framework for organizing cognitive, neurobiological, and intervention research, as in Figure 1.1.

The case for this approach is made in Chapter 3, which discusses classification and definition, and Chapter 4, which discusses assessment and identification. We argue that although LDs are heterogeneous, they are best defined by markers involving academic skills. Evidence suggests five major types of LD involving word recognition, reading fluency, and reading comprehension; mathematics; and written expression. These domains have been selected both because of their prominence in current definitions of LDs, and because most children and adults are identified as having LDs owing to unexpected underachievement or atypical development in these areas. In mathematics and written expression, less is known about the key academic skill deficits that would represent the marker variables in the classification. It is possible that other forms of LDs will be identified or that some of these domains will be further differentiated. A convergence of research on identification, assessment, and intervention will be required, which is occurring for these domains.

From a classification perspective, the central historical underpinnings of the construct of LDs are intrinsically linked to the concept of unexpected underachievement—the original idea was that LDs represent a group of individuals who should be able to achieve because they have intact sensory skills, adequate intelligence, an absence of emotional difficulties that interfere with learning, and have adequate opportunity to learn (Kirk, 1963). Hence, poor achievement is unexpected. With this approach, the failure to ensure that the instructional opportunities afforded the child are sufficient for learning academic skills has been a major culprit in the elusiveness of a definition of unexpected underachievement. Thus, in Chapter 3, we argue that classifications should ensure that those who are identified with LDs show evidence that they are demonstrably difficult to teach. *No person can be defined as learning disabled in the absence of evidence of a lack of adequate response to instruction that is effective with most students, and most efforts at definition incorporate appropriate instructional opportunities as an exclusionary criterion.* The issue is how to define adequate response to instruction, which is why we focus on serial curriculum-based assessments in Chapter 4 (Fuchs & Fuchs, 1998). We support a hybrid model of identification proposed by a consensus group of researchers (Bradley, Danielson, & Hallahan, 2002) that includes three components: (1) inadequate response to appropriate instruction; (2) poor achievement in reading, mathematics, and/or written expression; and (3) evidence that other factors (e.g., sensory disorders, mental retardation, limited proficiency in the language of instruction, inadequate instruction) are not the primary cause of low achievement.

From an assessment perspective, Chapter 4 suggests that identification should focus on academic achievement and response to instruction, especially because these types of assessments are directly linked to treatment and because academic therapies have the strongest evidence for efficacy. Assessment and identification must also involve evaluations of instructional response and the quality of instruction. Although Figure 1.1 includes multiple levels of analysis, a strong classification is based on a parsimonious set of markers that identify members into the different parts of the classification. Our discussion of academic skill deficits attempts to identify these markers, which should predict the cognitive and neurobiological factors. There are important interactions with the psychosocial and environmental variables that are critical for understanding intervention. Thus, adequate identification and intervention requires a focus on achievement, response to instruction, and other factors that impact the development of academic skills. These latter factors are typically used to exclude people from learning disabled classifications. However, without a focus on these factors, many children will be identified as learning disabled for whom the explanation of the disability is poor instruction and not unexpected underachievement. Although we recognize that cognitive processes are tightly linked with academic skill deficits, we find little evidence suggesting that assessment of these cognitive processes adds information that will facilitate intervention design; even the strengths and weaknesses in cognitive skills that some view as essential to the nature of LDs (e.g., phonological awareness) can be understood simply by assessing the achievement domains (e.g., word recognition). Routine assessment of cognitive skills is not indicated, just as the impressive research base on neuroimaging does not suggest a need for brain scans of each child suspected of LDs: the neural correlates are predicted by the task used to elicit brain activation (word reading, precise calculation, etc.), which should also predict the correlated cognitive processes. The ability to make these predictions and simplify the classification, identification, and assessment process signals the emergence of an evidence base in LDs and a classification with simple decision rules that moves people into treatment as quickly as possible.

In Chapters 5–9, we review each academic domain of LDs. In each of these chapters, we address (1) academic skill deficits that represent the achievement markers of the disability (e.g., word reading and spelling in dyslexia); (2) core cognitive processes correlated with the academic skills; (3) the epidemiology and developmental course; (4) neurobiological factors (brain structure and function, genetics) hypothesized to cause and/or contribute to the specific type of LD (when any LD has been identified); and (5) intervention research, including issues relevant to the purposes of treatment and the validity of different treatment protocols. The conduct of intervention research with individuals with LDs is complex and labor intensive. Several factors have consistently impeded attempts to study the effectiveness and the efficacy of different interventions in a well-controlled manner, not the least of which is the need to carefully define the types of LDs that are treated. As in the neurobiological research, this need is paramount and has been directly linked to progress across the field of LDs. For future research and treatment efforts to be as productive and informative as possible, they must be tied to an explicit classification.

The book concludes with Chapter 10, a review of current issues and a look toward the future. We focus on the need to continue to integrate research on LDs with normative research on the development of academic and cognitive skills. Closer links of neurobiological and instructional research are possible and promising. The quality of treatment research must continue to improve, and we identify factors that must be addressed in intervention studies. We summarize 10 principles that have emerged from research and should provide guidance to the field. Finally, we suggest from our perspective that the future of LDs is tied to the scientific process, and that the field must embrace the evolving process of scientific research and move away from unverified clinical intuition and anecdotes in order to provide a solid foundation for practice. Clinical experience is a fertile ground for hypothesis generation, but the inferences that emerge from experience must be empirically verified, particularly in identification practices and intervention. The issue remains: For whom do different factors converge to cause LDs, and how do different components of intervention relate to the various expressions of LD?

CAVEATS

Some caveats are in order. We present a particular approach to understanding LDs, which is based on a classification with its roots in academic achievement and which we use to account for the heterogeneity of LDs. Academic deficits are necessary, but not sufficient for a classification of LDs; without achievement as an anchor, it is difficult to validate the construct of LDs. We do not review research on students broadly defined as learning disabled when the form of academic impairment is not indicated, unless that approach predominates the instructional literature. In the absence of this type of specification, the groups are too heterogeneous to determine the relation with specific forms of LD.

We do not review research suggesting that LDs involving social or executive functions should be separately identified, because we do not feel that such approaches to identification result in effective classifications of LDs. Similarly, although we recognize that other approaches to defining "verbal" and "nonverbal" LDs have represented major contributions to the field (e.g. Johnson & Myklebust, 1967; Rourke, 1989), we do not explicitly organize our approach around this system for definition and classification. We do discuss some of these conceptual approaches in the context of the academic skills associated with them, such as the brief discussion of nonverbal LDs in Chapter 8 (mathematics LDs). The reader is encouraged to examine these approaches, such as the approach to the definition of "verbal" and "nonverbal" LDs developed by Rourke and colleagues (www.nld-bprourke.ca/index.html).

Given the enormous volume and complexity of literature on topics associated with treatment and instruction, our review of relevant research is necessarily selective rather than exhaustive. It was not possible to address research related to disorders of attention or to social and emotional difficulties—areas of development that are clearly problematic for many students with LDs. These influences are usually comorbid, that is, represent co-occurring difficulties as opposed to qualitatively different LDs. In terms of Figure 1.1, we do not provide an extensive discussion of the psychosocial and behavioral factors or a broad assessment of environmental factors (e.g., poverty) that impact on the development of children with LDs (for review, see Phillips & Lonigan, 2005). This is partly because there is little evidence that the phenotypic manifestations of academic difficulties vary by putative cause. We focus instead on intervention. Most psychosocial and environmental influences make the academic problems more severe, but do not produce qualitative variation; hence the importance of response to instruction in operationalizing unexpected underachievement (Chapter 3). Moreover, although various theoretical and conceptual models related to treatment are implicit in our review of interventions, as are specific intervention methods, we do not view the work emanating from these different sources and perspectives as necessarily contradictory and do not discuss these models in detail (see Lyon, Fletcher, Fuchs, & Chhabra, 2006). Rather, thoughtful integration of these models is resulting in more efficacious interventions for individuals with different types of LDs. It is clear that academic therapies that involve substantial exposure to reading, mathematics, and writing are most effective; older approaches to interventions that teach processes or focus on aspects of the disorder (e.g., vision) that are not directly tied to the academic skill do not result in improved outcomes for students with LDs. Further, the literature is replete with claims for instructional and treatment methods that are based on subjective, non-replicated clinical reports, testimonial information, and anecdotal statements on groups broadly defined as learning disabled. We have limited our discussion to empirical research that extends beyond testimony or evidence of efficacy in the absence of appropriate comparison groups or clearly defined groups of students with specific academic types of LDs. Finally, we attempted to review research from around the world, but our focus on history and policy is narrowly focused on the United States. We do not have good access to policy in other countries and do not always have good access to the many excellent studies completed by our international colleagues, especially in the intervention area.

Even with these stipulations, the range of research covered in this book is broad and there is wide variation in the quality of the studies and syntheses we have selected for discussion. We generally tried to select the strongest possible studies and syntheses for review. The quality of many of these pieces of information leads us to be optimistic about the continued development of both science and practice for LDs. As the example of dyslexia in Chapter 5 shows, LDs are unique among developmental disorders not only in the dramatic growth of knowledge across different domains, but also in the extent of vertical, cross-disciplinary integration that has occurred (Shavelson & Towne, 2002). In the future, we believe that this type of cross-disciplinary integration is essential to the development of a comprehensive model encompassing all forms of LDs, and offer this book in anticipation of continued development of an integrated understanding of LDs.

CHAPTER 2

History of the Field

Since the designation of LD as a disability in U.S. federal legislation in 1968, LDs now represent approximately one-half of all students receiving special education nationally (Donavon & Cross, 2002; President's Commission on Excellence in Special Education, 2002). Yet LDs have traditionally been among the least understood and most debated disabling conditions affecting students (Bradley et al., 2002; Fuchs & Fuchs, 1998; Lyon et al., 2001). Despite the idea advanced by some individuals that LDs constitute a unitary entity (Kavale & Forness, 2000), this observation is not supported by current research. To the contrary, converging scientific evidence shows that LDs represent a general category composed of disabilities in specific academic domains (Lyon, Fletcher, & Barnes, 2003a). Indeed, the heterogeneous nature of the disability was instantiated in U.S. federal regulations dating back to 1977 that organized the different types of LDs into seven areas: (1) listening comprehension (receptive language), (2) oral expression (expressive language), (3) basic reading skills (decoding and word recognition), (4) reading comprehension, (5) written expression, (6) mathematics calculation, and (7) mathematics reasoning.

These separate types of LDs frequently co-occur with one another and with deficits in social skills, emotional disorders, and disorders of attention. Thus, a student with LDs may have a problem in more than one area—a condition referred to as "comorbidity" (Fletcher et al., 1999). Although they are frequently misinterpreted as such, LDs are not synonymous with reading disability or dyslexia (Lyon, Shaywitz, & Shaywitz, 2003b). However, it is the case that much of the available information concerning LDs relates to reading disabilities (Lyon et al., 2001), and the majority of students with LDs (80–90%) demonstrate significant reading difficulties (Kavale & Reese, 1992; Lerner, 1989; Lyon et al., 2001). Moreover, two of every five students receiving special education in the United States were identified because of difficulties in learning to read (President's Commission on Excellence in Special Education, 2002).

The goal of understanding LDs is to provide the most effective instruction possible in order to ameliorate the disabling effects of the conditions. However, as many researchers and practitioners have learned, identifying and understanding the nature, causes, and correlates that should be considered when teaching children with LDs is difficult. As we discuss in this book, the accumulating evidence base on LDs is now playing a more explicit and prominent role in informing instruction than ever before. The field has progressed from simple explanations focusing on phenotypic behavioral and cognitive characteristics to more complex explanations that link cognitive, neurobiological, and instructional factors. From clinical and educational standpoints, the validity of the construct of LDs is directly linked to its ability to inform intervention decisions. As such, instruction is central to the concept of LDs as a disabling condition. If identifying students with LDs does not inform intervention and enhance communication among educators providing the instruction, then the concept would be virtually meaningless—except as a legal definition of a group of people with disabilities requiring civil rights protection.

To understand how these alternative perspectives have evolved, this chapter examines the historical underpinnings of LDs. Many sources are available that provide overarching reviews of the field's scientific, social, and political history and development (Doris, 1993; Hammill, 1993; Kavale & Forness, 1985; Morrison & Siegel, 1991; Rutter, 1982; Satz & Fletcher, 1980; Torgesen, 1991). These commentaries indicate that the field of LDs developed in response to two major needs. First, the emergence of the field was linked to a need to understand individual differences in learning and performance among children and adults displaying *specific* deficits in spoken or written language, while maintaining integrity in overall adaptive functioning. Unexpected patterns of strengths and *specific* weaknesses in learning were first noted and studied by physicians and psychologists, thus giving the biomedical and psychological orientation that has always characterized the field of LDs. Second, the LD movement developed as an applied field of special education driven by social and political forces, and from a need to provide services to youth whose learning characteristics were not being adequately addressed by the educational system. Each of these historical contexts is reviewed briefly.

LDs AND THE STUDY
OF INDIVIDUAL DIFFERENCES

Gall's Influence

Torgesen (1991) pointed out that interest in the causes and outcomes of interindividual and intraindividual differences in cognition and learning can be traced to early Greek civilization. However, the first work that has clear relevance to today's conceptualizations of LDs was conducted by Gall in the context of his work on disorders of spoken language in the early 19th century (Wiederholt, 1974). In describing the characteristics of one patient with brain damage, Gall recorded the following:

> In consequence of an attack of apoplexy, a soldier found it impossible to express in spoken language his feelings and ideas. His face bore no signs of a deranged intellect. His mind (*esprit*) found the answer to questions addressed to him and he carried out all he was told to do; shown an armchair and asked if he knew what it was, he answered by seating himself in it. He could not articulate on the spot a word pronounced for him to repeat; but a few moments later the word escaped from his lips as if voluntarily. It was not his tongue, which was embarrassed; for he moved it with great agility and could pronounce quite well a large number of isolated words. His memory was not at fault, for he signified his anger at being unable to express himself concerning many things, which he wished to communicate. It was the faculty of speech, alone, which was abolished. (quoted in Head, 1926, p. 11)

The relevance of Gall's observations to present conceptualizations of LDs was accurately summarized by Hammill (1993). Hammill postulated that Gall noted that some of his patients could not speak but could produce thoughts in writing, thus manifesting a pattern of relative strengths and weaknesses in oral and written language. In addition, Gall established that such patterns of strengths and weaknesses were a function of brain damage, and that brain damage could selectively impair one particular language capability but not affect others. Thus, the clinical roots were established in the area of brain injury for the present-day observation that many children with LDs manifest "specific" deficits rather than pervasive or "generalized" deficits. Finally, Gall argued that it was essential to rule out other disabling conditions, like mental retardation or deafness, that could impair a patient's performance. Within

this context, the origin for the "exclusion" component of current definitions of LDs is evident.

Early Neurology and Acquired Language Disorders

A number of other medical professionals also began to observe and report on patients demonstrating intraindividual strengths and weaknesses
that included specific deficits in linguistic, reading, and cognitive abilities. For example, Broca (1865) provided important observations that
have served to build the foundation of the "specificity" hypothesis in
learning disabilities. Broca (1865) reported that "expressive aphasia," or
the inability to speak, resulted from selective (rather than diffuse) lesions
in the anterior regions of the left hemisphere, primarily localized in the
second frontal convolution. The effects of a lesion in this area of the
brain were highly consistent in right-handed individuals and *did not* appear to affect receptive language ability (listening) or other nonlanguage
functions (e.g., visual perception, spatial awareness).

Similarly, Wernicke (1894) introduced the concept of a "disconnection
syndrome," predicting that the aphasic syndrome termed "conduction
aphasia" could result from a disconnection of the receptive (sensory)
speech area from the motor speech zone by a punctate lesion in the left
hemisphere. Wernicke's observations have also been relevant to theory
building in LDs. Wernicke reported that a complex function such as receptive language could be impaired within an individual who did not
display other significant cognitive or linguistic dysfunctions. Hence, the
concept of intraindividual differences in information processing was
born, primarily using observations and clinical studies with adults with
specific brain damage.

In the late 1800s and early 1900s, additional cases of unexpected
cognitive and linguistic difficulties within the context of otherwise normal functioning were reported. These cases were unique because they
did not seem to have the same neurological characteristics as acquired
disorders of language occurring with impairment of sensory or motor
functions. Kussmaul (1877) described a patient who was unable to read
despite having sufficient intellectual and perceptual skills. Additional reports by Hinshelwood (1895, 1917), Morgan (1896), and others (Bastian, 1898; Clairborne, 1906) distinguished a specific type of learning
deficit characterized by an inability to read against a background of normal intelligence and adequate opportunity to learn. Hinshelwood (1917)
described a 10-year-old youngster as follows:

> The boy had been at school three years and had got on well with every
> subject except reading. He was apparently a bright and in every respect

an intelligent boy. He had been learning music for a year and had made good progress in it. In all departments of his studies where the instruction was oral he had made good progress, showing that his auditory memory was good. He performs simple sums quite correctly, and his progress in arithmetic has been regarded as quite satisfactory. He has no difficulty in learning to write. His visual acuity is good. (pp. 46–47)

By the beginning of the 20th century, evidence from several sources contributed to a set of observations that defined a unique type of learning difficulty in adults *and* children—specific rather than general in presentation, and distinct from disorders associated with sensory handicaps and subaverage general intelligence. As Hynd and Willis (1988) have summarized, the most salient and reliable early observations of individuals with learning difficulties included the following: (1) the children had some form of congenital learning problem; (2) more male than female children were affected; (3) the disorder was heterogeneous with respect to the specific pattern and the severity of deficits; (4) the disorder might be related to a developmental process affecting primarily left-hemisphere central language processes; and (5) typical classroom instruction was not adequate in meeting the children's educational needs.

Orton and the Origins of Dyslexia

During the 1920s, Samuel Orton extended the study of reading disabilities with clinical studies designed to test the hypothesis that reading deficits were a function of a delay or failure of the left cerebral hemisphere to establish dominance for language functions. According to Orton (1928), children with reading disabilities tended to reverse letters such as *b/d* and *p/q*, and words such as *saw/was* and *not/ton*, because of the lack of left-hemispheric dominance for the processing of linguistic symbols.

Neither Orton's theory of reading disabilities nor his observation that reversals were symptomatic of the disorder has stood the test of time (Torgesen, 1991). However, Orton's writings were highly influential in stimulating research, mobilizing teacher and parent groups to bring attention to reading disorders and other LDs, and on the development of instructional techniques for teaching children with reading disabilities.

Moreover, Orton's influence on present-day conceptualizations of LDs can be seen indirectly in his early attempts to classify a range of language and motor disabilities in addition to reading disabilities (Doris, 1993). More specifically, in 1937, Orton reported a number of cases in which children of average to above-average intelligence manifested one of these six disabilities: (1) "developmental alexia," or difficulty in learning to read; (2) "developmental agraphia," or significant difficulty in learning to write; (3) "developmental word deafness," or a specific deficit in verbal understanding within a context of normal auditory acuity; (4) "developmental motor aphasia," or motor speech delay; (5) abnormal clumsiness; and (6) stuttering. Orton (1937) was the first to stress that reading disabilities manifested at a symbolic level appeared to be related to cerebral dysfunction rather than a specific brain lesion (as postulated by Hinshelwood and others) and could be identified among children with average to above-average intelligence.

The Straussian Movement and the Concept of Cerebral Dysfunction

Whereas Orton's contributions are linked primarily to the development of scientific and clinical interest in reading disabilities (particularly dyslexia), it was the work of Strauss and Werner (1943) and their colleagues (Strauss & Lehtinen, 1947) after World War II that led directly to the emergence of the general category of LDs as a formally recognized field (Doris, 1993; Rutter, 1982; Torgesen, 1991). This work built on earlier attempts to understand the behavioral difficulties of children who subsequently were described as hyperactive. In this series of clinical observations, children's overactivity, impulsivity, and concrete thinking were attributed to brain damage in the absence of physical evidence of injury to the nervous system.

Strauss and Werner expanded this concept in research involving children with mental retardation. They were particularly interested in comparing the behavior of children whose retardation was associated with known brain damage, with that of children whose retardation was not associated with neurological impairment but was presumably familial in nature. Strauss and Lehtinen (1947) reported that children with mental retardation and brain injury manifested difficulties on tasks assessing figure–ground perception, attention, and concept formation in addition to hyperactivity. However, children without brain damage but with mental retardation performed in a manner similar to children who were not mentally impaired and were less likely to show behavioral overactivity.

Within the context of these studies, Strauss's group subsequently observed what they believed were similar patterns of behavior and performance in children with average intelligence who displayed behavioral and learning difficulties. They attributed the behavior of all these groups of children to a syndrome they called "minimal brain injury" (MBI). From these studies, the concept of "minimal brain dysfunction" (MBD) emerged in the 1960s (Clements, 1966), with an emphasis on the

Straussian thesis that MBI or MBD could be identified solely on the basis of behavioral signs, even when physical and neurological examinations were normal.

> When no mental retardation exists, the presence of psychological disturbances can be discovered by the use of some of our qualitative tests for perceptual and cognitive disturbances. Although the [physical] criteria may be negative, whereas the behavior of the child in question resembles that characteristic for brain injury, and even though the performances of the child on our tests are not strongly indicative of brain injury, it may still be reasonable to consider a diagnosis of brain injury. (Strauss & Lehtinen, 1947, p. 112)

The Straussian movement had a profound influence on the development of the field of LDs (Doris, 1993; Hammill, 1993; Kavale & Forness, 1985). Torgesen (1991) concluded that three concepts emerging from the Straussian movement provided a rationale for the development of the field of LDs separately from other fields of education: (1) Individual differences in learning could be understood by examining the different ways that children approach learning tasks (the processes that aid or interfere with learning); (2) educational procedures should be tailored to patterns of processing strengths and weaknesses in the individual child; and (3) children with deficient learning processes may be helped to learn normally by employing teaching methods that focus on their processing strengths rather than their weaknesses. Expanding on this list, Kavale and Forness (1985) included (1) The locus of an LD is within the affected individual, and thus represents a medical (disease) model; (2) LDs are associated with (or caused by) neurological dysfunction; (3) the academic problems observed in children with LDs are related to psychological processing deficits, most notably in the perceptual–motor domain; (4) the academic failure of children with LDs occurs despite the presence of normal intelligence; and (5) LDs cannot primarily be due to other handicapping conditions.

Cruickshank, Myklebust, Johnson, and Kirk and the Concept of LDs

Among the most significant behavioral scientists involved in the early conceptualization and study of LDs were William Cruickshank, Helmer Myklebust, Doris Johnson, and Samuel Kirk, all of whom propelled the field away from a focus on etiology toward an emphasis on learner characteristics and educational interventions to address learning deficits. For example, Cruickshank and his colleagues (Cruickshank, Bice, & Wallen, 1957) studied and recommended modifications in classroom environments to reduce stimuli hypothesized to be distracting for children with learning and attention deficits. Helmer Myklebust and Doris Johnson at Northwestern University conducted numerous studies of the effects of different types of language and perceptual deficits on academic and social learning in children. They were also among the first to develop well-designed intervention procedures for the remediation of disabilities in skills related to school learning (Johnson & Myklebust, 1967). However, it was Samuel Kirk who proposed the term "learning disabilities" in a 1963 conference devoted to exploring problems of perceptually handicapped children. Kirk (1963) stated:

> I have used the term "learning disabilities" to describe a group of children who have disorders in the development of language, speech, reading, and associated communication skills needed for social interaction. In this group, I do not include children who have sensory handicaps such as blindness, because we have methods of managing and training the deaf and blind. I also excluded from this group children who have generalized mental retardation. (pp. 2–3)

By 1963 the new field was moving toward the formal legislative designation of LD as a specific disability with entitlements for civil rights protections and special services. This movement was based largely on the arguments of Kirk and others that children with LDs (1) had different learning characteristics than children diagnosed with mental retardation or emotional disturbance; (2) manifested learning characteristics that resulted from intrinsic (i.e., neurobiological) rather than environmental factors; (3) demonstrated learning difficulties that were "unexpected," given the children's strengths in other areas; and (4) required specialized educational interventions. Note that in this insightful definition, no mention is made of intelligence. Rather, the focus is on social interaction and "normal" adaptive behavior. Exclusionary conditions are identified on the basis of differential intervention needs, not simply defining LDs in terms of what conditions are not LDs. What is interesting is that the field received its initial momentum on the strength of clinical observation and advocacy.

THE INFLUENCE OF ADVOCACY ON DEFINITIONS AND THE RECOGNITION OF THE FIELD

Not uncommonly, in both the educational and public health domains, LDs were initially and formally identified as disabilities on the basis of advocacy rather than systematic scientific inquiry. In fact, in the United

States, the majority of scientific advances are typically stimulated by vocal critics of the educational or medical status quo. It is rare that a psychological condition, disease, or educational problem is afforded attention until political forces are mobilized by parents, patients, or other affected individuals expressing their concerns about their quality of life to their elected officials. Clearly, this was the case in the field of LDs, in which parents and child advocates successfully lobbied Congress to enact legislation in 1969 through the Education of the Handicapped Act (Public Law 91-230). This law authorized research and training programs to address the needs of children with specific LDs (Doris, 1993).

The diagnostic concept of LDs gained significant momentum during the 1960s and 1970s. As Zigmond (1993) explained, the proliferation of children diagnosed as having LDs during these two decades was related to multiple factors. First, the label "LDs" was not a stigmatizing one. Parents and teachers were more comfortable with the term than with etiologically based labels such as "brain injuries," "MBI," and "perceptual handicaps." Moreover, receiving a diagnosis of an LD did not imply low intelligence, behavioral difficulties, or sensory handicaps. On the contrary, children with LDs manifested difficulties in learning *despite* "normal" adaptive behavior and intelligence, and intact hearing, vision, and emotional status. The fact that youngsters with LDs displayed strong intelligence gave parents and teachers hope that learning difficulties could be surmounted, given that the right set of instructional methods, conditions, and settings could be identified. Advocacy efforts fueled a series of consensus conferences, two of which are noteworthy: one on MBI and the other on LDs. Both attempted to identify a single overarching diagnostic category that could define the disabilities widely believed to hamper the educational and behavioral performance of many children.

MINIMAL BRAIN DYSFUNCTION

In the 1960s, the twin strands of individual differences and social and political advocacy joined together through a common endeavor to define unexpected behavioral difficulties and underachievement dependent on factors intrinsic to the child. The first significant effort involved the development of a definition of MBI in 1962. A formal definition of a syndrome called "minimal brain dysfunction" was formulated in a meeting between the Easter Seals Society and what is now the National Institute of Neurological Disorders and Stroke:

> The term "minimal brain dysfunction syndrome" refers to children of
> near average, average, or above average general intelligence with certain

learning or behavioral disabilities ranging from mild to severe, which are associated with deviations of function of the central nervous system. These deviations may manifest themselves by various combinations of impairment in perception, conceptualization, language, memory, and control of attention, impulse, or motor function. (Clements, 1966, pp. 9–10)

This definition essentially substituted the term "dysfunction" for "injury," recognizing the etiological implications of terms like "injury." It stressed that MBD was a heterogeneous category, encompassing both behavioral and learning difficulties. As noted earlier, this definition stipulated that brain dysfunction could be identified solely on the basis of behavioral signs. However, the definition of MBD was controversial (Rutter, 1982; Satz & Fletcher, 1980). Educators objected to the concept, despite the fact that this definition was based on over half a century of clinical observation and research in clinical neurology, as well as empirical support from emergent psychophysiological methods to study brain function (Dykman, Ackerman, Clements, & Peters, 1971). To the educational community, MBD was closely connected to a medical model and implied that psychologists and physicians would have to work in schools in order to make a diagnosis. Others found the concept fuzzy and too broad (Rutter, 1982). The latter concern was magnified in the 1970s with the development of checklists for MBD that included more than 30 symptoms (Peters, Davis, Goolsby, & Clements, 1973). These symptoms ranged from difficulties with academic skills to aggressive, acting-out behavior. The syndrome encompassed such a broad range of symptoms that the treatment implications of identifying a child with MBD were unclear (Rutter, 1982; Satz & Fletcher, 1980).

American Psychiatric Association

When the third edition of the *Diagnostic and Statistical Manual of Mental Disorders* (DSM-III) was published by the American Psychiatric Association (1980), the concept of MBD was dropped and the learning and behavioral characteristics were separately defined as "specific developmental disorders" and "attention deficit disorder." This division aptly solved the classification problem of the comorbidity of learning and attention disorders that plagued those interested in MBI and MBD. Although many children with LDs also meet criteria for attention-deficit/hyperactivity disorder (ADHD), these are separate disorders (Rutter, 1982). However, both require intervention. Heritability, neurobiological correlates, and intervention needs are different, so unifying them as a single syndrome did not facilitate research or practice.

U.S. Federal Definition of LDs

Not surprisingly, the development of the definition of MBD led to reactions among educators and other professionals working in schools. In 1966, the U.S. Office of Education organized a meeting in which the participants formally defined Kirk's (1963) concept of "learning disability" as follows:

> The term "specific learning disability" means a disorder in one or more of the basic psychological processes involved in understanding or in using language, spoken or written, which may manifest itself in an imperfect ability to listen, speak, read, write, spell, or to do mathematical calculations. The term includes such conditions as perceptual handicaps, brain injury, minimal brain dysfunction, dyslexia, and developmental aphasia. The term does not include children who have learning disabilities, which are primarily the result of visual, hearing, or motor handicaps, or mental retardation, or emotional disturbance, or of environmental, cultural, or economic disadvantage. (U.S. Office of Education, 1968, p. 34)

The resemblance of this 1966 definition of LD to the 1962 definition of MBD is striking (Satz & Fletcher, 1980). Reflecting more than 60 years of work, the notion of MBD as an "unexpected" disorder not attributable to mental deficiency, sensory disorders, emotional disturbance, or cultural or economic disturbance was retained. Etiological terms were dropped and replaced by educational descriptors. The definition acknowledged intrinsic factors within a child and intended to be inclusive of minimal brain dysfunction and other formulations derived from neurology and psychology (Doris, 1993; Rutter, 1982; Satz & Fletcher, 1980). However, the pivotal importance of this definition is that it continues to serve as the U.S. federal statutory definition of LDs. It has persisted through a series of parental and professional advocacy efforts that led to the provision of special education services for children with LDs. This occurred initially through the 1969 Learning Disabilities Act. The statutory definition of LDs in the 1969 Act appeared in the Education for All Handicapped Children Act of 1975 (Public Law 94-142) and is currently in IDEA 2004. This definition has endured despite the fact that it does not specify any inclusionary criteria for LDs. It essentially says that LDs are heterogeneous, reflect problems with cognitive processing, and are not to be commingled with other disorders that represent exclusionary conditions. In a sense, LDs became legitimized and codified in U.S. public law mostly on the basis of what they were not.

The absence of inclusionary criteria became an immediate problem in 1975, with passage of Public Law 94-142 and the expectation that the states would identify and serve children with LDs. In response to this problem, the U.S. Office of Education (1977) published recommendations for procedures for identifying LDs that included the notion of a discrepancy between IQ and achievement as a marker for LDs, as follows:

> a severe discrepancy between achievement and intellectual ability in one or more of the areas: (1) oral expression; (2) listening comprehension; (3) written expression; (4) basic reading skill; (5) reading comprehension; (6) mathematics calculation; or (7) mathematic reasoning. The child may not be identified as having a specific learning disability if the discrepancy between ability and achievement is primarily the result of: (1) a visual, hearing, or motor handicap; (2) mental retardation; (3) emotional disturbance; or (4) environmental, cultural, or economic disadvantage. (p. G1082)

The use of IQ–achievement discrepancy as a marker for LDs has had a profound impact on how LDs are conceptualized. There was some research at the time validating an IQ–achievement discrepancy model (Rutter & Yule, 1975), which has not stood up over time (Fletcher et al., 2002). However, researchers, practitioners, and the public continue to assume that such a discrepancy is a marker for specific types of LDs that are unexpected and categorically distinct from other forms of underachievement. Some researchers continue to use IQ–achievement discrepancy as a key aspect of the identification process (Kavale & Forness, 2000), despite the fact that the evidence base for its validity as a central feature of LD classification is weak to nonexistent (see Chapter 3). But the impact of IQ–achievement discrepancy was clearly apparent in the regulations concerning LD identification in the 1992 and 1997 reauthorizations of IDEA. The statute has maintained the definition of LDs formulated in the 1966 meeting, and the regulations maintained the 1977 procedures until the 2004 reauthorization.

Other Definitions of LDs

The federal definition of LDs has been widely criticized (Fletcher et al., 2002; Kavale & Forness, 1985; Lyon, 1987, Lyon et al., 2001; Senf, 1987). As Torgesen (1991) has pointed out, this definition has at least four major problems that render it ineffective: (1) It does not clearly indicate that LDs are a heterogeneous group of disorders; (2) it fails to recognize that LDs frequently persist and are manifested in adults as well as children; (3) it does not clearly specify that, whatever the cause of LDs, the "final common path" consists of inherent alterations in the way information is processed; and (4) it does not adequately recognize that persons with other handicapping or environmental limitations may have an LD *concurrently* with these conditions. Other formal attempts to tighten the federal definition of LDs have not fared significantly better, as can be seen in the revised definition produced by the National Joint Committee on Learning Disabilities (NJCLD, 1988; see also Hammill, 1993):

> *Learning disabilities* is a general term that refers to a heterogeneous group of disorders manifested by significant difficulty in the acquisition and use of listening, speaking, reading, writing, reasoning, or mathematical abilities. These disorders are intrinsic to the individual, presumed to be due to central nervous system dysfunction, and may occur across the life span. Problems in self-regulatory behavior, social perception, and social interaction may exist with learning disabilities but do not by themselves constitute a learning disability. Although learning disabilities may occur concomitantly with other handicapping conditions (for example, sensory impairment, mental retardation, social and emotional disturbance) or with extrinsic influences (such as cultural differences, insufficient or inappropriate instruction), they are not the result of these conditions or influences. (p. 1)

Although the NJCLD definition addresses the issues of heterogeneity, persistence, intrinsic etiology, and comorbidity discussed by Torgesen (1991), it continues to reflect a vague and ambiguous description of multiple and heterogeneous disorders. These types of definitions cannot be easily operationalized or empirically validated and do not provide clinicians, teachers, or researchers with useful information to enhance communication or improve predictions. There are no inclusionary criteria, and the definition is based on exclusion. Given this state of the field, many scholars have called for a moratorium on the development of broad definitions and advocate definitions that address LDs only in terms of coherent and operational domains. For instance, Stanovich (1993) has stated:

> Scientific investigations of some generically defined entity called "learning disability" simply make little sense given what we already know about heterogeneity across various learning domains. Research investigations must define groups specifically in terms of the domain of deficit (reading disability, arithmetic disability). The extent of co-occurrence of these dysfunctions then becomes an empirical question, not something decided a priori by definition practices. (p. 273)

Both the DSM-IV (American Psychiatric Association, 1994) and the *International Classification of Diseases*, 10th revision (ICD-10; World

Health Organization, 1992), have defined, classified, and coded learning disorders and specific developmental disorders of academic skills into specific deficit domains. For example, DSM-IV provides criteria for the diagnosis of "reading disorder" (315.00), and ICD-10 provides identification criteria under the term "specific reading disorder" (F81.0). DSM-IV and ICD-10 refer to disabilities in mathematics as "mathematics disorder" (315.1) and "specific disorder of arithmetical skills" (F81.2), respectively. Finally, disabilities involving written language skills are classified and coded by DSM-IV as "disorder of written expression" (315.2) and by ICD-10 as "specific spelling disorder" (F81.1). These definitions implicitly support the heterogeneity and exclusion components of most definitions.

Interestingly, the definitions invoke IQ–achievement discrepancy as an inclusionary criterion. But the definitions in DSM-IV and ICD-10 are essentially the same definitions applied to each domain, thus lacking any real specificity. The problems with the federal definition of LDs also apply to the DSM-IV and ICD-10 definitions. Regardless of whether one approaches the task of defining LDs in a general fashion as has been traditionally done at the federal level, or whether one seeks to define domain-specific LDs (e.g., reading disability) as advocated by Stanovich (1993), the definitional process must be informed by and constructed within a classification system that ultimately has communicative and predictive power (Chapter 3). The logic underlying the development of such a classification system is that identification, diagnosis, treatment, and prognosis cannot be addressed effectively until the heterogeneity across and within domain-specific LDs is addressed, and until subgroups are delineated that are theoretically meaningful, reliable, and valid. Of utmost importance is the validity of the three classification hypotheses (discrepancy, heterogeneity, exclusions) implicit in most definitions of LDs.

2004 Revision of the U.S. Regulatory Definition of LDs

In the 2004 reauthorization of IDEA, the U.S. Congress passed statutes that permitted alterations of the 1977 regulations, indicating specifically that (1) states could not require districts to use IQ tests for the identification of students for special education in the LD category, and (2) states had to permit districts to implement identification models that incorporated response to instruction (RTI) (IDEA, 2004). In addition, the statute clearly indicated that children could not be identified for special education if poor achievement was due to lack of appropriate instruction in reading or math, or to limited proficiency in English. In response to the statute, the Office of Special Education and

Rehabilitative Services (OSERS) within the U.S. Department of Education (2006) published federal regulations in response to IDEA 2004 to revise rules for the identification of LDs. What is noteworthy is that the statute and regulations are based on the converging scientific evidence bearing on the limited value of IQ–achievement discrepancies in identifying LDs, while at the same time underscoring the value of RTI in the identification process. Although issues surrounding the validity of IQ–achievement discrepancies and RTI are discussed in detail in Chapter 3, the regulations relevant to LDs are summarized here. In essence, regulations indicate that states:

1. May not require local education agencies (LEAs) to use a discrepancy model for determining whether a student has LDs.
2. Must permit the use of a process that determines if the student responds to scientific research-based intervention.
3. May permit other alternative research-based procedures.

Although a number of advocacy and practitioner groups questioned specific provisions of the regulations, what is encouraging is that all organizations have acknowledged the critical importance of using research to guide policies and practices concerning students with LDs, which is clearly reflected in the IDEA 2004 statutes and regulations. Equally significant in the new statute and regulations is the more explicit recognition that LDs should not be identified in the absence of evidence of appropriate instruction. The statute indicates that LDs may not be identified if the cause of poor achievement is inadequate instruction in reading or math, or limited proficiency with English by requiring:

1. Evidence of appropriate instruction in reading and math in general education.
2. Data-based documentation at repeated intervals of the student's response to this instruction.

This information must be provided to parents and included in team decisions determining whether the child has an LD, that the LD is a disabling condition, and that special education services are warranted. Thus, the IDEA 2004 statute moves toward the accumulating research base on LDs by reducing the focus on IQ tests and emphasizing the critical role of instruction both for preventing LDs and for their identification.

CONCLUSIONS

The field of LDs emerged from a genuine social and educational need. LDs constitute a diagnostic category of interest to clinical practice, law, and policy. Historically, parents, educators, and other advocates for children have successfully negotiated a special education category subsuming LDs as a means of protecting civil rights and procedural safeguards in law (Lyon & Moats, 1997; Zigmond, 1993). In many respects, however, LDs have been legitimized and codified in public law on the basis of what they are not, that is, through a focus on definition by exclusion. Moreover, the concept of LDs is based on what is now a century of attempts to define it as an overarching classification applicable to a wide segment of childhood difficulties involving learning (and behavior). Only in the past 30 or so years have systematic research efforts emerged that make progress toward understanding the causes, developmental course, treatment conditions, and long-term outcomes of LDs a reality. Despite significant research advances, many of these efforts have not led to more precise definitions and interventions for those with LDs. However, the revisions in the 2004 reauthorization of IDEA could ensure that policies and practices will be based on converging scientific evidence.

If the field of LDs is to progress and result in positive outcomes, it has little choice. The reification of historically unsupported assumptions about LDs that collapse under scientific scrutiny may hinder the successful application of what we have learned from the significant advances in research that have occurred over the past 30 years. This is unfortunate. The groups of advocates who successfully implemented essential educational reforms legitimizing the concept of LDs and helped make a systematic research program possible may be continuing to support components of the definition that are outdated, indefensible, and not aligned with research. In doing so, they may be promulgating identification and intervention practices that are not effective, making it difficult to implement practices that have emerged from research (Fletcher et al., 2003; Lyon et al., 2001). These practices have the potential to ameliorate some of the adverse long-term outcomes often associated with LDs (Bruck, 1987; Satz, Buka, Lipsitt, & Seidman, 1998; Spreen, 1989).

CHAPTER 3

Classification, Definition, and Identification of Learning Disabilities

No single problem has plagued the study of LDs more than the problem of definition. This problem emerged early in U.S. public policy efforts to address LDs, and the persistent lack of definitional clarity has impeded the accurate identification of children and adults in need of services in special education and other services for people with disabilities. Furthermore, this lack of clarity has interfered with the provision of accommodations for high-stakes accountability and college aptitude tests, the selection of people with LDs for research studies, individual eligibility for insurance, social security, and other entitlements, and the development of specialized interventions. As Chapter 2 illustrates, the evolution of LDs into an entity warranting special attention in public policy and research had much to do with attempts in the 1960s to define a group of students who displayed "unexpected" academic underachievement. At the same time, these early efforts sought to differentiate LDs from their historical antecedents, epitomized by the MBD hypothesis.

Despite more than a century of efforts, definition issues remain inadequately resolved, though some progress has been made. There is no better arena for highlighting definition issues than educational policy. As we discussed in Chapter 2, in the 2004 reauthorization of the U.S. Individuals with Disabilities Education Act (IDEA), the definition of LDs was fiercely debated. On the basis of their review of the converging scientific evidence, both the U.S. House and Senate concurred in rewriting the IDEA statutes to allow states to move away from regulations that based identification of LDs on aptitude–achievement models and toward models that explicitly incorporated response to instruction as a component of the eligibility process. Despite the evidentiary support for this change in policy, substantial resistance to policy modifications have come from individuals and groups concerned that changes in current practice could lead to reduced services for individuals with LDs. As with any change in educational policy, such resistance was not unexpected.

At the heart of the definition problem is a lack of understanding of the criteria by which different disorders are classified so that the resulting categories have both internal and external validity. For this reason, in this chapter we approach the definition issue from a classification perspective, reviewing evidence for the reliability and validity of four different models: aptitude–achievement discrepancy, low achievement, intraindividual differences, and response to instruction (RTI). We also review the evidence for the validity of the different exclusionary conditions observed in most definitions of LDs.

CLASSIFICATION IN RESEARCH AND PRACTICE

What Are Classifications?

Classifications are systems that permit a larger set of entities to be partitioned into smaller, more homogeneous subgroups based on similarities and dissimilarities in attributes thought to define different aspects of the phenomenon of interest. When entities are assigned, or identified, to subgroups, the process represents an operationalization of the definitions emerging from the classification. Diagnosis (or identification) occurs when the operational definitions are used to determine membership in one or more subgroups. This process occurs in biology when plants and animals are assigned to species; in medicine when diseases are organized into categories based on etiology, symptoms, and treatment; and in LDs when a determination is made that a child's difficulties in school represent an LD as opposed to a behavior problem, oral language problem, or mental retardation. Even deciding that a child needs academic interventions is a decision that reflects an underlying classification (children who need or do not need intervention; Morris & Fletcher, 1988).

Although the terminology describes groupings, we define groupings as decisions made about how individuals are related on correlated dimensions that define the subgroups. The decisions can appear arbitrary and are subject to measurement error. Thus, it is critical to formally assess the validity and reliability of the subgrouping. Valid classifications do not exist solely because subgroups can be created. Rather, the subgroups making up a valid classification can be differentiated according to variables (i.e., external validity) not used to establish the subgroups (Skinner, 1981). Validity, however, hinges on evidence that the classification is not dependent on the method of classification, can be replicated in other samples, and permits identification of the majority of entities of interest (i.e., internal validity or reliability). Reliable and valid classifications facilitate communication, prediction, and treatment, although different classifications may be better for some of those purposes than others (Blashfield, 1993).

For LDs, classification occurs in identifying children as needing intervention; as learning disabled or as typically achieving; as learning disabled as opposed to mentally retarded or having ADHD; and, within LDs, as reading rather than math impaired. By virtue of exclusionary criteria, LDs are hypothesized to represent a subgroup of people with *unexpected* underachievement. LD is differentiated from *expected* underachievement due to emotional disturbance, economic disadvantage, linguistic diversity, and inadequate instruction (Kavale & Forness, 2000). These levels of classification represent hypotheses that should be evaluated for the reliability of the hypothetical model and for validity by reference to variables that are different from those used to establish the classification and assign individuals to subgroups.

Why Are LDs Difficult to Define?

There are two major issues that make LDs difficult to define (Fletcher, Denton, & Francis, 2005a; Francis et al., 2005a).The first is that, as a construct, LD represents an unobservable latent variable that does not exist apart from attempts to measure it. As such, LD has the same status as other unobservable constructs, such as IQ, achievement, or ADHD. The second involves the dimensional nature of LDs (i.e., the common observation that the traits representing LDs exist on a continuum and do not represent discrete categories; Ellis, 1984).

LD Is an Unobservable Construct

We alluded to the latent construct representing LDs in Chapter 2, noting the efforts to identify a group of children as underachieving despite the absence of circumstances that produce low achievement. These efforts represented attempts to assess *unexpected underachievement,* typically conceptualized as individuals unable to master academic skills despite the absence of known causes of poor achievement (sensory disorder, mental retardation, emotional disturbances, economic disadvantage, linguistic diversity, inadequate instruction).

Many efforts at definition and identification have been attempts to measure this attribute, which epitomizes the LD construct. The primary approach to identification has been the measurement of unevenness in academic or cognitive development as a marker for the "unexpected-ness" of LDs, along with the exclusion of other causes of underachievement that would be "expected" to produce underachievement. Thus, the appeal of aptitude–achievement discrepancies is the relatively simple task of assessing IQ and academic achievement to determine if a discrepancy exists between the two domains. If the score on an achievement test is significantly lower than the score obtained on an IQ measure, then it is hypothesized that the learning difficulties are in fact unexpected, because the IQ score is viewed as a measure of "learning potential," and discrepancies occur only when the exclusions have been eliminated.

Unfortunately, the evidence for this hypothesis is weak and the measurement of unexpected underachievement is not a simple task. By establishing definitions of LDs and using these definitions to assess people for the presence or absence of the unobservable latent variable, all efforts at measurement will be imperfect and inconsistent because of differences in how the construct is measured, leading to differences in who is identified with an LD. We can observe what is measured, such as reading, math, and/or cognitive processes. Each of these observable measures indicates, albeit imperfectly, the latent variable of LD. The measurement is imperfect because no single measure captures all the components of the construct and each measurement contains a certain amount of error. The critical issue is the effect of these imperfect measurements on the reliability and validity of the overarching classification that is the basis for identifying LD. This is the essence of classification research.

LDs Are Dimensional

The second issue is the dimensional nature of LDs. Most of the research on LDs, particularly those affecting reading, shows that they occur along a continuum of severity rather than presenting as an explicit dichotomous category delineated by clear cut-points on the achievement distribution. The psychometric markers of LDs, such as achievement test scores, appear normally distributed in most population-based studies (Jorm, Share, Matthews, & Matthews, 1986; Lewis, Hitch, & Walker, 1994; Rodgers, 1983; Shalev, Auerbach, Manor, & Gross-Tsur, 2000; S. E. Shaywitz, Escobar, B. A. Shaywitz, Fletcher, & Makuch, 1992; Silva, McGee, & Williams, 1985). This conclusion is not without controversy. Some studies of children with LDs in reading have suggested that the distribution of achievement test scores is not normal and have identified a natural cut-point where a separate distribution of nondyslexic poor readers can be identified (Miles & Haslum, 1986; Rutter & Yule, 1975; Wood & Grigorenko, 2001). In the Rutter and Yule (1975) studies, the separate distribution, or "hump," has been attributed to an inadequate ceiling on the reading test (van der Wissell & Zegers, 1985) and to the inclusion of a large number of brain-injured children with IQ scores in the deficient range (Fletcher et al., 2002). The studies by Miles and Haslum (1986) and Wood and Grigorenko (2001) do not provide enough details for evaluation of their findings. Thus, most studies support Stanovich's (1988) contention that LDs occur along a continuum of reading ability and are similar to medical disorders such as hypertension and obesity that occur along a continuum (Ellis, 1984; S. E. Shaywitz, 2004).

Findings supporting the dimensional nature of LDs are consistent with studies applying methods from behavioral genetics, which have not identified qualitatively different genetic constellations associated with the heritability of reading and math disorders (Fisher & DeFries, 2002; Grigorenko, 2001, 2005; Plomin & Kovas, 2005). As these are dimensional traits that exist on a continuum, there would be no expectation of natural cut-points that differentiate individuals with LDs from those who are underachievers, but not identified with LDs; the distribution is simply a continuum of severity (S. E. Shaywitz et al., 1992).

If we simply dealt with the average performances of groups with and without LDs, as in research, the dimensional nature of LDs (and the imperfection of measurements of the construct) would not be a major problem because the errors of measurement would be reflected in the variability around the mean. However, it is necessary to identify individuals who have or do not have LDs (and we rarely talk of degrees of LD except in terms of severity, which is also a continuous concept), making it necessary to categorize what are inherently normal distributions of some attribute serving as an indicator of LD (e.g., reading or math).

In research, LD is commonly defined according to a cut-point (e.g., reading below the 20th percentile), and students scoring below this point are grouped into the "LD group," while those above the point are categorized as the "not LD group." U.S. public policy applied this procedure to schools by stipulating the use of aptitude–achievement definitions, which resulted in states setting cut-points on the bivariate distribution of IQ and achievement. The use of a cut-point, particularly when the score is not criterion referenced and the score distributions have been normalized, is a major problem when the underlying attribute is continuous. The problem occurs in part because of the measurement error of any test. Because of measurement error, any cut-point will lead to instability in the identification of specific individuals for the category. Scores will fluctuate around the cut-point with repeat testing, even for a decision as straightforward as demarcating low achievement or mental retardation (Francis et al., 2005a). This fluctuation is not the result of repeat testing, nor is it a matter of selecting the ideal cut-point. Simply put, no *single* score perfectly captures a student's ability in a specific domain at a single point in time. Thus, it is common in the identification of LDs to add other criteria, such as an absence of other disorders that cause low achievement, to try to improve the accuracy of the assessment of the latent construct.

Subdividing a normal distribution to create groups has been criticized in the measurement literature (Cohen, 1983). The group structure is often arbitrary when the distributions are dimensional in nature and may constrain the variability within groups and reduce the range of measurement. The subdivision thus distorts the relative importance of the underlying dimensions to performance on other measures, leading to reduced power in statistical comparisons, as well as inaccurate results due to the failure to allow for the correlation between different dimensions. Because individuals around the cut-point are similar, the error around the cut-point is not a major issue. The amount of error related to the cut-point could influence the size of the effect, but this issue also involves the correlations of the dependent and independent variables. If the effect size is the major focus of the research, there is little reason for the use of a subdivision of the measured attribute, and any questions could be addressed with correlation methods (Stuebing et al., 2002). However, it is necessary to determine the severity of the LD to identify those in need of services, accommodations, and better treatment from society. Therefore, LDs can never be defined solely on the basis of cut-points on psychometric procedures, particularly if the attribute is measured only once, which magnifies the effect of the error of measurement (Francis et al., 2005a).

Many of the issues involving different models for identifying children with LDs reflect confusion about the relation of classification, definition, and identification. The relation is inherently hierarchical in that the definitions derived from a classification yield criteria for identifying members of the subcomponents of the classification. Definitions of LDs originate from an overarching classification of childhood disorders that differentiate LDs from mental retardation and various behavior disorders, such as ADHD. This classification yields definitions and criteria based on attributes that distinguish LDs from mental retardation and ADHD. These criteria can be used to identify children as members of different subgroups within the classification model.

MODELS OF CLASSIFICATION FOR LDs

In the rest of this chapter, we address the reliability and validity of the four primary models proposed for the identification of individuals with

LDs: (1) aptitude–achievement discrepancy; (2) low achievement; (3) intraindividual differences; and (4) RTI. In evaluating these models, we assumed that a valid classification must identify individuals who represent a subgroup with unexpected underachievement. The pattern of differences among low achievers identified as learning disabled or not learning disabled in each model should lead to a unique set of characteristics in those identified as learning disabled. Assessing the validity of the classification should evaluate how well the definition produces a unique group of low achievers when variables are used that were not part of the approach to identification.

Aptitude–Achievement Discrepancy

Although the most common approach to determining aptitude–achievement discrepancy is the identification of a discrepancy between the results of an IQ test and a test of achievement, there is disagreement as to which IQ and achievement tests should be used. We focus initially on discrepancies between a composite measure of IQ and reading achievement, typically word reading. We then review issues related to the proposed use of a verbal IQ measure, nonverbal IQ measure, and non-IQ measure, such as listening comprehension. We also review other domains that do not necessarily involve LDs, but for which similar models have been proposed. Our focus is on whether external variables validate the hypothesized classification.

Prior to considering the research on these different approaches, it is important to note that the use of an aptitude measure assumes that such tests assess, to some degree, a person's capacity for learning. This is an assumption that has its origins in the earliest development of IQ tests and one that has been debated since their inception (Kamin, 1974). It is beyond the scope of this book to review this debate, except to note that this assumption is inherent in the use of any aptitude measure and widely questioned. As stated by Cyril Burt (1937): "Capacity must obviously limit content. It is impossible for a pint jug to hold more than a pint of milk and it is equally impossible for a child's educational attainment to rise higher than his educable capacity" (p. 477). This view of aptitude assessment in which IQ limits a child's learning potential has been termed "milk and jug" thinking (Share, McGee, & Silva, 1989) because of the unproven assumption that IQ sets an upper limit on educational outcomes.

Cognitive, Achievement, and Behavioral Correlates of IQ Discrepancy

Over the past 20 years, research has tried to establish whether cognitive, behavioral, and achievement variables that are not currently used to define children as IQ–achievement discrepant or low-achieving could differentiate between these two groups. These studies, reviewed by Aaron (1997), Siegel (1992), Stuebing et al. (2002), and Stanovich (1991), usually found small but statistically significant differences between IQ–achievement discrepant children with poor reading skills and children with no such discrepancy, but equally poor reading skills. However, the more important issue is not whether such groups of children are different, but how much they differ and whether the differences are meaningful.

Two meta-analyses have synthesized research on cognitive correlates of poor reading in groups variously defined as having IQ–achievement discrepancy and as low-achieving but nondiscrepant. In the first meta-analytic study, Hoskyn and Swanson (2000) coded 19 studies that met stringent IQ and achievement criteria. They computed effect sizes from studies in which cognitive skills were compared in groups of children with poor reading abilities that differed in whether there was a significant discrepancy relative to IQ. It is conventional to conceptualize effect sizes in terms of small, medium, and large effects (Cohen, 1983). An effect size difference of 0 indicates complete overlap of the two groups. Effect sizes over 0.20 are considered small; those over 0.50 are considered medium; and those over 0.80 are considered large.

Figure 3.1 shows the average effect size and the confidence intervals for eight representative domains. A positive effect size indicates that the IQ–achievement discrepancy group had higher average scores; a negative effect size indicates higher average scores by the low achievement group. Figure 3.1 shows negligible to small differences for measures of reading real words (–0.02), automaticity (0.05) and memory (0.12), small effects for phonology (0.27) and reading pseudowords (0.29), but larger differences on measures of vocabulary (0.55) and syntax (0.87). The authors concluded that most cognitive abilities assessed in the meta-analysis, especially those closely related to reading, showed considerable overlap between the two groups, leading them to question the validity of IQ–achievement discrepancy. This overlap occurred despite the attempt by Hoskyn and Swanson (2000) to select studies in which low achievement was associated with low IQ scores. Some studies included children with IQ scores in the deficient range.

In the second study, Stuebing et al. (2002) synthesized 46 studies that compared groups composed of poor readers who met explicit criteria for IQ–achievement discrepancy or for nondiscrepant low achievement. The 46 studies met multiple criteria for inclusion and exclusion but were more liberal than those examined by Hoskyn and Swanson (2000), especially in allowing IQ to range freely in both groups. The most important criteria required (1) explicit discrepancy criteria to form

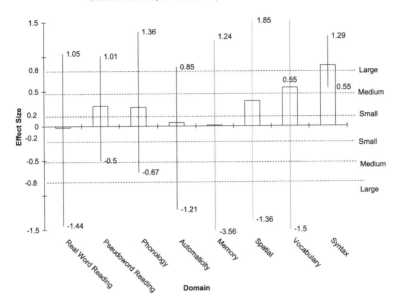

FIGURE 3.1. Effect sizes and 95% confidence intervals for selected domains from Hoskyn and Swanson (2000). The effect size is represented by the box and the confidence interval is represented by the lines on both ends of the box. An effect size of 0 indicates complete overlap in the groups. Effect sizes of 0.2 are considered small; 0.5 are considered medium; and 0.8 are considered large.

the discrepant group and (2) an indication that the low-achieving, nondiscrepant group did not include individuals who might have IQ–achievement discrepancy or typical achievement in reading. Variables used to form groups were not used to estimate effect sizes in addressing validity, as the definitions ensured large group differences on group formation variables. In addition to effect sizes in cognitive ability, Stuebing et al. (2002) also assessed achievement and behavior domains. Aggregated effect sizes were negligible for the behavior (–0.05, 95% confidence interval = –0.14, 0.05) and achievement (–0.12, 95% confidence interval = –0.16, –0.07) domains. A small effect size difference was found for the cognitive ability domain (0.30, 95% confidence interval = 0.27, 0.34), showing higher scores in the IQ–achievement discrepant group. However, the significance of this difference is questionable, given that this group had IQ scores that averaged about one standard deviation higher than those of the group with nondiscrepant low achievement.

When the achievement domain was broken down because of statistical evidence for heterogeneity in the effect size estimates (Figure 3.2),

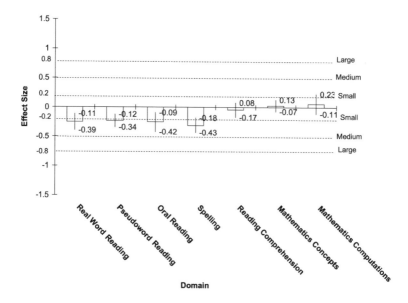

FIGURE 3.2. Effect sizes and 95% conference intervals for academic domains in Stuebing et al. (2002). The effect size is represented by the box and the confidence interval is represented by the lines on both ends of the box. An effect size of 0 indicates complete overlap in the groups. Effect sizes of 0.2 are considered small; 0.5 are considered medium; and 0.8 are considered large.

those tasks that involved reading real words (–0.25), and pseudowords (–0.23), oral reading (–0.25), and spelling (–0.31) showed small effect sizes indicating poorer performance by the group with IQ–achievement discrepancy. Tasks involving reading comprehension (–0.04), mathematics concepts (0.03) and computations (0.06), and writing (–0.08; not shown in Figure 3.2) yielded negligible effect sizes. Because many tasks used word recognition as the measure of poor reading, the small effect sizes for reading real words, spelling, and oral reading may reflect their similarity to the types of tasks used to define poor reading in other studies.

Figure 3.3 summarizes effect sizes for tasks in the cognitive domain. As in the Hoskyn and Swanson (2000) meta-analysis, cognitive abilities closely related to reading did not differentiate the two groups with poor reading: phonological awareness (–0.13), rapid naming (–0.12), verbal memory (0.10), and vocabulary (0.10). Thus, the core cognitive skills that are most closely related to reading disabilities (see Chapters 5–7) do not significantly discriminate children with IQ–achievement discrepancy from children with low achievement and no discrepancy. Not surpris-

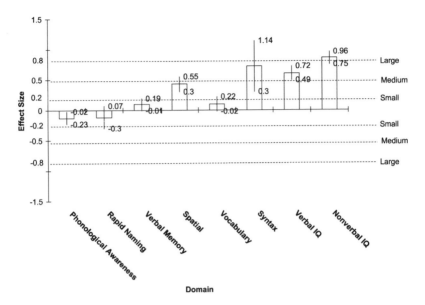

FIGURE 3.3. Effect sizes and 95% conference intervals for cognitive skills from Stuebing et al. (2000). The effect size is represented by the box and the confidence interval is represented by the lines on both ends of the box. An effect size of 0 indicates complete overlap in the groups. Effect sizes of 0.2 are considered small; 0.5 are considered medium; and 0.8 are considered large.

ingly, since these measures are similar to those used to define the groups, measures of IQ not used to define the groups demonstrated medium to large effect sizes (range = 0.60–1.01). Measures of cognitive skills involving spatial skills (0.43) and syntax (0.72), and other domains not shown in Figure 3.3, yielded small to medium effect sizes, showing better performance by the IQ–achievement discrepant group. These tasks are similar to those used in many IQ tests. The finding for syntax in both studies is based on a small number of comparisons.

Other analyses indicated that the size of the effects in different studies could be predicted by the IQ and reading tasks used to define the groups. In other words, sampling variation across studies explains the effect size differences that emerge across studies. Following the lead of other researchers (Hoskyn & Swanson, 2000; Siegel, 1992; Stanovich & Siegel, 1994; Sternberg & Grigorenko, 2002), Stuebing et al. (2002) concluded that LD classifications based on IQ–achievement discrepancy have weak validity. The difference is that this conclusion is based on an empirical synthesis of multiple studies–not on a single study or review of multiple studies.

Development and Prognosis

There is little evidence that the long-term development of reading skills in children defined as IQ–achievement discrepant is different from that in children defined as low achieving but nondiscrepant. In a previous study, Rutter and Yule (1975) reported that children in the former group showed more rapid development of academic skills than those in the latter group. However, the reading and spelling skills of the low-achieving but nondiscrepant children were lower at baseline. As children were not randomly assigned to the two groups, the greater advances may reflect regression to the mean. In a subsequent study of a large longitudinal cohort in New Zealand, Share et al. (1989) attempted to replicate these findings using similar definitions and alternative methodologies that would tease out the relationship of IQ and reading over time. They found no relation of IQ and reading achievement within age bands of 7, 9, 11, and 13 years. Moreover, IQ scores were not predictive of change in reading skills over time. Share et al. (1989) concluded that IQ is not a relevant explanatory variable for predicting the development of children with reading difficulties.

Francis, Shaywitz, Stuebing, Shaywitz, and Fletcher (1996) examined the question of prognosis, using data from the Connecticut Longitudinal Project (S. E. Shaywitz et al., 1992, 1999). Children in grade 3 were defined as meeting an IQ–achievement discrepancy or nondiscrepant low achievement definition in reading. They compared the growth of reading skills, using yearly assessments of reading in grades 1–9. The results, shown in Figure 3.4 through grade 12 (S. E. Shaywitz et al., 1999), demonstrated no differences between the two groups with reading difficulties in the rate of growth over time or the level of reading ability at any age, despite the average 18-point higher IQ score characterizing the discrepant group. S. E. Shaywitz et al. (1999) reported that more than 70% of those who read poorly in grade 3 read poorly in grade 12 despite the fact that many of these children received special services through special education and other resources. Other longitudinal studies also failed to demonstrate differences in long-term prognosis (Flowers, Meyer, Lovato, Wood, & Felton, 2001) or the precursors of poor reading (Wristers, Francis, Foorman, Fletcher, & Swank, 2002) in comparisons of poor readers defined as discrepant or low achieving.

Intervention Outcomes

Several studies have examined the outcomes of reading interventions in relationship to different indices of IQ or IQ–achievement discrepancy.

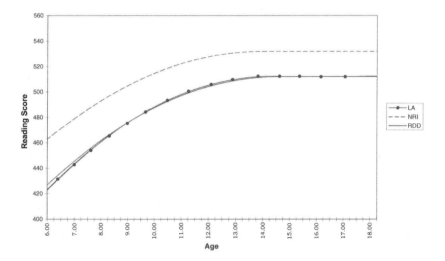

FIGURE 3.4. Growth in reading skills by children in grades 1–12 in the Connecticut Longitudinal Study based on the reading cluster of the Woodcock–Johnson. The children were identified at grade 3 as not reading impaired (NRI); reading disabled according to a 1.5 standard error discrepancy between IQ and reading achievement (RDD); or having low reading achievement with no discrepancy (25th percentile; LA). There is no difference in the long-term growth of the RDD and LA groups. From Fletcher et al. (2002, p. 193). Copyright 2002 by Lawrence Erlbaum Associates. Reprinted by permission.

Aaron (1997) reviewed earlier studies that sometimes included comparisons of groups defined as having an IQ–achievement discrepancy and as low achieving but having no such discrepancy. He found that both groups made little progress in their reading development, even with remedial placements. More recent studies have explicitly examined this hypothesis in remedial or prevention interventions. Most studies do not identify a strong relation, particularly an interaction that would demonstrate differential effects of the intervention across levels of IQ (Foorman et al., 1997; Foorman, Francis, Fletcher, Schatschneider, & Mehta, 1998; Hatcher & Hulme, 1999; Mathes et al., 2005; Stage, Abbott, Jenkins, & Berninger, 2003; Torgesen et al., 1999, 2001; Vellutino, Scanlon, & Lyon, 2000; Vellutno, Scanlon, Small, & Faneule, 2006). One exception was a remedial study of children with reading difficulties in grades 2–5 (Wise, Ring, & Olson, 2000). In this study, Full Scale IQ predicted about 5% of the variance in word-reading outcomes on one measure of word reading, but this effect was not apparent on other measures of word reading or assessments of phonological processing ability. Summarizing the results of their study of IQ–achievement discrepancy and reading outcomes, Vellutino et al. (2000) concluded that

> the IQ–achievement discrepancy does not reliably distinguish between disabled and non-disabled readers. Neither does it distinguish between children who were found to be difficult to remediate and those who are readily remediated prior to initiation of remediation, and it does not predict response to remediation. (p. 235)

Some of these studies found that levels of IQ predicted reading comprehension outcomes (Wise et al., 2000; Hatcher & Hulme, 1999; Torgesen, Wagner, & Rashotte, 1999). However, the subtests that make up a Verbal IQ scale represent a general verbal comprehension factor closely related to vocabulary (Fletcher et al., 1996a; Sattler, 1993; Share, Jorm, MacLean, & Matthews, 1984). As vocabulary is a component of IQ and correlated with reading comprehension skills, it is not surprising that Verbal IQ predicts reading comprehension. However, the relevant construct is not IQ but vocabulary (Sternberg & Grigorenko, 2002). Consider that if measures of phonological processing were included as IQ subtests, it is unlikely that any child with word recognition problems would meet an IQ–achievement discrepancy definition; such a child's IQ would, on average, be much lower.

Neurobiological Factors

The IQ–achievement discrepancy hypothesis has been explicitly addressed in research on genetic factors in LDs, and implicitly in neuroimaging research. Pennington, Gilger, Olson, and DeFries (1992) used a twin sample to create a non-disabled group and three groups with a reading disability: one with IQ-achievement discrepancy, one with no such discrepancy, and a mixed discrepant–nondiscrepant group. Pennington et al. found no evidence for differential genetic etiology based on type of definition. In a subsequent study from a Colorado group with a larger sample, Wadsworth, Olson, Pennington, and DeFries (2000) subdivided twin pairs with and without reading disabilities according to higher (> 100) and lower (< 100) IQ scores. Although the overall heritability of reading skills was 0.58, children with reading disabilities and lower IQ scores had a heritability estimate of 0.43, as compared with 0.72 for the higher IQ group. These statistically significant differences in heritability are nonetheless small; Wadsworth et al. (2000) required almost 400 pairs of twins in order to detect the difference.

There are also studies of children with reading disabilities that utilize functional imaging methods, such as functional magnetic resonance imaging (fMRI) and magnetic source imaging (MSI) (see Chapter 5). Although no study has a sample that is large enough to actually compare children with and without IQ—achievement discrepancy who read poorly, it is noteworthy that no study includes only those children with discrepancy. There is no evidence from these studies that these two groups of children have different neuroimaging profiles. In particular, studies that permit examination of individual brain activation profiles, especially MSI, show no differences in brain maps from children who read poorly with and without IQ–achievement discrepancy.

Alternative Approaches to Aptitude–Achievement Discrepancy

Are IQ indices or assessments of listening comprehension better measures of aptitude? Some have advocated the use of nonverbal IQ measures (e.g., performance IQ; PIQ) because this type of measure is less confounded by language, and many students with LDs have language difficulties. Scores on nonverbal IQ measures are believed to better reveal a student's aptitude for learning (Perfetti, 1985; Rutter & Yule, 1975). Alternatively, Hessler (1987) and Berninger et al. (2003a) suggested that a verbal measure of IQ was a better aptitude assessment because difficulty in learning to read should represent a discrepancy relative to language potential. Here the distinction is essentially between students who do not learn to read, despite adequate verbal skills, and those whose reading difficulties are part of the constellation of language problems. Finally, others have argued that a listening comprehension measure is a better index of aptitude for learning to read because a reading disability should represent a discrepancy between listening comprehension and reading comprehension (Spring & French, 1990).

There is no support for the greater validity of these approaches. Fletcher et al. (2005a) summarized evidence pertaining to alternative approaches to operationalizing aptitude and achievement for students who are poor readers and found negligible to small effect sizes across measures. For example, in Fletcher et al. (1994), effect sizes in relation to word recognition were 0.14 for Full Scale IQ and Verbal IQ, and 0.22 for Performance IQ. Stanovich and Siegel (1994) found inconsistent and small differences on cognitive measures, mostly outside the language domain, based on the use of Verbal IQ versus Performance IQ. Like Aaron, Kuchta, and Grapenthin (1988), Fletcher et al. (1994) found small differences between discrepant and nondiscrepant poor readers based on a discrepancy between listening comprehension and reading comprehension (effect size = 0.20). Badian (1999) found that these definitions were unstable over time.

IQ–Achievement Discrepancy and Math Disabilities

Fletcher (2005) compared IQ–achievement discrepant and low-achieving groups of math-impaired children who did not show evidence of word recognition problems on cognitive variables involving attention, language, problem solving, concept formation, and visual–spatial processing. The results showed that the discrepant group had higher performance levels on all variables. The group that had nondiscrepant low achievement in math was notably poorer in vocabulary despite average reading skills. The critical issue, as for reading disabilities, is not that the groups differ. Differences in level of performance are expected because IQ tests are used to define the groups; one group has higher IQ scores, and IQ is moderately to highly correlated with each of the measures (e.g., vocabulary) used to evaluate the children. More significant is the *pattern* (shape) of differences between the groups. Testing the profiles for differences in pattern did not yield a statistically significant difference, and the effect size was negligible (0.06). As we have shown in the reading area (Fletcher et al., 1994), eliminating variability due to a difference in vocabulary—a proxy for IQ in many studies—eliminates most of the differences in level of performance apparent between the two math groups. The differences appear to be a product of the definitions, and the correlates of poor math achievement do not appear to vary once the differences induced by the definition are taken into account. The differences in vocabulary between those with IQ–achievement discrepancy and nondiscrepant low achievement in math and reading most likely reflect a higher correlation between reading and vocabulary than between vocabulary and math. Mazzocco and Myers (2003) also found little validity for the use of IQ–achievement discrepancy in defining math LDs.

IQ and Reading Comprehension Disabilities

The role of IQ in defining the reading comprehension subgroup has emerged differently in studies of poor comprehenders from the way it has in studies of those with dyslexia. There are few studies that use IQ–achievement discrepancies to define groups of poor comprehenders. Thus, the issue of IQ or IQ–achievement discrepancy has had little impact on research on reading comprehension disability. Some studies of reading comprehension have used IQ as an outcome measure or covariate rather than as an inclusionary criterion for identifying disability. For example, children with specific reading comprehension difficulties show phonological skills and nonverbal intelligence similar to those of typically achieving children, but their verbal IQ scores are lower (e.g.,

Stothard & Hulme, 1996). These findings suggest that more general verbal processing difficulties underlie the reading comprehension disability in some children with good decoding but poor comprehension, highlighting the difficulties that would emerge if IQ were controlled in studies of poor comprehenders. As vocabulary and other lexical measures are related to both reading comprehension and verbal IQ, the lower verbal scores are hardly surprising (Fletcher et al., 1996a). However, in a recent study of typically achieving readers, verbal IQ was found to account for only a small amount of the variability in reading comprehension skills (Oakhill, Cain, & Bryant, 2003). After verbal intellectual skills were accounted for in different models, significant unique variance in comprehension was predicted by text integration skills, metacognitive monitoring, and working memory.

IQ–Achievement Discrepancy and Speech–Language Disorders

The federal definition of LDs includes disorders of oral expression and listening comprehension. These disorders can also be represented as disorders of expressive and receptive language, which constitute a separate category in special education under IDEA. A consensus group convened by the National Institute of Deafness and Communication Disorders concluded that the practice of using IQ scores to identify children with these disorders was not supported by research and practice (Tager-Flusberg & Cooper, 1999). This conclusion was based on an emerging database on the validity of "cognitive referencing," the term for discrepancy identification used in this area (Casby, 1992). In this database, the most convincing evidence came from an epidemiological study by Tomblin and Zhang (1999). The investigators used measures of nonverbal IQ and oral language ability to create three groups of children from a large epidemiological sample: a group with no impairment; a group with specific language impairment (IQ > 87 and composite language skills < 1.25 standard deviations below age); and a group with general delay (IQ < 87 and composite language skills < 1.25 standard deviations below age). Comparisons of the three groups on different language measures showed consistent differences between the nonimpaired group and both language-impaired groups. However, differences between the two language-impaired groups were also apparent: "Children with general delay closely parallel the specifically language-impaired group except that the children with general delay were more impaired and noticeably poorer on the test involving comprehension of sentences (grammatical understanding)" (p. 367). Tomblin and Zhang (1999) questioned whether this latter difference in grammatical understanding is specific to either group, noting that "current diagnostic methods and standards for specific language impairment do not result in a group of children whose profiles of language achievement are unique" (p. 367).

PSYCHOMETRIC FACTORS IN DISCREPANCY MODELS

Thus far, we have addressed the *validity* of the IQ–achievement discrepancy approach to identification, failing to find much evidence supporting the validity of definitions and identification procedures based on aptitude–achievement discrepancies. The reasons for these weak validity results undoubtedly stem from issues concerning the *reliability* of any test-based model for identifying individual students with LDs. Although these problems have been well documented for various approaches to the estimation of discrepancy, many of the same issues will affect the use of a definition based on low achievement. Such problems involve the measurement error of the tests, the unreliability of difference scores, and the use of cut-points to subdivide a normal distribution.

REGRESSION TO THE MEAN

Approaches to IQ–achievement discrepancy that are based on regression methods adjusting for the correlation of IQ and achievement are superior to other methods when two tests are involved (Bennett & Clarizio, 1988; Reynolds, 1984–1985). IQ and achievement test scores are moderately correlated, so the failure to adjust for this correlation leads to regression to the mean. Regression effects indicate that when individuals are chosen because of low performance on one test, they will, on average, score closer to the mean on the second test. This phenomenon results in overidentification of LDs at upper levels of IQ and underidentification at lower levels of IQ. A regression approach adjusts for the correlation of IQ and achievement, thus correcting this problem.

LOWER RELIABILITY OF DISCREPANCY SCORES

Discrepancy models involve the estimation of a score that reflects the difference between two tests. It is well known that difference scores are typically lower in reliability than the measures used to compute the difference (Bereiter, 1967). The low reliability of difference scores can be exacerbated because they artificially constrain the variance in scores (Rogosa, 1995), as in the case when IQ and achievement scores are used to identify the lower-performing segment of the population.

CUT-POINTS

We described the problems associated with the use of cutoff scores to subdivide a normal distribution. The empirical effects of this subdivision were studied by S. E. Shaywitz et al. (1992), who found that definitions based on IQ–achievement discrepancy were especially unstable from grades 1 to 3, but were more stable from grades 3 to 5. However, this study did not examine definitions of low achievement. In a systematic study of this issue, Francis et al. (2005a) used simulated data and actual data from the Connecticut Longitudinal Study to evaluate the stability of classifications based on definitions of IQ–achievement discrepancy and nondiscrepant low achievement. If the groups formed by either definition represented meaningful subdivisions of the achievement distribution, some degree of stability over time would be expected. The results of the simulations showed that groups formed by imposing cut-points based on either definition of LDs were unstable over time, even when the simulations were designed with high reliability of measurement and to minimize individual change. Similar instability was apparent in longitudinal data from the Connecticut Longitudinal Study, in which 39% of children designated as having LDs in grade 3 using different definitions changed group placement with repeated testing in grade 5.

It is not surprising that different approaches to aptitude–achievement discrepancies are not likely to produce valid classifications, because the underlying psychometric model is the same and the measures are moderately correlated. Individuals who cluster around a cut-point are more similar than different, so differences in identification reflect the differences in the correlation of the two tests with achievement. Thus, the slope of the regression line will shift, depending on the correlation of the aptitude and achievement measures regardless of how the constructs are assessed or the domain in which the discrepancy is computed. In Figure 3.5 (Fletcher et al., 2005a), the regression line is steeper for Verbal IQ than Performance IQ because of the higher population correlation of reading (.69) and Verbal IQ than for reading and Performance IQ (.40). The difference in slopes and in measures shifts individuals at the edges of the regression cut-point on one IQ measure to either a discrepant or low-achieving subgroup when the other IQ measure is used. Because the correlation of IQ and reading is lower, effect sizes would be larger for Performance IQ than Verbal IQ (see Fletcher et al., 1994). Nonetheless, collapsing across IQ-discrepancy and low achievement definitions, 80% of the sample is consistently identified as LD, simply shifting from one LD group to another. Changing the IQ measure moves the observations left or right across the cut-point, but does not move them up or down

Effect of IQ–Achievement Correlation on Classifications

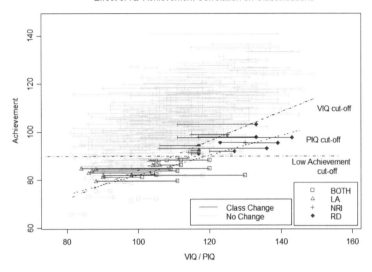

FIGURE 3.5. Regression lines based on the population correlations of the Woodcock–Johnson III Basic Reading Skills score with Performance IQ and Verbal IQ. Higher correlations are reflected in steeper slopes, so that different decisions about group membership are made because of slight shifts in slopes. Individual observations are connected and show significant movement around the cut-points demarcating those who meet both low achievement and discrepancy (Both) definitions, only low achievement (LA) definitions, only discrepancy (RD) definitions, and not reading impaired (NRI). From Fletcher et al. (2005a, p. 548). Copyright 2005 by PRO-ED. Reprinted by permission.

because the achievement measure is the same. These shifts are displayed in Figure 3.5 by a line that connects pairs of observations. An observation that does not change in the identified group has the same symbol connected by a faint horizontal line; observations that change groups have two different symbols that are connected by a dark horizontal line. As Figure 3.5 shows, observations with IQ scores that are most different and that are located near the cut-point are most likely to shift, reflecting both measurement error and differences between how the construct of aptitude is assessed by Verbal and Performance IQ.

Conclusions: Aptitude–Achievement Discrepancy

The aptitude–achievement classification hypothesis lacks strong evidence for external validity across multiple domains. The psychometric evidence shows that classifications based on cut-points have problems with reliability. Thus, the IQ–achievement discrepancy classification hypothesis has weak validity and will not produce differences among subgroups that represent different forms of underachievement. Discrepancy models cannot possibly produce a clearly unique set of underachievers because they are underidentified, tests have measurement errors that are magnified by the computation of difference scores, and individuals around the cut-points are too similar. Models based on aptitude–achievement discrepancies do not appear to identify a unique group of underachievers and therefore do not adequately operationalize the construct of LDs.

Low Achievement Models

A commonly proposed alternative to aptitude–achievement discrepancies involves identifying individuals as learning disabled based on absolute low achievement (Siegel, 1992). In reviewing this proposal, an immediate problem is that identification of LDs based solely on low achievement essentially equates LDs with low achievement. Because the purpose of the LD construct is to identify a unique group of low achievers whose underachievement is unexpected, it is questionable as to whether such an approach could ever identify individuals with LDs without additional criteria. At a minimum, it would be necessary to rule out other causes of low achievement. However, it would also be difficult to identify unexpected underachievement without measuring achievement, especially because the strongest evidence for the validity of the construct of LD comes from studies that include low achievement as part of the definition.

Validity

Models based on the use of achievement markers have a great deal of validity (see Fletcher et al., 2002, 2003; Siegel, 1992). If groups are formed such that the participants do not meet the criteria for mental retardation and have achievement scores that are below the 20th percentile (an arbitrary designation), comparisons show that subgroups of underachievers emerge that can be validly differentiated on external variables and help demonstrate the viability of the construct of LDs. Consider, for example, Figure 3.6. This figure displays actual profiles for three groups of students in grades 2 and 3 who participated in a classification study by the Yale Center for Learning and Attention Disorders (S. E. Shaywitz, 2004). These children represent groups who have isolated problems in

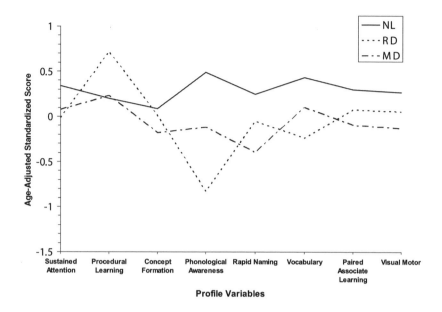

FIGURE 3.6. Profiles across different cognitive tests for children who are impaired only in reading (RD) and in math (MD) relative to typical achievers (NL). The groups differ in shape and elevation, suggesting three distinct groups.

the domains of word recognition and math, along with a comparison group of typically achieving children. The students with disabilities were defined according to several different approaches to identification, including discrepancies relative to Verbal IQ, Performance IQ, or Full Scale IQ, as well as a low-achieving definition that simply required performance below the 26th percentile on either word recognition or math calculations, and an IQ score (Verbal IQ, Performance IQ, Full Scale IQ) of at least 80.

To validate the implicit hypothetical classification of LDs in reading versus math, the children received assessments of cognitive skills that were not used to create the LD subgroups. These measures included assessments of problem solving, concept formation, phonological awareness, rapid naming, vocabulary development, verbal learning, and visual motor skills. As Figure 3.6 shows, the three groups are distinct in the pattern and level of performance, indicating that the implicit classification of LDs in reading versus math is supported in terms of the cognitive correlates, along with clear evidence that children defined with LDs in reading and math domains differ from typically achieving students. As will be seen in subsequent chapters, these groups differ in both the neural correlates of reading and math performance and the heritability of reading and math disorders (Plomin & Kovas, 2005). These achievement subgroups, which by definition include children who meet either low achievement or IQ–achievement discrepancy criteria, differ in response to instruction: Effective interventions are specific to the academic domain, so that teaching math to children whose problem is in reading (and vice versa) would be ineffective. Such findings support a low achievement classification, especially because comparing IQ–achievement discrepant and low-achieving children within the reading and math groups does not yield large or meaningful differences in any of these external variables.

Despite this evidence for validity, simply utilizing a low achievement definition, even when different exclusionary criteria are applied, does not operationalize the true meaning of "unexpected underachievement." Although such an approach to identification is deceptively simple, it is arguable whether the subgroups that remain represent a unique group of underachievers. For example, how well are underachievers whose low performance is attributed to LDs differentiated from underachievers whose low performance is attributed to emotional disturbance, economic disadvantage, or inadequate instruction (Lyon et al., 2001)? To use the example of word recognition, there is little evidence that these subgroups vary in terms of phonological awareness or other language tasks, response to intervention, or even neuroimaging correlates. In this respect, the validity is weak because the underlying construct of LDs is not adequately assessed. Although additional criteria are needed, simply adding a single aptitude measure *decreases* reliability and does not increase the validity of a low achievement definition.

Reliability

The measurement problems that emerge when a specific cut-point is used for identification purposes in IQ–achievement discrepancy definitions affect *any* psychometric approach to the identification of LDs (see Figure 3.5). To reiterate, LDs are essentially a dimensional trait, or variation on normal development. These problems are more significant when the test score is not criterion referenced or when the score distributions have been smoothed to create a normal univariate distribution. Regardless of normality, measurement error attends any psychometric procedure and affects cut-points in a normal distribution (Shepard, 1980). More data points are needed to improve the reliability of the assessment of each individual's position relative to the cut-point, which is why models based on a single attempt to establish status on a normal distribution are often underidentified.

Intraindividual Differences Model

Models based on the assessment of cognitive strengths and weaknesses continue to be proposed to identify individuals with LDs. It is well established that LDs are associated with specific impairments in cognitive processes and that there is variability in the cognitive strengths and weaknesses displayed by individuals with LDs. An intraindividual differences model proposes to use this pattern of strengths and weaknesses as a marker to identify unexpected underachievement. Thus, this model moves beyond the assumption of aptitude–achievement discrepancy models in looking for a marker for learning capacity; rather, these models operationalize unexpected underachievement as unevenness in development as indicated by performance across a battery of cognitive or neuropsychological tests. The person with LDs is one with strengths in many areas but weaknesses in some core cognitive processes that lead to underachievement.

There is little research that specifically addresses the reliability and validity of classification models based on intraindividual differences in cognitive skills. However, few studies show that assessing cognitive skills is either necessary or sufficient for identifying LDs (Reschly & Tilly, 1999). Nonetheless, proponents of this view call for better classifications that more clearly delineate the different profiles associated with LDs. They often argue that cognitive deficits are an inherent part of LDs and that knowledge of strengths and weaknesses can facilitate treatment planning. Some even argue that cognitive assessments can separate underachievement that is due to intrinsic, constitutional factors from underachievement due to social and economic factors (Hale, Naglieri, Kaufman, & Kavale, 2004).

Validity

Along this vein, Hale et al. (2004) indicate that there is research suggesting cognitive differences between learning disabled and low-achieving populations, concluding "that some of these children have disabilities and some are low-achieving, but discriminating between the two would be difficult without objective individual measurement" (p. 9). We reiterate that major meta-analyses of the aptitude–achievement model have not found evidence for this assertion (Hoskyn & Swanson, 2000; Stuebing et al., 2002). Hale et al. (2004) also suggest that assessment of cognitive processes will assist in the determination of whether the cause is neurobiological, environmental, or attributable to some other cause. As we review below, there is little evidence showing that achievement difficulties in children who are economically disadvantaged, second language learners, or emotionally disturbed vary with putative cause (Kavale, 1988). To illustrate, word recognition problems in individuals with attributes associated with LD, emotional disturbance, or poverty will be reliably associated with cognitive difficulties in phonological awareness and rapid naming of letters. It does not seem likely that an assessment of phenotypic characteristics permits the sorting of the causes of underachievement.

A major assumption of this model is that classifications based on intraindividual differences in cognitive skills will lead to enhanced treatment of children with LDs. This assumption is not supported, as there is little evidence that instruction addressing strengths and weaknesses in cognitive skills is related to intervention outcomes (Fletcher et al., 2003; Reschly & Tilly, 1999). Training cognitive processes in the absence of an emphasis on content does not usually translate into the related academic area, which begs the question: Why teach to the process? For example, training phonological awareness skills with no letter component typically leads to improvements in phonological awareness, but these improvements do not apply to reading (National Reading Panel, 2000). In the area of math, Naglieri has evaluated the utility of the Cognitive Assessment System (CAS; Naglieri & Das, 1997) as an assessment that leads to differential instruction for students with math problems. Naglieri and Johnson (2000) assessed 19 children with the CAS and identified a subgroup with significantly lower scores in Planning ($n = 3$). They compared with this subgroup a subgroup of 6 students who were lower on one of the other CAS scales and another subgroup of 10 with no weaknesses. Students with planning difficulties benefited more from an intervention emphasizing planning than the other two subgroups. However, in a larger study, Kroesbergen, Van Luit, and Naglieri (2003) identified 267 students with LDs in math. An evaluation of the effects of intervention revealed no relation between the CAS subgroup and outcome.

Reliability

Another major issue involves low-achieving individuals with relatively flat cognitive profiles. Presumably such individuals are not learning disabled. However, the severity of an achievement problem is correlated with profile flatness due to the lack of independence of different tests used to construct the profile (Morris, Fletcher, & Francis, 1993). Individuals with increasingly severe academic problems will show increasingly flat profiles on cognitive tasks (and achievement measures) in direct correspondence to severity. If the criterion is evidence of a discrepancy in cognitive processing skills, such an approach may exclude the most severely impaired because these individuals are less likely to show discrepancies owing to the intercorrelation of the tests (Morris et al., 1993, 1998). Thus, this model introduces other psychometric issues into identification, especially those that involve the analysis of profiles.

RTI Models

All the approaches reviewed so far are based on assessments administered at a single time point. If the same assessments were used multiple times during the year, which would be necessary to increase their reliability for assessing individuals around a cut-point (Francis et al., 2005a), they would be unwieldy and impractical. In discussing aptitude–achievement models, Shepard (1980) proposed that students receive four aptitude–achievement assessments in order to reliably assess a student's position relative to the cut-point. An approach to identification that takes 12 or so hours of assessment is not likely to have much appeal. The intraindividual differences approach attempts to address this problem by using multiple tests at the same time point, looking for recurrent discrepancies in similar tests within a profile. However, the measures of processing skills used in an intraindividual differences model have reliabilities that are usually lower than norm-referenced IQ and achievement tests, thus magnifying the problem of reliably identifying profile variations.

Models incorporating RTI typically involve identification based in part on mass screening of all students and repeated probe assessments of the same core area, such as reading or math, in students who demonstrate risk characteristics. RTI models are dynamic and base identification on the assessment of ability change. By tying multiple assessments to specific attempts to intervene with a student, the construct of unexpected underachievement can be operationalized in part on the basis of an inadequate response to instruction that is effective with most individuals (Fuchs & Fuchs, 1998; Gresham, 2002). Those who do not benefit adequately from increasingly intense instruction could be identified as having an LD. Such models have been proposed in several recent consensus reports that address LD identification (Bradley et al., 2002; President's Commission on Excellence in Special Education, 2002), most notably in a recent report of the National Research Council (Donavon & Cross, 2002). These reports suggest that one criterion for LD identification is that the student does not respond to appropriate instruction and high-quality intervention.

There are many models of RTI, which were developed initially from public health models of disease prevention (Vaughn, Wanzek, Woodruff, & Linan-Thompson, in press) and first utilized in school-wide education models designed to prevent behavior problems in children (Donavon & Cross, 2002). For implementations in schools, it is better to think of RTI as a process and not a single model, with considerable variation in how the process is implemented. The goal is not just to identify students as learning disabled or for special education, but also to enhance educational opportunities for all children and to prevent disabilities. Essential to the effective implementation of an RTI process are (1) reliable and valid measures that are sensitive to intervention and can be administered multiple times (Stecker, Fuchs, & Fuchs, 2005), (2) validated intervention protocols for targeted outcomes such as word recognition and comprehension (Vaughn, Linan-Thompson, & Hickman, 2003a), and (3) school-level models delineating a coordinated system of screening, intervention, and placement (Vaughn et al., in press). The intervention protocols are sometimes standardized, as in the examples of multitiered reading interventions described in Chapter 5. Other implementations use a problem-solving process that simply tries to implement a variety of strategies that address the difficulties experienced by a student with an academic subject or behavior. This reflects an empirical approach to the discovery of "what works," which is focused largely on improvements in the behaviors that may lead to identification (Reschly & Tilly, 1999). Common to any RTI model is the view that what is paramount in considering LDs is how to treat them to ensure better outcomes for all students. For LDs, identification is not a test-to-diagnosis model in which identification must occur in order to intervene; rather, RTI incorporates instruction into the definition of LDs.

Models that utilize an RTI process do not radically represent new classifications of LDs. Like the other models reviewed in this chapter, RTI models retain the concepts of unexpected underachievement and discrepancy, but base them on assessments of learning and progress over time (Fletcher et al., 2003). For example, the initial decision regarding whether a child is discrepant from school and/or parent expectations essential to this model is a discrepancy classification (Ysseldyke & Marston, 1999). The decision is fraught with the same difficult issues that the more traditional normative classification systems possess. If children are from a very low performing school, does that mean they are not poor readers if their performance is in line with school expectations? Similarly, if children are from a very high functioning school, should parental expectations that their child be an outstanding reader represent the basis for such decisions? Even if one uses curriculum-based measurements (CBM) as an alternative to more traditional norm-referenced psychometric measures, there is always the decision of whether a child has or has not achieved the specified academic skill or ability level for his or her group. The decision reflects a classification problem because of the need to define the comparison group, the academic skills/abilities to be evaluated, and the criteria for progress. The decision involves a discrepancy that is based on multiple assessments over time. Thus, unexpected underachievement is quantified in part on the basis of a discrepant response to instruction based on multiple assessments. This provides a distinct advantage over status models. The underlying classification is based on responder status, and identification involves stipulating criteria for sorting individuals into those who respond and do not respond.

Validity

The introduction of serial assessments has an advantage beyond any statistical advantage it may confer for the estimation of an individual's true status. Specifically, the introduction of serial assessments brings learning and the measurement of change to the forefront in conceptualizations of LDs. The collection of serial assessments under specified conditions of effective instruction simultaneously focuses the definition of LD on a failure to learn, where learning can be measured more directly. Moreover, the specific instructional elements and the conditions under which they are implemented can be described, thereby providing a clearer basis for the expectation of learning and the unexpectedness of any failure to learn. Finally, focusing on multiple assessments in an RTI model has the advantage of clearly tying the identification process to the most important component of the construct of LD, which is unexpected underachievement. Models that incorporate RTI may identify a unique group of inadequate responders who can be clearly differentiated from other low achievers in terms of cognitive correlates, prognosis, and even neurobiological factors. Moreover, there is evidence from research implementations and school-based implementations that RTI models lead to enhanced student outcomes and lower rates of referrals for special education (Burns, Appleton, & Stenhouwer, 2005a; VanDerHeyden & Burns, 2005).

Studies of children defined as responders and nonresponders across different methods clearly show large differences in cognitive skills. For example, Stage et al. (2003), Vellutino, Scanlon, and Jaccard (2003), and Vaughn et al. (2003a) found that inadequate responders to early intervention differed from responders in both preintervention achievement scores and pre-intervention cognitive tasks. Inadequate responders typi-

cally had more severe deficits in both reading-related factors (e.g., phonemic awareness, fluency) and reading skills. In recent imaging studies
involving both early intervention and remediation of older students
(Fletcher, Simos, Papanicolaou, & Denton, 2004), we likewise found
that individuals who were nonresponders showed more severe reading
difficulties prior to intervention. The differences in neuroimaging correlates between those who responded to intervention and those who did
not respond to intervention were more dramatic. We have found that
nonresponders persist with a brain activation pattern that generally
demonstrated a failure to activate left hemisphere areas known to be involved in the development of reading skills. In fact, nonresponders
showed predominant right hemisphere activity much like that observed
in children and adults with identified reading disabilities.

Reliability

Are RTI approaches that involve multiple assessments over time psycho-
metrically more reliable than traditional approaches to LD identification? An approach based on multiple measures over time has the potential to reduce the difficulties encountered with reliance on a single
assessment at a single time point. Certainly the reliability of the multiple
assessment approach is greater than if a single assessment is used to form
a discrepancy, inasmuch as typically the discrepancy will be a poorer
(i.e., less reliable) measure of the true difference than are the observed
measures of their respective underlying constructs. Focusing on successive measurements over time has the effect of moving the identification
process from "ability–ability" comparisons (two different abilities compared at one point in time) to "ability–change" models (same ability
over time). Such approaches have the potential to ameliorate the difficulties associated with ability–ability discrepancies, whether univariate or
bivariate, because they involve the use of more than two assessment time
points. Generally, the more information that is brought to bear on any
eligibility or diagnostic decision, the more reliable the decision, although
it is certainly possible to create counterexamples by combining information from irrelevant or confounding sources. Such irrelevancies are not
likely to be introduced by assessing the same skill over time as in a
model that incorporates RTI, when that skill was previously deemed relevant to assess at a single time point.

Conceptually, the study of change is made *more* feasible by the collection of multiple assessments because the precision by which change
can be measured improves as the number of time points increases
(Rogosa, 1995). When assessments at more than two time points are collected, the reliability of estimated change can also be estimated directly

from the data, and the imprecision inherent in individual estimates can be used to provide improved estimates of growth parameters for individual students as well as for groups of students. If change is not linear, the use of four or more time points can map the form of growth. And for those who favor status models over change or learning models, it remains possible to use the intercept term in the individual growth model as an estimate of status. This intercept will provide a more precise estimate of true status at any single point in time than would any single assessment.

These approaches are not without difficulty. The introduction of serial assessments has not eliminated the necessity of indirect estimation of the parameters of interest, representing change over time. Models based on RTI also involve imperfect measures that include measurement error (Fletcher et al., 2003). However, this problem is reduced because of the use of multiple assessments and the borrowing of precision from the entire collection of data to provide a more precise estimate of the growth parameters of each individual. Thus, it becomes possible to estimate a child's "true" status more precisely, as well as to estimate the rate of skill acquisition and to use these estimates as indicators of LD. In addition, this approach to estimation will make assumptions about the distribution of errors of measurement. In some cases, errors might be assumed to be uncorrelated. Again, this assumption must be examined in terms of its importance to inferences about individual status and rates of learning. In many cases, the inclusion of multiple assessment time points will allow this assumption to be relaxed, and the correlation among errors of measurement can be estimated and taken into account in forming inferences about individual status and rates of learning.

Perhaps the most significant problem with RTI models is the need to consider other factors in identifying those with LDs (Fuchs & Fuchs, 2006). There is still a need to identify individual children as learning disabled, and some consideration of cut-points is necessary unless the entire process devolves to clinical judgment. Models that include RTI do not solve the issue of the dimensional versus categorical nature of LD. Determining cut-points and benchmarks, for example, will continue to be an arbitrary process until cut-points are linked to functional outcomes (Cisek, 2001), an issue never really addressed in LD identification for *any* identification model. However, models that include RTI have the promise of incorporating functional outcomes because they are tied to intervention response. They also suggest ways in which other criteria can be meaningfully incorporated into identification. In the next section, we discuss the use of criteria that by definition preclude identification of LDs.

EXCLUSIONARY FACTORS

Most definitions of LDs have prominent components that indicate what conditions lead to underachievement that is "expected underachievement." Stipulating that LDs are not due to mental retardation, sensory disorders, or linguistic diversity is reasonable, as children with these characteristics have different intervention needs. A person whose primary language is a minority language should not be identified as learning disabled unless it can be demonstrated that the difficulties producing the reading or math problem are a pervasive characteristic across languages. There are also issues with distinctions between mental retardation and LDs that make the precise demarcation unclear, but information beyond IQ tests is essential for identifying mental deficiency (MacMillan & Siperstein, 2002).

Other exclusions stem from policy decisions that involve the need to avoid the mixing of special education and compensatory education funds, as well as the existence of other eligibility categories in IDEA to support children with special needs (e.g., mental retardation, emotional disturbance). The original exclusionary criteria were not meant to preclude children from placement, but to better classify each child's difficulties— on the assumption that when economic disadvantage, emotional disturbance, and inadequate instruction are the primary causes of underachievement, different interventions are needed.

In the other exclusionary areas, determining the primary "cause" when the evidence is largely behavioral has proven to be a difficult proposition. The cognitive correlates of academic difficulties in children with achievement deficiencies attributed to emotional disturbance, inadequate instruction, and economic disadvantage do not appear to be different according to these putative causes. Moreover, the intervention needs, responses to interventions, or mechanisms whereby interventions work do not appear to vary according to these factors (Fletcher et al., 2005a; Lyon et al., 2001). As such, these distinctions are not strongly related to the types of intervention programs that are likely to be effective, especially in reading. Of particular concern is the idea that inadequate instruction precludes identification of LDs, when in fact it may cause LDs. Later in this section, we examine specifically exclusion due to socioeconomic disadvantage and lack of opportunity for learning.

Emotional and Behavioral Difficulties

Most definitions of LDs exclude individuals whose poor achievement is due primarily to emotional and behavioral difficulties. This assessment is

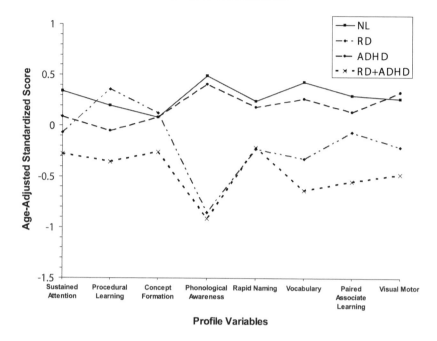

FIGURE 3.7. Profiles of cognitive performance by children with only reading disability (RD), only attention-deficit/hyperactivity disorder (ADHD), both RD and ADHD (RD + MD), and typically achieving children (NL). ADHD results in more severe RD, but the shape differences are not significant between the two reading-impaired groups. From Fletcher (2005, p. 310). Copyright 2005 by PRO-ED. Reprinted by permission.

difficult to make, largely because LDs co-occur with disorders of attention (ADHD) (Barkley, 2006; Fletcher et al., 1999b) and other social and emotional problems. Determining which disorder is primary is difficult, as those who struggle may develop behavioral difficulties that are secondary to lack of success in school. Thus, many children have co-occurring, or *comorbid*, learning and behavioral difficulties. As Figure 3.7 shows for the area of reading, the two types of disorders are distinct and separable (Fletcher et al., 1999b; Wood, Felton, Flowers, & Naylor, 1991). LDs involving word recognition are consistently associated with deficits in phonological awareness regardless of the presence or absence of ADHD, whereas the effects of ADHD on cognitive functioning are variable, with primary deficits noted in executive functions (Barkley, 1997). Furthermore, ADHD appears relatively unrelated to phonological awareness tasks (Fletcher et al., 1999; Wood et al., 1991). A child who meets

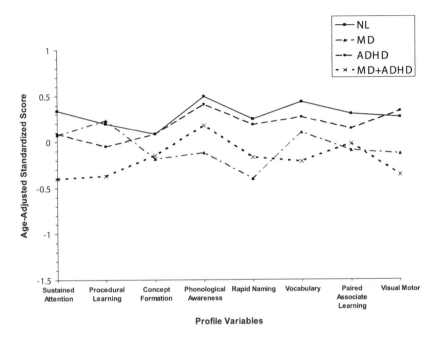

FIGURE 3.8. Profiles of cognitive performance by children with only math disability (MD), only attention-deficit/hyperactivity disorder (ADHD), both MD and ADHD (MD + ADHD), and typically achieving children (NL). ADHD results in more severe MD, but shape differences are not significant between the two math-impaired groups. From Fletcher (2005, p. 311). Copyright 2005 by PRO-ED. Reprinted by permission.

the criteria for both an LD in reading and ADHD shows characteristics of both.

In studies examining comorbidity of math disabilities and ADHD (Figure 3.8), the groups overlap more than groups with reading disabilities and ADHD. This likely reflects the role of executive functions (strategy use, procedural learning) and working memory in both math disabilities and ADHD. But the disorders are separable on dimensions involving attention and behavior (Fletcher et al., 2002), with individuals who meet criteria for both disorders showing characteristics of both. Finally, disorders of written language and math are especially common in children identified as having ADHD (Barkley, 1997). Nonetheless, reading problems are also common (Fletcher et al.,1999). In most instances, these appear to be comorbid associations: A child with disabilities involving ADHD and a domain-specific LD appears like a child with ADHD through the behavioral lens, and like a child with LDs through the cognitive lens. However, when both forms of disability are apparent, the cognitive and academic deficits invariably appear more severe (Figures 3.7 and 3.8).

Researchers have also reported that children with reading disabilities present with co-occurring social-emotional difficulties (Bryan, Burstein, & Ergul, 2004). In some clinical studies, these difficulties appear to be secondary to difficulties in learning to read. For example, of the 93 adults in a clinic population with LDs, the majority of whom displayed reading problems, 36% had received counseling or psychotherapy for low self-esteem, social isolation, anxiety, depression, and frustration (Johnson & Blalock, 1987). Likewise, others (Bruck, 1987; Cooley & Ayers, 1988) have reported that many of the emotional problems displayed by readers with LDs reflect adjustment difficulties resulting from labeling or academic failure. Despite these studies of highly selected populations, meta-analyses of the relations of LDs and social skills found little evidence for specific deficits in children broadly defined as having LDs (Zeleke, 2004) or for the effectiveness of interventions addressing these problems (Kavale & Mostert, 2004) unless such a student had low self-esteem before the study began (Elbaum & Vaughn, 2003). Many of these studies were not well controlled for other factors related to social skills, such as ADHD and socioeconomic status (SES). The common failure to specify the subgrouping of LDs into reading versus math disabilities is unfortunate, as there is evidence that children with math disabilities are more impaired than those with reading disorders, especially if other nonverbal processing skills are also impaired (Rourke, 1989, 1993). Other studies find that reading problems are associated with higher rates of internalizing and externalizing psychopathology, even in nonclinical samples (Willcutt & Pennington, 2000). In this latter study, the comorbid association of reading disabilities and ADHD could explain much of this relationship. When ADHD was controlled, externalizing disorders were no longer linked but relationships with internalizing symptoms persisted, especially in girls with reading disabilities. Finally, recent large-scale clinical trials show that improving reading and math instruction in programs that provide positive behavioral support reduces subsequent behavioral difficulties in first-graders followed into middle school. The most significant path is from achievement to behavior, so poor achievement clearly leads to behavioral difficulties (Kellam, Rebok, Mayer, Ialongo, & Kalodner, 1994). Altogether, these findings illustrate the significant need to identify and intervene early with those children who are at risk for academic failure, given the substantial social and emotional consequences that can occur if the disabilities are not remediated. The findings do not support the idea of excluding individuals from identification as learning disabled if they show evidence for emotional, behavioral, or social difficulties.

Economic Disadvantage

Although most current definitions of LDs state that the academic deficits encompassed by the disorder cannot be attributed to economic disadvantage and cultural factors (including race or ethnicity), limited information exists regarding how race, ethnicity, and cultural background might influence school learning in general and the expression of different types of LDs in particular. For example, Wood et al. (1991) conducted a longitudinal study of specific LDs (in reading) within a random sample of 485 children selected in the first grade and followed through the third grade (55% European American, 45% African American). Wood et al. (1991) found that the effects of race were, in fact, important as well as highly complicated. For example, at the first-grade level, race did not appear to be an influential variable in reading development once vocabulary ability was accounted for. That is, once a child's age and level of vocabulary development were known, race did not provide any additional predictive power to forecasting first-grade reading scores. However, by the end of the third grade, race had become a significant predictive factor ($p = .001$) even when the most powerful predictors—first-grade reading scores—were also in the prediction equation. Specifically, by the end of the third grade, African American children were having significantly greater difficulties in learning to read. In attempting to understand this race effect, Wood and his group assessed a number of additional demographic factors, including parental marital status, parental education, parental status as welfare recipient, SES, the number of books in the home, and occupational status. Their findings were clear: The presence of any or all of these demographic variables in the prediction equation "did not remove the race effect from its potency as an independent predictor of third grade reading" (Wood et al., 1991, p. 9).

A major issue is that many of the conditions that are excluded as potential influences on LDs interfere with the development of cognitive and linguistic skills that lead to the academic deficits that in turn lead to LDs (Phillips & Lonigan, 2005). Parents with reading problems, for example, may find it difficult to establish adequate home literacy practices because of the cumulative effects of their reading difficulties (Wadsworth et al., 2000). Children who grow up in economically disadvantaged environments are behind in language development when they enter school (Hart & Risley, 1995). This delay will interfere with the development of reading and math skills. Moreover, interventions that address the early development of these skills seem to promote academic success in evaluative studies of Title I programs, as well as intervention studies in which alphabetic forms of instruction have been shown to be advantageous for economically disadvantaged children (Foorman et al., 1998; National Reading Panel, 2000). Thus, the mechanisms and practices that promote reading success in advantaged populations appear to be similar to those that promote reading success or failure in disadvantaged populations. There is little evidence that the phenotypic representation of reading disabilities varies according to SES. Children at all SES levels appear to have reading problems predominantly (but not exclusively) because of word-level difficulties apparent in the beginning stages of reading development (Foorman et al., 1998; Wood et al., 1991). As Kavale (1988) and Lyon et al. (2001) have pointed out, the basis for excluding disadvantaged children from the LDs category has more to do with how children are served than with empirical evidence demonstrating that characteristics of reading failure are different in groups with LDs as opposed to those who are economically disadvantaged.

Inadequate Instruction

Exclusion based on the opportunity to learn and the provision of appropriate instruction in general education makes sense if there has been no effort to teach a child. But this notion is often expanded to include children whose instruction has not been adequate. Although children's failure to respond to appropriate instruction is a very strong indication of a disability, the cognitive problems associated with their LDs parallel those exhibited by children who do not respond to adequate instruction. The two types of children are equally disabled. Of the different exclusionary criteria for LDs, instructional factors are the least frequently examined but perhaps the most important. The opportunity-to-learn exclusion presumed that the field has a good understanding of what constitutes adequate instruction. This was not the case at the time the federal definition was adopted. Recent consensus reports (Snow, Burns, & Griffin, 1998; National Reading Panel, 2000) make it clear that we do know a lot about teaching children to read. At least in reading, which accounts for most forms of LDs, consideration of the students' response to high-quality intervention needs to become part of the definition of LDs, representing a major impetus for RTI models (Gresham, 2002; Fuchs & Fuchs, 1998). Why should the complex identification criteria and expensive due-process procedures of special education be used before an attempt is made to provide intervention early in a child's development? A child's failure to respond to high-quality intervention may be the best way to operationalize the notion of opportunity to learn.

Conclusions: Exclusionary Factors

Approaching the exclusion hypothesis from the perspective of classification research shows little evidence supporting exclusions based on economic disadvantage and lack of opportunity to learn. This reflects the difficulties of differentiating forms of low achievement that are presumably "specific" or "unexpected" from those that can be attributed to other causes where low achievement is expected. This does not mean that the concept of LDs is not valid or that the exclusions should not be used, particularly since many children can be served under other categories in IDEA or other approaches to providing services (e.g., compensatory education). These exclusions must be seen as policy-based determinations to facilitate service delivery and to avoid mixing of funds, not as classification factors that have strong validity.

CONCLUSIONS: AN INTEGRATED MODEL

Following the recommendations introduced by the Learning Disabilities Summit convened by the U.S. Office of Special Education Programs (Bradley et al., 2002), we recommend a hybrid model that combines features of low achievement and RTI models. Bradley et al. proposed three sets of criteria for identifying students with LDs. The first is the student's response to instruction, which should be based on designations of the child as "at risk"; serial curriculum-based assessments of the academic domain of concern; and evaluations of the quality of the instruction. Second, if a child demonstrates an inadequate response to instruction, norm-referenced assessments should occur specifically in the achievement domain. These assessments help establish the child's normative level of achievement, verify the findings from the CBM assessments, and ensure that all academic domains have been evaluated (see Chapter 4). Finally, the child should receive some type of comprehensive evaluation that extends beyond the evaluation of the achievement domain. This evaluation should be relatively brief and should not be based on any type of standard battery. Rather, there should always be concerns about comorbid conditions in the child considered for LDs, which would necessitate, at a minimum, parent and teacher behavioral rating scales. In addition, other questions that emerge as to the causes of underachievement should be evaluated, including the possibility of mental retardation, speech and language impairments, and behavioral difficulties. Finally, there should always be evaluations of home, language, and social factors that may produce underachievement. There is rarely any need for extensive cognitive evaluations, but there may be instances in which inadequate responders would benefit from additional cognitive assessments attempting to determine the reason for lack of response (e.g., severe phonological awareness difficulties). Thus, we are recommending a model that is based essentially on a hybrid involving RTI, intraindividual differences in the achievement domains from both a low achievement and intraindividual perspective, and consideration of exclusionary factors. A hybrid model should permit the isolation of a group of inadequate responders, for which the integrity of instruction is assured, and that epitomize the construct of unexpected underachievement.

The differences in a model that incorporates RTI versus traditional models based on referral and assessment can be clearly identified in Figure 3.9. In this figure, the traditional approach does not involve progress monitoring or the concept of mass screening, which is apparent in the new model. The ideal of multiple treatments and modifying instruction based on progress is implicit in the traditional model, but explicit in the new model. The traditional model sets aside special education as a sepa-

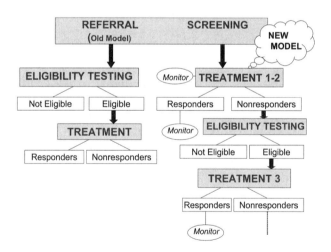

FIGURE 3.9. A comparison of a traditional model for identification and a model based on RTI. On the left side, the student is typically referred for an eligibility evaluation. The student is either eligible or not eligible; if eligible, the student receives intervention that is evaluated at 1 to 3 years. In an RTI model, all children are screened; those at risk receive progress monitoring assessments and immediate intervention. If there is not adequate response to different interventions, beginning in general education, increasingly intense interventions are provided. Lack of adequate response may result in referral to special education and a dramatically different eligibility evaluation. Progress is monitored at all stages so that intervention can be adjusted in short-time intervals. Figure courtesy of Maureen Dennis.

rate service; the new model usually links general and special education. In the end, the real test of the new model will involve whether different types of students are identified with LDs in relation to the traditional model. Some may argue that the two models should be competed in some type of randomized study. Such a study would be expensive and difficult to achieve, given the complexity of both models. From a classification perspective, historical controls for efficacy should be sufficient, provided it is possible to determine whether students identified as LD under these models are different. We hypothesize that individuals identified in the model incorporating RTI will be harder to teach and will show poorer response to even high-quality instruction, that they will have stronger heritability of reading problems and brains that show less activation in areas known to be critical for different LDs, and will have more severe cognitive processing problems. Hence, there will be little debate about whether LDs are disabilities and less discussion about their reality.

CHAPTER 4

Assessment of Learning Disabilities

The review of classification models in Chapter 3 leads directly to an approach to the clinical assessment of people for whom LD is an issue (Fletcher, Francis, Morris, & Lyon, 2005b; Fuchs & Fuchs, 1998). The tests and procedures selected for any assessment stem from a classification model and the constructs it specifies. If the classification is based on an aptitude–achievement discrepancy model, the primary tools would be the tests used to measure aptitude (e.g., IQ or listening comprehension) and achievement tests of reading, math, and written language. If the classification reflects a low achievement model, aptitude would not be measured in favor of a focus on achievement. Classifications based on an intraindividual differences model would utilize cognitive processing measures or neuropsychological tests. If a model incorporates RTI, assessments of the quality of instruction, along with curriculum-based measurement (CBM) to assess response to that instruction, would be required.

In the hybrid model we proposed, an evaluation of LD requires an assessment of RTI, norm-referenced assessments of achievement, and an evaluation of contextual factors and associated conditions that may explain the achievement problem and, most important, suggest alternative intervention needs that differ from those that directly address achievement issues through instructional methods.

TEST AND TREAT VERSUS TREAT AND TEST

This approach to assessment of LDs is different from the traditional test-to-diagnosis approaches that have dominated the assessment domain for many years (see Figure 3.9). In the approach to identification we propose, LDs are not "diagnosed" on the basis of a battery of psychometric tests administered on a single occasion. Rather, LDs are identified only after a specific attempt is made to systematically instruct the person. An obvious question is whether LDs can be identified in the absence of intervention or even outside of schools. We suggest that ensuring adequate opportunity to learn is indeed a prerequisite to the identification of LDs regardless of setting, so that traditional test-to-diagnosis approaches can, at best, identify the person as being "at risk" for LDs. But a single assessment will not lead to reliable identification if the approach is based on cutoff scores or based on a related approach.

The goal of any evaluation should be to intervene as soon as possible with a person who is struggling to achieve. In schools, screening for reading problems can be done on a large scale, as advocated in the National Research Council consensus report on minority overrepresentation in special education (Donovan & Cross, 2002) and implemented in states like Texas (Foorman, Fletcher, & Francis, 2004). Those who are identified as being at risk should have their progress monitored with CBM and receive increasingly intense, multitiered interventions that may eventuate in identification for special education if the student responds inadequately to intervention and meets additional criteria (Vaughn & Fuchs, 2003). This approach, central to an RTI model, prioritizes establishment of a disability over establishment of a disorder in a "treat-and-test" model. In most disability eligibility systems, disability status depends on both the presence of a disorder *and evidence that the disorder interferes with adaptive functions*, so there is evidence that the disorder is *disabling*. Evaluating instructional response is one way to operationalize the disability component of an evaluation for LDs.

If an evaluation of federal guidelines is conducted independently (i.e., outside of schools in mental health or psychoeducation clinics or other similar settings), the basis should still reside in the hybrid model described in Chapter 3 (Bradley et al., 2002). In clinic situations, it may be necessary to initially establish evidence of low achievement. Evidence of low achievement should lead to concerns about intervention, not about assessments of IQ or cognitive processing skills to "diagnose" LDs. Professionals who conduct assessments related to LDs should have a working knowledge of educational interventions and a relationship with professionals in or out of school who can provide intervention and measure RTI in people with achievement difficulties. There is no point in assessing students for LDs just to make a diagnosis. If necessary, the professional can independently evaluate progress in conjunction with more frequent assessments of progress obtained by the intervention source.

HETEROGENEITY OF LDs

Prior to discussing evaluations of RTI, achievement, and contextual factors, the question of the relevant domains of LDs should be addressed. This question reflects long-term issues concerning the heterogeneity of LDs—the fact that the construct of LDs can be rooted in impairment in any one of several different domains of achievement. LDs are clearly domain specific, meaning that disabilities involving reading, math, and written expression are different in phenotypic characteristics and intervention needs. Although many people with LDs have impairment in more than one of these domains, there are prototypes for subgroups of people with disabilities isolated to the domains of reading and math. This heterogeneity alone makes difficult the proposition that LDs can be subsumed under a single overarching conceptualization.

There are prototypes that epitomize other groups that would make up the domains of a hypothetical classification of LDs. However, these domains are not consistently reflected in the 1977 U.S. federal definition of LDs. In discussing this issue, Fletcher et al. (2002) noted that two of the categories in the 1977 U.S. federal definition of LDs (Chapter 2) involving domains of oral expression and listening comprehension are also addressed in the speech and language category. The reason for this duplication is that these conditions are described in the U.S. statutory definition (Chapter 2). Even if listening comprehension is not regarded as a component of receptive language, it closely parallels reading comprehension in children who do not show word-reading disabilities (Chapter 7).

The organization of the other five domains (basic reading, reading comprehension, math calculations, math concepts, and written expression) is not consistent with the subgroups that consistently emerge in research studies. Difficulties are not identified in "reading fluency," and "math concepts" does not represent the domain actually addressed in education and in intervention studies. Consistent with Chapter 8, it may be better to identify "problem solving" as a relevant domain of math skills.

Table 4.1 lists five subgroups consistently identified in research. These subgroups include three forms of reading disabilities, involving word recognition (Chapter 5); fluency (Chapter 6); and comprehension (Chapter 7); math disabilities (Chapter 8); and disorders of written expression, involving spelling, handwriting, and expression (Chapter 9). The research base is weakest in identifying the academic skill deficits that lead to identification of math disabilities—computations, problem solving, and so on. Moreover, it is not clear whether math difficulties associated with reading difficulties are different or reflect a comorbid association (see Chapter 8). Math and writing fluency may also be important

TABLE 4.1. Subgroups Forming a Hypothetical Classification of LD

LD type	Component academic deficits
Reading disability	Word recognition and spelling
Reading disability	Comprehension
Reading disability	Fluency and automaticity
Mathematics disability	Computations, problem solving
Written expression disability	Handwriting, spelling, and/or composition

domains, but there is little evidence presently suggesting that disorders involving fluency of reading, math, and writing are distinct. It is always possible that future research will identify other subgroups for this hypothetical classification.

The evidence that supports these domains is summarized in the respective chapters that follow. For assessment purposes, these domains of achievement must be considered. Assessments of RTI with CBM are best developed for word recognition, reading fluency, math, and spelling. It is possible to assess comprehension with CBM measures using cloze or maze tests, but the format provides a limited assessment of reading comprehension, which in itself is difficult to assess because it reflects so many underlying processes. All of these domains can be assessed using norm-referenced tests. The difficulties in assessing complex skills such as reading comprehension and written expression are major reasons underlying our suggestion that norm-referenced assessments of the achievement domain are important for identifying LDs.

As we indicated in Chapter 1, some argue that LDs extend beyond achievement domains, the most obvious example being social skills. Many individuals with LDs do have problems with social skills. In some instances this represents a comorbid disorder, as in the example of ADHD. In other instances, problems with social skills seem to reflect the same underlying processes that lead to achievement difficulties, epitomized by the hypothesis of a nonverbal LD. This proposed form of LD is characterized by a constellation of deficits in math procedures, reading comprehension, and social skills, and other cognitive, motor, and sensory functions (Rourke, 1989). Some children with LDs clearly have problems with social skills, motor skills, perceptual abilities, oral language, and other areas that do not directly involve achievement. Consider, however, that many people with problems in these areas do not have achievement problems. In arguing that achievement deficits are necessary but not sufficient, we are suggesting that classifications that include LDs are not viable without some type of marker that reliably indicates the presence of LDs (Stanovich, 1991, 2000).

In the next sections, we discuss the three essential components needed to evaluate and identify people with LDs, including the evaluation of RTI (including the evaluation of intervention integrity), the evaluation of achievement, and the evaluation of contextual factors and associated conditions.

EVALUATING LDs

Monitoring Progress

If a child is screened or tested for achievement deficits and a problem is identified, progress should be monitored in relation to instruction. We emphasize screening because we believe that rapid identification of students with achievement difficulties is essential and should lead directly to intervention and progress monitoring. Even if screening is performed with norm-referenced assessments, these tests should be readministered at least twice during the school year as one method of assessing the efficacy of the intervention plan. The rate of development of a child who is at risk and responding to intervention should be accelerated relative to normative expectations, indicating that the achievement gap is closing (Torgesen, 2000). Progress can be monitored on a frequent basis, with the use of short fluency-based probes assessing word reading accuracy and fluency, math, and spelling. It is more difficult to monitor the progress of reading comprehension and composition because these domains will show less rapid change, and progress-monitoring tools for these types of problems have not been adequately developed. Methods for assessing progress over longer periods of time will be necessary.

Figure 4.1 provides a CBM graph showing program development and progress for a child in grade 3 mathematics. Each dot represents performance on one occasion on one alternate form of a CBM test that systematically sampled the grade 3 curriculum. In this example, Stephen's teacher can look across rows of the skills profile to see, for example, that applied computation has gone from (1) not attempted, to (2) attempted but not mastered, to (3) partially mastered, then back to (4) attempted but not mastered after the winter break, to (5) partially mastered again, to (6) probably mastered in March–April.

Most norm-referenced tests have alternate forms, but are not suitable for administration every 1–3 weeks, which is necessary for frequent monitoring of progress. Thus, CBM assessments have been developed to permit frequent assessments (Stecker et al., 2005). These measures are often used by an instructor to assess RTI, but could also be completed by a diagnostician or other testing professional. With progress-monitoring assessment, children read a short passage appropriate for grade level, complete math computations, or spell words for 1–6 minutes. The num-

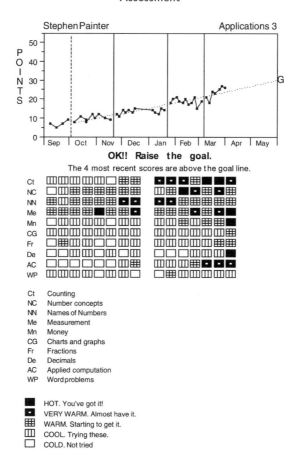

FIGURE 4.1. A CBM graph showing program development and progress for "Stephen Painter" in the grade 3 mathematics concepts and applications curriculum. Each dot represents performance on one occasion on one alternate form of a CBM test that systematically sampled the grade 3 curriculum. The vertical dotted line denotes the setting of the goal (also see G at year's end); the dotted vertical line indicates the rate of progress required to achieve the year-end goal; and the solid vertical lines show when the teacher revised the instructional program in an attempt to boost the rate of progress. The last set of data points reveals a stronger rate of growth (the four most recent scores are all above the goal line), so the decision was to increase the goal. The boxes at the bottom represent mastery of the skills taught in the grade 3 curriculum. The first stack of boxes shows no mastery (i.e., no dark boxes); in mid-April, Stephen had mastered three skill areas (measurement, money, decimals); had probably mastered two additional skills (counting, applied computation); and had partially mastered four more skills (number concepts, names of numbers, charts/graphs, fractions), leaving only word problems as attempted but not mastered. Stephen's teacher could look across rows of the skills profile to see, for example, that applied computation had gone from (1) not attempted, to (2) attempted but not mastered, to (3) partially mastered, then back to (4) attempted but not mastered after the winter break, to (5) partially mastered again, to (6) probably mastered in March–April.

ber of accurately read words, correct math problems, or correctly spelled items would be graphed over time and compared against benchmarks representing expected outcomes. These measures can also be used for screening to determine level of risk and to provide a baseline for the evaluation of RTI.

Progress-monitoring assessments are about more than testing—they are an integral part of good intervention strategies. Although research supports the efficacy of a variety of instructional methods for promoting academic achievement among students with LDs (Swanson et al., 2003), the heterogeneity of this population, combined with the severe and multifaceted nature of their needs, results in a rate of unresponsiveness to validated interventions that is high, ranging between 10 and 50%, depending on the intervention and the criteria for "inadequate response." For this reason, academic outcomes for students with LDs can be enhanced substantially when student progress is systematically monitored while validated interventions are being implemented. With progress monitoring, teachers and others gauge the extent to which an individual student is responding to an instructional intervention. When response is inadequate, teachers can quickly revise the program and then monitor the impact of those revisions.

Progress monitoring can be done using a variety of methods. In terms of a norm-referenced test, it is possible to employ widely used tests such as the Test of Word Reading Efficiency (Torgesen et al., 1999a) or the Woodcock–Johnson Achievement Battery (Woodcock, McGrew, & Mather, 2001). With such tests, alternate forms can be used repeatedly to model student improvement as a function of intervention, but only at relatively long intervals of time (usually several months). There are alternate forms for frequent CBM data collection, many of which have been reviewed by the National Center for Student Progress Monitoring (www.studentprogress.org). As the reviews by this Center indicate, CBM procedures vary considerably in the extent of reliability data, and the number of forms, grades, and academic domains for which they are available. However, research substantiates that some forms of CBM provide reliable and valid information about how well students are progressing and show that when CBM is used to determine when revisions to student programs are needed, better end-of-year academic outcomes result than when CBM is not used.

CBM efficacy studies have examined the effects of alternative data-utilization strategies, showing that CBM enhances instructional planning and student learning by helping teachers set ambitious student goals, by assisting in determining when instructional adaptations are necessary to prompt better student growth, and by providing ideas for potentially effective teaching adjustments. With respect to goal setting,

Fuchs, Fuchs, and Hamlett (1989b) explored the contribution of goal-raising guidelines within CBM decision-making rules. Teachers were assigned randomly to, and participated in, one of three treatments in mathematics for 15 weeks: (1) no CBM, (2) CBM without a goal-raising rule, and (3) CBM with a goal-raising rule. The goal-raising rule required teachers to increase goals whenever the student's actual rate of growth exceeded the growth rate anticipated by the teacher. Teachers in the CBM goal-raising condition raised goals more frequently (for 15 of 30 students) than teachers in the non-goal-raising conditions (for 1 of 30 students). Moreover, concurrent with teachers' goal-raising behavior was differential student achievement on pre–post standardized achievement tests. The effect size comparing the pre–post change of the two CBM conditions (i.e., with and without the goal-raising rule) was 0.52 standard deviation units. Consequently, using CBM to monitor the appropriateness of instructional goals and to adjust goals upward whenever possible is one way in which CBM can be used to assist teachers in their instructional planning.

Another key way in which CBM can be used to enhance instructional decision making is in assessing the adequacy of student progress and determining whether instructional adaptation is necessary. When actual growth rate is less than expected growth rate (slope of the goal line), the teacher modifies the instructional program to promote stronger learning. Fuchs, Fuchs, and Hamlett (1989c) estimated the contribution of this CBM decision-making strategy with 29 special educators who implemented CBM for 15 school weeks with 53 students with mild/moderate disabilities. Teachers in a "CBM—measurement only" group measured students' reading growth as required but did not use the assessment information to structure students' reading programs. Teachers in the "CBM—change the program" decision-rule group measured student performance and used the assessment information to determine when to introduce programmatic adaptations to enhance growth rates. Results indicated that although teachers in both groups measured student performance, important differences were associated with the use of the "change the program" decision rule. As indicated on the Stanford Achievement Test—Reading Comprehension Subtest, students in the "change the program" decision-rule group achieved better than a no-CBM control group (effect size = 0.72), whereas the "measurement only" CBM group did not (effect size = 0.36). Moreover, the slopes of the two CBM treatment groups were significantly different, favoring the achievement of the "change the program" group (effect size = 0.86). As suggested by these findings and results of other researchers (e.g., Wesson, 1991), collecting CBM data, in and of itself, exerts only a small effect on student learning. To enhance student outcomes in important ways, teachers need to use the CBM data experimentally to build effective programs for students with LDs.

For helping teachers determine when adjustments are required in students' programs and for identifying when goal increases are warranted, the CBM total scores are used. In addition, by inspecting the graph of performance indicators over time (see Figure 4.1), teachers may formulate ideas for potentially effective instructional adaptations. For example, a flat or decelerating slope might generate hypotheses about lack of maintenance of previously learned material or about motivational problems. Nevertheless, to obtain rich descriptions of student performance, alternative ways of summarizing and describing student performance are necessary. Because CBM assesses performance on the year's curriculum at each testing, rich descriptions of strengths and weaknesses in the curriculum can be generated.

The effects of CBM diagnostic profiles were investigated in three studies, one in math (Fuchs, Fuchs, Hamlett, & Stecker, 1991b), one in reading (Fuchs, Fuchs, & Hamlett, 1989d), and one in spelling (Fuchs, Fuchs, Hamlett, & Allinder, 1991a). In each investigation, teachers were assigned randomly to one of three conditions: (1) no CBM, (2) CBM with goal-raising and change-the-program decision rules, and (3) CBM with goal-raising and change-the-program decision rules along with CBM diagnostic profiles. In all three studies, teachers in the diagnostic profile treatment group generated instructional plans that were more varied and more responsive to individuals' learning needs. Moreover, they effected better student learning as measured on change between pre- and posttest performance on global measures of achievement. Effect sizes associated with the CBM diagnostic profile groups ranged from 0.65 to 1.23. This series of studies demonstrated how structured, well-organized CBM information about students' strengths and difficulties in the curriculum helps teachers to build better programs and effect greater learning.

Research has also provided evidence of CBM's overall utility in helping teachers plan more effective programs (e.g., L. S. Fuchs, Deno, & Mirkin, 1984; Fuchs et al., 1991a; Shapiro, Edwards, & Zigmond, 2005; Wesson, 1991). To illustrate this database, we describe one study in reading. Fuchs et al. (1984) conducted a study in the New York City public schools. Teachers participated for 18 weeks in a contrast group or in a CBM treatment group, where they measured students' reading performance at least twice weekly, scored and graphed those performances, and used prescriptive CBM decision-making rules for planning the students' reading programs. When teachers employed CBM to plan reading programs, their students achieved better than when teachers used conventional monitoring methods on the Passage

Reading Test and the decoding and comprehension subtests of the Stanford Diagnostic Reading Test, with respective effect sizes of 1.18, 0.94, and 0.99. This suggests that, despite exclusive focus on passage reading fluency for progress monitoring, teachers planned more comprehensive reading programs involving fluency, decoding, and comprehension.

In sum, a large set of controlled investigations provides corroborating evidence of dramatic effects on student outcomes in reading, spelling, and math when teachers rely on CBM to inform instructional planning. When this form of progress monitoring is used to assess the effects of validated interventions on individual students with LDs and to revise programs responsively to those data, positive academic outcomes for students with LDs are more likely.

Evaluating Interventions

The CBM assessments should also be accompanied by observations of the integrity of the implementation of the intervention, including the nature of and the amount of time spent on supplemental instruction, especially if the child does not appear to be making progress. School psychologists are often well prepared in this area of assessment. Although a psychologist operating outside of schools may not be in a position to implement CBM or to personally evaluate the integrity with which the intervention is implemented, such assessments should be expected, especially if the referral is to a private academic therapist.

Identifying Inadequate Response

When CBM data are systematically collected, a variety of approaches can be used to establish whether the person's response is adequate. Although it is apparent that "responsiveness" exists on a continuum and firm cutoff scores are not likely to encompass every student of concern, specific criteria provide guidelines for identifying students in need. The literature identifies different approaches to defining adequate response to instruction. Some indices are based on progress-monitoring assessments that permit computation of slope and intercept functions relative to a comparison group that could be school based or have some other normative basis. Fuchs and Fuchs (1998) and Speece and Case (2001) have reported that indices based on both slope and intercept are more predictive of long-term outcomes than slope or intercept alone, the rationale being that a student could begin an intervention well below benchmark standards, but have a very positive response that would be masked by the intercept or an end-of-year benchmark alone.

Others have relied primarily on end-of-year benchmarks (Torgesen, 2000), computing the number of students who read below a benchmark, typically an age-adjusted standard score below the 25th or 30th percentile. Finally, another common benchmark sets a criterion based on passage reading fluency. First graders, for example, should read 35–40 words per minute depending on the difficulty level of the text. It is useful to examine multiple criteria. However, examinations of slope should be included because the question is about change (progress), and the number of data points needed to estimate change increases the reliability of identification of inadequate response. Because an estimate of change always includes an intercept function that addresses level of function, both the slope and absolute level of performance can be examined with CBM. Fuchs and Fuchs (1998) proposed the use of both slope and final status for identifying inadequate response, suggesting that a student must demonstrate a "dual discrepancy" in which the slope and final level are both at least one standard deviation below those of peers or some type of norm-referenced standard. Figure 4.2 presents different trajectories based on a growth mixture analysis (Fuchs, Compton, Fuchs, Hamlett, & Bryant, 2006a). For the analysis, 27 weekly curriculum-based computation assessments were collected from October to April of first grade (n = 225). The analysis yielded four trajectory classes. Students with low intercept and low slope were significantly more likely to be classified as disabled in math at the end of second grade (defined as performance below the 10th percentile on the Wide Range Achievement Test–Arithmetic), as compared with students with high intercept (regardless of slope) and as compared with students with low intercept but with high slope. As Figure 4.2 shows, final status by itself permits some students to be classified as inadequate responders, despite significant progress, because the initial level of performance was very low. Despite strong growth, the students remained below the benchmark at the end of the intervention. Focusing only on the benchmark might suggest that the intervention was ineffective, when examination of the slope suggests that it would be premature to abandon the intervention. Alternatively, examining only the slope permits some students to be identified as inadequate responders even though they complete the intervention meeting the norm-referenced or benchmark criteria, suggesting positive future outcomes. By simultaneously considering slope of improvement and final status, the dual discrepancy approach permits the identification of inadequate response classification only when a student (1) fails to make adequate growth and (2) completes the intervention below the normalized or benchmark criteria. Additional work is required to examine and compare alternative methods for identifying LD within an RTI system, but the dual discrepancy approach appears most promising.

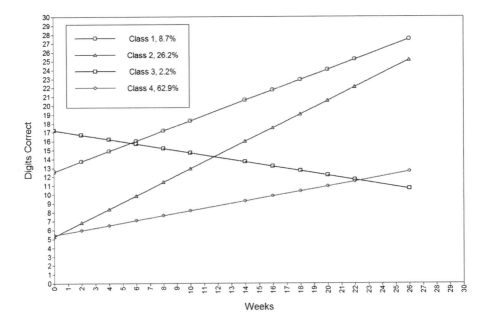

FIGURE 4.2. Four trajectory classes derived from using growth mixture modeling of 27 weekly curriculum-based computation assessments in first grade (Fuchs, Compton, Fuchs, Hamlett, & Bryant, 2006a). Students with low intercept and low slope were significantly more likely to be classified as having a mathematical disability (MD) at the end of second grade, as compared with students with high intercept (regardless of slope) and as compared with students with low intercept but with high slope.

Evaluating Achievement Domains

There are many norm-referenced achievement tests that can be incorporated into the assessment of LDs. Table 4.1 suggests five major achievement subgroups representing people who are primarily impaired in (1) word recognition, (2) reading fluency, (3) reading comprehension, (4) mathematics computations/problem solving, and (5) written expression, including spelling, handwriting, and/or composition. These patterns were established through research Rourke and Finlayson (1978), Siegel and Ryan (1989), Stothard and Hulme (1996), and Chapters 5–9 provide extensive discussion of the evidence for these subgroups. Many individuals have difficulties in multiple domains, making a complete evaluation of academic achievement necessary for anyone considered for LDs. Table 4.1 also identifies the academic skill deficits that represent the primary achievement markers of each form of LD.

Fletcher et al. (2005b) proposed the use of tests from the same achievement battery because the same cohorts would be used to develop the norms. This constancy facilitates comparisons across tests. However, more important than the battery from which these tests are selected are the constructs that are measured and the quality of the indicators of these constructs. Based on Table 4.1, the important constructs are word recognition, reading fluency, reading comprehension, math computations and problem solving, and written expression.

Table 4.2 maps the constructs and their assessment with the Woodcock–Johnson Achievement Battery–III (WJ; Woodcock et al., 2001) or the Wechsler Individual Achievement Test–II (WIAT; Wechsler, 2001), both frequently employed to assess LDs. There are also other norm-referenced assessments that can be used instead of, or to supplement, the WJ or WIAT, some of which we mention below. For example, spelling can be used to screen for written expression and handwriting difficulties.

Because many people have problems in multiple academic domains, the *pattern* of academic strengths and weaknesses across these tests is an important consideration (Fletcher et al., 2002; Fletcher et al., 2005b; Rourke, 1975). The evaluation can be conducted hierarchically and not all tests need to be given to each person. A majority of people with significant academic problems in which LDs may eventually be a concern have difficulty with word recognition skills. This typically produces problems across the domains of reading, so that assessments beyond the core tests are usually not necessary. Isolated problems with reading comprehension and written expression occur more infrequently. If the problem is specifically math, using assessments in addition to the WJ or WIAT is helpful in ensuring that the deficiency is not just a matter of attention or other difficulties.

TABLE 4.2. Woodcock–Johnson–III (WJ) and Wechsler Individual Achievement Test–II (WIAT) Subtests in Relation to Academic Skill Deficits

	Core tests	
Academic skill deficit	WJ subtest	WIAT subtest
Word recognition	Word Identification	Word Reading
	Word Attack	Pseudoword Decoding
Reading fluency	Reading fluency	—
Reading comprehension	Passage Comprehension	Reading Comprehension[a]
Math computations	Calculations	Numerical Operations
Math problem solving	Applied Problems	Math Reasoning
Spelling	Spelling	Spelling

Note. Adapted from Fletcher, Francis, Morris, and Lyon (2005b). Copyright 2005 by the American Psychological Association. Adapted by permission.
[a]Also assesses fluency.

Word Recognition

Both the WJ and WIAT include subtests requiring oral reading of lists of real words and pseudowords allowing measurement of the person's sight word knowledge and capacity for sounding out words. Most achievement batteries assess recognition of actual words typically ordered for difficulty, which is the essential component for any assessment related to LDs in this domain. Fletcher et al. (1996) found these measures of reading accuracy to be highly correlated, assessing a similar latent variable (e.g., Wide Range Achievement Test–III [Wilkinson, 1993] and the Gray Oral Reading Test—Fourth Edition [GORT-IV; Wiederholt & Bryant, 2001]).

Reading Fluency

Reading fluency measures are also typically highly correlated. We have found that the reading fluency subtest from the WJ is highly correlated with other fluency measures despite the fact that it asks the child to answer some questions while reading a series of passages for 3 minutes. The WIAT assesses reading speed during silent reading comprehension. Neither of these measures is as straightforward as the fluency assessments from the Test of Word Reading Efficiency (Torgesen et al., 1999a), which involves oral reading of real words and pseudowords on a list, or the Test of Reading Fluency (Deno & Marston, 2001) which requires text reading. Grade-appropriate CBMs are also reasonable approaches to assessing reading fluency. All of these measures are quick, efficient, and widely used. The key to assessing reading fluency is to have text read orally, so that fluency can be measured in terms of words read correctly per minute. Thus, the GORT–IV includes a score for fluency of oral text reading.

Reading Comprehension

Reading comprehension is difficult to assess (Francis et al., 2005b). It is important to attend to the nature of the material the person reads as well as the response format. Tests assessing reading comprehension vary what the child reads (sentences, passages, genre [narrative, expository]), response format (cloze, open-ended questions, multiple choice, think aloud), memory demands (answering questions with and without the text available), and the depth of assessment of the abstraction of meaning (vocabulary elaboration vs. knowledge, inferencing, and activation of background knowledge). If the issue is comprehension and the source contains elements beyond the child's word recognition or fluency skills, a single test is rarely adequate and multiple measures that assess reading comprehension in different ways may be needed.

To illustrate, measures like the WJ Passage Comprehension subtests can only be considered screens for achievement in reading comprehension. This cloze-based assessment requires a child to read a sentence or passage and fill in a blank with a missing word. Similarly, the WIAT does not require reading of significant amounts of text. The problem is that many children who struggle to comprehend text in the classroom will not experience difficulties with the reading materials in the WJ or WIAT because the level of complexity does not parallel what children read in the classroom. A good assessment of reading comprehension requires the reading of significant amounts of complex text. For people for whom comprehension is an issue, assessments using the Group Reading Assessment and Diagnostic Education (GRADE; Williams, Cassidy, & Samuels, 2001), GORT–IV (Wiederholt & Bryant, 2001), or one of the group-based reading comprehension tests like the Iowa Test of Basic Skills (Hoover, Hieronymous, Frisbie, & Dunbar, 2001), or the Stanford Achievement Test–10th edition (Harcourt Assessment, 2002), is essential. If a person has had these kinds of assessments in school, the results can be reviewed as part of the evaluation. It is important not to rely only on group tests because the person may not have exerted adequate effort or paid attention, or may have engaged in other behaviors that invalidated the test.

Mathematics

Table 4.2 identifies the Calculations subtest of the WJ and the Numerical Operations subtest of the WIAT, representing paper-and-pencil tests of math computations. Poor performance on these calculation tasks reliably predicts variation in cognitive skills associated with math difficulties depending on other academic strengths and weaknesses (Rourke, 1993). The problem is that math difficulties have multiple sources. Poor performance on these tests could reflect problems with fact retrieval and phonological memory if word recognition is comparably lower. In contrast, if word recognition is significantly higher than math performance, the problems may stem from difficulties with procedural knowledge. In any person, poor performance can reflect attention difficulties (Fuchs et al., 2006b) especially in children with comorbid ADHD. The Arithmetic (math computations) subtest of the WRAT-III is useful because it is timed and the problems are less organized, making it more susceptible to attention and executive function difficulties. The key is math computations in a paper-and-pencil format, which is how difficulties in math are typically manifested in children who do not have reading problems.

If an assessment of math problem solving is needed, which we would complete only if math were an overriding concern, the WJ Applied Problems or WIAT Math Reasoning subtest can be used. These tests introduce word problems that are difficult for children with reading difficulties.

As in reading, assessments of fluency can be helpful, although there is no evidence suggestive of a math fluency disorder. The WJ Math Fluency subtest could be used as a supplemental measure. This is a timed assessment of single-digit arithmetic facts that may be helpful for identifying children who lack speed in basic arithmetic skills, which can lead to difficulties in mastering more advanced mathematics.

Written Expression

The most difficult domain to assess is written expression, partly because what constitutes a disorder of written expression is not well established. Does a disorder of written expression primarily involve spelling, handwriting, or composition? Problems with handwriting and spelling will constrain composition, so these domains are related (Berninger, 2004). Table 4.2 identifies spelling, which should be assessed as it may represent the primary source of difficulty with written expression for many children, especially those with word recognition difficulties. An analysis of spelling errors can be informative in understanding whether the problem is with the phonological component of language or with the visual form of letters (i.e., orthography; Rourke, 1993). Asking people to complete spelling tasks also permits an informal assessment of handwriting.

The WJ and WIAT have measures of written expression. The utility of these measures is not well established. From a construct view, significant construction and writing of passages is not really required. In students for whom text writing is a major issue, assessments with a measure like the Thematic Maturity subtest of the Test of Written Language (Hammill & Larsen, 2003) may be essential. As in reading and math, assessments of fluency of writing can be informative, as they can predict the quality of composition (Berninger & Hart, 1993). Thus, measuring fluency with a measure like the WJ Writing Fluency subtest may be useful, particularly for screening purposes.

Achievement Patterns

Characteristic patterns will emerge across norm-referenced tests that can help identify the type of LD and indicate specific kinds of intervention. For each of the five types of LDs in Table 4.1, there are interventions with evidence of efficacy that should be utilized in or out of a school setting (see Chapters 5–9). The goal is not to diagnose LDs, which is not feasible in a one-shot evaluation, for the psychometric and conceptual reasons outlined in Chapter 3, but to identify achievement difficulties that can be addressed through intervention. If the testing professional is knowledgeable about these patterns, very specific intervention recommendations, as well as the need for other assessments, can be provided.

Table 4.3 summarizes six achievement patterns that are well established in research (Fletcher et al., 2005b) that tie directly to the hypothetical classification in Table 4.1 and the core assessments in Table 4.2. It should be understood that the cut-point is deliberately set high in order to minimize false negative errors (missing people with significant problems). The cut-points are not hard-and-fast decision rules, nor are the levels of discrepancy across domains firm. The patterns are the important dimension (Rourke, 1975). We are not indicating that 25% of all children have an LD, only that scores below the 25th percentile are commonly associated with low performance in school, assuming the cut-point is reliably assessed. Response to validated intervention should be also be assessed to determine the presence of an LD.

The patterns in Table 4.3 help distinguish students with word recognition difficulties, who are typically also impaired in spelling and reading comprehension, from those who have adequate reading and spelling skills but struggle with math. We recognize that some students have difficulties in reading and spelling but do well in math, whereas other students have problems in all of these domains. There is considerable research supporting this distinction, representing a group likely with comorbid reading and math difficulties, which are often more severe than when the reading or math problem occurs in isolation (see Chapter 8). Similarly, students who have well-developed word recognition and spelling skills, but who struggle with math, are clearly different from students whose primary problem is in the word recognition domain (Rourke, 1993). The discrepancy in word recognition versus math skills is one of the best single indicators of a nonverbal learning disability (Pelletier, Ahmad, & Rourke, 2001; Rourke, 1993). Table 4.3 also identifies students who specifically have reading fluency and comprehension difficulties. There are also suggestions for examining variations in reading comprehension, decoding, and spelling, largely in relation to intervention.

Identifying LDs must take into account factors that extend beyond test scores (see Figure 1.1). As we describe in the next section, the decision process should focus on what is needed for intervention. This requires an assessment of contextual variables and the presence of comorbid disorders that will influence decisions about what sort of plan will be most effective for an individual child. Low achievement is related to many contextual variables, which is why the flexibility in special education guidelines allows interdisciplinary teams to base decisions on factors that go beyond test scores. The purpose of assessment is ultimately to develop an intervention plan.

TABLE 4.3. Achievement Patterns Associated with Intervention

1. Word recognition and spelling < 90; math computations one-half standard deviation higher than word recognition and spelling and at least 90. This is a pattern characterized by problems with single-word decoding skills and better arithmetic ability. Reading comprehension will vary depending on how it is assessed, but is usually impaired. Children with this pattern have significant phonological processing problems and often have strengths in spatial and motor skills (Rourke & Finlayson, 1978).

2. Reading fluency < 90 and word recognition one-half standard deviation higher will reflect a problem in which accuracy of word reading is less of a problem than automaticity of word reading (Lyon et al., 2003a). The most reliable correlate is rapid automatized naming of letters.

3. Reading comprehension < 90 and 7 points below word recognition. This pattern often reflects problems with vocabulary and receptive language, working memory, and attention, with strengths in phonological processing (Stothard & Hulme, 1996).

4. Math computations < 90, word recognition and spelling > 90 and at least 7 points higher. Children with difficulties that involve only math show this pattern, which is associated with problems with executive functions/attention, working memory, motor and spatial skills; phonological processing and vocabulary are often strengths (Rourke & Finlayson, 1978). If spelling is also < 90, this is essentially the same pattern with a more significant motor problem.

5. Spelling < 90. This pattern reflects (1) motor deficits in a young child or (2) residuals of earlier phonological language problems that have been remediated or compensated in older children and adults. The pattern is common in adults with a history of word recognition difficulties. Fluency is often impaired.

6. Word recognition, reading fluency, reading comprehension, spelling, and arithmetic < 90. This pattern represents a problem with word recognition and math characterized by pervasive language and working memory problems more severe than in children with poor decoding and better development of math skills (Rourke & Finlayson, 1978). It is likely a comorbid association of word recognition and math difficulties.

Note. The patterns are based on relations of word recognition, reading fluency, reading comprehension, arithmetic, and spelling. Any score below the 25th percentile (standard score = 90) is assumed to indicate at least mild impairment. A difference of one-half standard deviation is assumed to be important (± 7 standard score points). These patterns are unrelated to IQ scores. The patterns are prototypes; the rules should be loosely applied. Data from Fletcher, Foorman, et al. (2002) and Fletcher, Francis, Morris, and Lyon (2005).

Assessing Contextual Factors and Related Conditions

The evaluation of contextual factors and associated conditions that help explain low achievement is necessary in order to adequately plan intervention. The general principle is to assess for these factors in the same way that a factor or condition would be assessed if the possibility of the factor or condition was present in the absence of concerns about LDs. Parent and teacher rating scales of behavior and academic adjustment, along with parent-completed developmental and medical history forms, should be routinely obtained. Many behavioral difficulties present comorbidly with LDs and sometimes explain the achievement difficulty (Fletcher et al., 1999a). These potentially comorbid factors need to be assessed and treated. Simply referring a child for educational interventions without treating these factors will increase the probability of a poor RTI. Similarly, it is not likely that treating a child for a behavioral disorder, such as ADHD, will result in improved levels of achievement in the absence of educational intervention, so evaluations of academic achievement should always be completed when assessing children. Thus, the possibility of these factors and conditions should be routinely screened with multiple informants. If the problem is both an academic and a behavioral one, the joint occurrence usually represents two areas of difficulty, both requiring intervention.

In other domains, assessments are done depending on the question. If mental retardation is suspected, IQ, adaptive behavior, and related assessments consistent with this classification can be administered. However, a person with achievement scores in reading comprehension or math within two standard deviations of the mean (i.e., inconsistent with traditional legal definitions of mental retardation) or development of adaptive behavior obviously inconsistent with mental retardation is unlikely to demonstrate levels of performance on IQ tests consistent with mental retardation. A score at levels consistent with mental retardation would not be interpreted as indicating mental retardation in the absence of adaptive behavior deficits or strengths in reading comprehension or math that extend beyond the development of basic skills.

Some children with low IQ scores may have oral language disorders requiring speech and language intervention that will require referral and additional evaluation. Such problems are also commonly seen in LDs, and oral language disorders increase the risk for developing academic problems (Bishop & Snowling, 2004). Simple assessments with vocabulary measures will help identify children in whom overall language development is an issue and also help screen children who may benefit from more formal assessments of intelligence. Again, these problems typically extend beyond the academic domain and represent additional areas that require intervention.

The other major considerations are factors related to English language learners. People who are struggling to read in their nonnative language should not be considered learning disabled unless there is clear evidence that the problems also occur in the native language. It may be necessary to administer formal tests of language proficiency and academic skill development in the native language and in English to evaluate this possibility. This question does not need to be routinely assessed in children whose language exposure is exclusively English, but can be a major issue in areas where significant segments of the population are not native English speakers.

CONCLUSIONS

Based on our evaluation of models in Chapter 3, we proposed a hybrid model that incorporated features of RTI, low achievement, and intraindividual difference models for the identification of children as learning disabled. We did not suggest extensive assessments of cognitive, neuropsychological, or intellectual skills in order to identify children as learning disabled because of the lack of evidence that such assessments contribute to intervention or that discrepancies on those tests provide information not apparent in profiles of achievement tests (see Chapter 3). This approach to assessment assumes that the person is old enough that there is an expectation that reading, math, and written expression skills have begun to develop. It is entirely appropriate to administer cognitive or neuropsychological tests to children below such ages, particularly in an effort to identify risk characteristics. Even these assessments should be relatively brief and targeted to specific academic areas (e.g., phonological awareness and letter–sound knowledge in kindergarten as predictors of reading ability). Once the person achieves an age at which word recognition, math, and written expression skills are expected to be developed, there is little independent variability that is contributed by cognitive or neuropsychological tests. In general, LDs should not be identified in preschoolers. Even in grade 1, the reliability of identification will be lower because of maturational issues and the limited floors of many achievement tests in this age range (S. E. Shaywitz et al., 1992).

The heart of the identification model and approach to assessment is the focus on the measurement of RTI. Although some may see our model as appropriate only for schools, there is little evidence that evaluating a person in a single status assessment based on IQ–achievement discrepancy, low achievement, or patterns on cognitive and neuropsychological tests leads to better intervention. Such assessments do not have direct implications for treatment; if the "diagnosis" is based on a single assessment, it may not be adequately reliable. More important, as soon as it is apparent that the person has an achievement problem, intervention begins; resources expended on "diagnosis" should be expended on intervention. *People should not be identified as learning disabled until a proper attempt at instruction has been made.* Serial monitoring of RTI with CBM and the integrity of instruction should be completed before children are identified as learning disabled. However, because of the need for more research on what constitutes appropriately intensive intervention, estimation of slope and intercept effects, and decisions that have to be made about cut-points to differentiate adequate and inadequate responders (Gresham, 2002), RTI cannot be the sole criterion for identification. Nonetheless, there appears to be considerable validity in approaches that incorporate RTI, not the least of which is the likely possibility that inadequate responders represent "unexpected underachievement," epitomizing the essential construct of LDs (Fletcher et al., 2003).

Assessments must be derived and linked to an overarching classification of childhood learning and behavioral difficulties. Academic skill deficits represent *markers* for an underlying classification that distinguish the LD prototype from, for example, a behavioral disorder like ADHD. If the classification and assessment is expanded to mental retardation, the key for differentiating mental retardation from LD (or ADHD) is not just the IQ test score; rather, the major issue is the development of adaptive behavior. For mental retardation, deficits in adaptive behavior are pervasive; for LDs, adaptive behavior represents a relatively narrow range of deficits (Bradley et al., 2002). A classification of LDs, mental retardation, and ADHD (as an example of a behavior disorder) requires markers for achievement, attention-related behaviors, and adaptive behavior. The assessment should focus on the marker variables that identify members of different subgroups in the classification. In the absence of these types of markers, which stem from an overarching classification, people with problems are simply "disordered." There is no need for assessment of any kind, because the same interventions would be applied to everyone. When the assessment of LD is tied to levels and patterns of achievement and RTI, an evidence base for differential interventions focused on learning in specific academic domains emerges that provides strong evidence for the validity of the concept of LD. It becomes possible to clearly articulate how LDs should be classified, identified, and differentiated from other disorders. Such classification models lead directly to evidence-based approaches for assessment and identification, and to intervention, which are addressed in the next five chapters.

CHAPTER 5

Reading Disabilities

Word Recognition

In the previous chapter we discussed the evidence for different subgroups of LDs based on variations in reading, math, and written expression. Chapters 5 through 9 discuss each of the six domains of LDs in turn, beginning with disorders involving word recognition and then proceeding to domains involving reading fluency (Chapter 6), reading comprehension (Chapter 7), math (Chapter 8), and written expression (Chapter 9). In each chapter, we discuss issues related to definition, epidemiology, developmental course, academic skill deficits, core cognitive processes, neurobiological factors, and intervention. The current chapter is longer than the other chapters, partly because there is more research on LDs involving word recognition, but also reflecting the fact that disorders at the word level are the most common form of LD. But we also use this chapter to highlight many of the issues involved in conducting research and treating LDs, again because such issues have emerged most commonly for LDs that involve word recognition.

ACADEMIC SKILL DEFICITS

Word Recognition

Word-level reading disability (WLRD) is synonymous with "dyslexia," a form of LD that has been described throughout the 20th century as "word blindness," "visual agnosia for words," and "specific reading disability" (Doris, 1993). Thus, the major academic skill deficit characterizing children with dyslexia is a difficulty in single-word decoding (Olson, Forsberg, Wise, & Rack, 1994; Perfetti, 1985; S. E. Shaywitz, 2004;

Stanovich, 1986). This deficit leads to a profound disturbance of reading ability that pervades different domains of academic achievement. Comprehension is dependent on one's ability to decode rapidly and recognize single words in an automatic and fluent manner. Stanovich (1994) has noted: "Reading for meaning (comprehension) is greatly hindered when children are having too much trouble with word recognition. When word recognition processes demand too much cognitive capacity, fewer cognitive resources are left to allocate to higher-level processes of text integration and comprehension" (p. 281).

Given the converging evidence documenting the importance of word recognition, it is not surprising that the ability to read single words accurately and fluently has been the most frequently selected research target in the study of LDs in reading. Again, this is not to diminish the role of reading comprehension as an academic skill to be taught and acquired. However, word recognition is not only a prerequisite behavior to comprehension; it is also a more narrowly circumscribed behavior and is not related to the numerous nonreading factors typically associated with comprehension (Wood et al., 1991). Therefore, it offers a more precise developmental variable for study. Many of the advances in reading research have resulted from the focus on definitions using word recognition, as opposed to simply lumping together children as having "LDs" or combining children with different kinds of reading difficulties. Indeed, the focus on specific domains of reading (word recognition, fluency, comprehension) is specifically responsible for many of the advances in understanding the causes of LDs and the effective methods for intervention that are described in subsequent sections of this chapter.

Spelling

The other academic skill deficit characteristic of WLRD (dyslexia) is a spelling deficit. Not only is it difficult for individuals with WLRD to decode words, it is also difficult for them to spell (encode) words either in isolation or in context. We return to the issue of spelling in Chapter 9 as part of our discussion of writing. However, although spelling (like word reading) is a multidetermined skill and does not simply boil down to phonological processing, in people with dyslexia it is likely that the same phonological processing difficulties that cause word reading difficulties also cause spelling problems. The distinction between word reading and spelling, however, is important, because there are individuals for whom spelling, but not word recognition, is a problem. These patterns are especially apparent in the identification of LDs in people who use languages that have more transparent relationships between phonology and orthography, such as German or Spanish (Wimmer & Mayringer, 2002).

Here slow reading fluency emerges as a central academic skill deficit even when spelling is adequate. This issue is addressed more fully in Chapter 6 as part of the discussion of reading fluency difficulties.

CORE COGNITIVE PROCESSES

With the marker variables thus identified, there continues to be some debate about the nonreading factor or factors (e.g., linguistic, perceptual, temporal processing speed) that account for deficits in single-word reading. Two different perspectives continue to exist. The first and more influential school of thought proposes that deficits in word recognition are primarily associated with, or caused by, one primary nonreading factor (i.e., phonological awareness, rapid temporal processing). The second is that deficits in the ability to read single words rapidly and automatically are referable to multiple factors (e.g., phonological awareness, rapid naming, verbal short-term memory), thus giving rise to hypothesized subtypes of reading disabilities. Any theory of dyslexia, however, must explain the key academic skill deficits, which are word decoding and encoding (Share & Stanovich, 1995; Vellutino et al., 2004).

Phonological Awareness

The predominant core cognitive correlate of dyslexia (and word recognition) involves deficiencies in phonological awareness, a metacognitive understanding that the words we hear and read have internal structures based on sounds (Blachman, 1997; Liberman & Shankweiler, 1991; Share & Stanovich, 1995). Speech sounds, or phonemes, are the smallest parts of speech that make a difference in the meaning of a word. They are described by their phonetic properties, such as their manner or place of articulation, and their acoustic features or patterns of sound waves. English is an alphabetic language containing 44 phonemes. As in any alphabetic language, the unit characters (letters) that children learn in order to read and spell words are keyed to the phonological structure of the words (Liberman & Shankweiler, 1991; Lukatela & Turvey, 1998). A child's primary task in the early development of reading and spelling in an alphabetic language is to develop an understanding of the alphabetic principle—the realization that speech can be segmented into phonemes and that these phonemes are represented in printed forms (Blachman, 1997; Liberman, 1971; Lyon, 1995). However, this awareness that words can be divided into segments of sound is a very difficult task for many children. The difficulty lies in large part in the fact that speech, unlike writing, does not consist of separate phonemes produced one after another "in a row over time" (Gleitman & Rosen, 1973, p. 460). Instead, the sounds are "coarticulated" (overlapped with one another) to permit rapid communication of speech, rather than sound-by-sound pronunciation. This property of coarticulation—critical for speech, but possibly harmful to the beginning reader and speller—is explained by Liberman and Shankweiler (1991) as follows:

> The advantageous result of co-articulation of speech sounds is that speech can precede at a satisfactory pace—at a pace indeed at which it can be understood. . . . Can you imagine trying to understand speech if it were spelled out to you letter by painful letter? So co-articulation is certainly advantageous for the perception of speech. But a further result of co-articulation, and a much less advantageous one for the would-be reader, is that there is, inevitably, no neat correspondence between the underlying phonological structure and the sound that comes to the ears. Thus, though the word "bag" . . . as three phonological units, and correspondingly three letters in print, it has only one pulse of sound. . . . Beginning readers can understand, and properly take advantage of, the fact that the printed word *bag* has three letters, only if they are aware that the spoken word "*bag*," with which they are already quite familiar, is divisible into three segments. They will probably not know that spontaneously, because as we have said, there is only one segment of sound, not three, and because the processes of speech perception that recover the phonological structure are automatic and quite unconscious. (pp. 5–6)

The awareness of the phonological structure of language is the basis for the accurate recognition of known words necessary for basic reading, reading comprehension, spelling, and written expression (Liberman & Shankweiler, 1991; Rayner et al., 2002; Share & Stanovich, 1995). When phonological awareness develops and the child understands the alphabetic principle, word recognition is mastered early in the reading process; the critical issues are then the automaticity of these processes and the development of comprehension ability, both of which develop along with accuracy, but have longer developmental trajectories. When the child does not understand the relation of sound and print, word recognition will be delayed. The longer the child struggles to learn to read words, the more likely it is that a severe reading disability will emerge as the child cannot access print. Developing fluency and accessing comprehension abilities becomes increasingly difficult as the child loses exposure to sight words and the opportunity to access books. It is not surprising that, at this point in time, the most common form of LD in reading involves word recognition ability.

There is substantial support for this relationship and its pivotal importance not only in learning to read, but also as a proximal cause of WLRD (Shankweiler & Crain, 1986; Share & Stanovich, 1995; S. E. Shaywitz, 2004). Learning to read in nonalphabetic languages, or in languages with a more transparent relation of phonology and orthography, still has a significant relation with phonological processing (Goswami, 2002).

Other Cognitive Processes

In addition to problems with phonological awareness, two other cognitive processes are related to word recognition difficulties. These are rarely formulated as core processes exclusively of phonological processing; their role has usually been formulated in terms of whether other cognitive processes contribute unique variance to reading outcomes (Wolf & Bowers, 1999) or are simply explained by phonological processing deficits (Shankweiler & Crain, 1986).

Rapid Naming

The first process is rapid automatized naming of letters and digits. Many individuals with dyslexia not only have difficulties in manipulating the sound structures of language, but also show difficulties on tasks that require them to name letters or digits (or even objects) as rapidly as possible. Wolf and Bowers (1999) argued that the deficit in rapid naming is independent of the phonological processing, and there is support for this hypothesis. For example, Schatschneider, Fletcher, Francis, Carlson, and Foorman (2004) found that phonological awareness and rapid naming of letters are both predictive of word recognition skills at the end of first grade, based on kindergarten assessments. Bowers and Wolf (1993) argued that naming speed deficits reflected the operation of a timing mechanism that influences the temporal integration of phonological and visual components of printed words. They specifically attempted to relate naming speed deficits to the processing of orthographic patterns in words.

Structural equation studies that model the growth of reading and reading-related skills over time have found that phonological awareness and rapid naming abilities uniquely predict reading skills over time (Wagner, Torgesen, & Rashotte, 1994; Wagner, Torgesen, Rashotte, & Hecht, 1997). However, Wagner et al. (1997) suggested that, because of the high correlation of phonological awareness and rapid naming assessments at the latent variable level, both were determined by phonological processing. Such an interpretation is consistent with the phonological limitation hypothesis of dyslexia (Shankweiler & Crain, 1986).

The relation of rapid naming deficits and reading in individuals with dyslexia remains controversial. A recent review of the evidence concerning the relation of naming speed and dyslexia (Vukovic & Siegel, 2006) concluded that there was little evidence supporting rapid naming difficulties as an isolated deficit specific to individuals with WLRD, stating that "the existing evidence does not support a persistent core deficit in naming speed for readers with dyslexia" (p. 25). In contrast, a twin study by Petrill, Deater-Deckard, Thompson, DeThorne, and Schatschneider (2006a) found that phonological awareness and rapid naming were moderately correlated, but factorially distinct at a latent variable level, and that both contributed uniquely to word recognition outcomes. However, whereas phonological awareness had both genetic and shared environmental influences, the contribution of rapid naming was primarily genetic. They concluded "that serial naming speed is phenotypically separable from phonological awareness and could constitute a second, etiologically distinct source of variance in reading skills" (p. 120). Many studies of general populations have shown that rapid naming of letters contributes independent variance to word reading even when phonological processing is controlled (Schatschneider et al., 2004). However, whether this relation holds *specifically* within people with dyslexia is unclear (Vukovic & Siegel, 2006).

Regardless of whether rapid serial naming is a task in the phonological domain, Wolf and Bowers (1999) would probably agree that rapid naming is more strongly related to *fluent* reading of single words and text than it is to accurate word reading; in English-speaking countries where the bulk of studies have been conducted, lack of accurate reading is the primary problem that characterizes individuals with dyslexia. This is less apparent in countries such as Germany where dysfluent word reading and poor spelling occur with accurate word reading; rapid naming predicts fluency in German children (Wimmer & Mayringer, 2002). We return to this issue in Chapter 6, but note for now that rapid naming of letters is more strongly related to fluency assessments than it is to accuracy assessments (Schatschneider et al., 2004). Moreover, once phonological processing is controlled, many cognitive factors appear related to abilities even as discrete as word recognition skills. Such correlations do not indicate a causal role, and more research needs to be completed.

Phonological Memory

The other cognitive process that is significantly related to word recognition skill and to dyslexia involves working memory for verbal and/or acoustic (sound-based) information. In Wagner et al. (1997) and Schatschneider et al. (2004), different phonological memory tests were not found to contribute unique variance once phonological processing was included in the model. However, there are many comparisons of different verbal working memory tasks between people with dyslexia and those in a typically achieving control group, with working memory problems commonly observed (Siegel, 2003). The question is whether the working memory problems are independent of phonological processing.

Oakhill and Kyle (2000) suggested that the nature of the task may be particularly important. They compared performance on a short-term memory task that emphasized storage capacity with performance on a working memory task that emphasized both storage and processing capacity. The researchers found no evidence that the short-term memory task accounted for significant independent variance on the measures of phonological awareness. However, working memory predicted independent variability on a phonological awareness test that clearly invoked working memory. Because virtually any assessment of phonological awareness involves some working memory component, it may be very difficult to assess phonological awareness without requiring a working memory component, which may be why such tasks do not contribute independent variability in many multivariate studies.

A Causal Link?

Regardless of the interpretation, there is substantial evidence for a causal relation of phonological processing and success in learning to read words. The strength of this causal relationship is commonly challenged. For example, Castles and Coltheart (2004) questioned whether there was a causal link, arguing that the available literature was largely correlational and did not provide adequate control of different skills to support an unequivocal link of phonological awareness with word recognition ability. In a response, Hulme, Snowling, Caravolas, and Carroll (2005) argued that the balance of evidence did support a causal link. They also noted that learning to read depended on broader language skills, and that strict attempts to causally link phonological awareness with reading ability were inherently weakened because reading itself is a multicomponent system.

Other Unitary Processes

VISUAL MODALITY

There is a long history of identifying single factors in the etiology of dyslexia and other reading disabilities, much of which was reviewed in

Vellutino (1979) and Vellutino et al. (2004). This is clearly seen, for example, in the attempt to tie *visual–perceptual difficulties* to reading disabilities, a characteristic of much of the literature in the 1960s and 1970s (Vellutino, 1979). However, although it is common to observe the presence of difficulties with copying or matching geometric designs in comparisons of children who are disabled and nondisabled in reading, there is little evidence that the spatial processing problems per se are linked to reading disorders (Vellutino et al., 2004).

At the same time, children with reading disabilities have problems that extend beyond the reading process. They are often observed to have comorbid difficulties involving math or attention, or other cognitive and motor difficulties that are frequently interpreted as clinically relevant in psychometric evaluations. This pattern was clearly apparent in the older neuropsychological studies, which commonly focused on the emergence of a difference between groups as explanatory of the disorder (Doehring, 1978). Thus, the history of behavioral research on children with reading disabilities is characterized by various attempts to compete and compare single causal factors (Benton & Pearl, 1978). These studies invariably beg the question of how the presence of a particular factor in children with reading difficulties explains the reading problem; such research sometimes leads to convoluted theories in which the presumably causal factor is related to the reading process. Visual–perceptual theories are classic examples of generalizing from a group difference or correlation to cause.

This same trend is apparent in more contemporary studies that attempt to relate *low-level sensory deficits* in either the auditory or visual modality to dyslexia. In the visual area, there are studies using psychophysical methods involving visual persistence, contrast and flicker sensitivity, and the detection of motion thresholds; these studies are often interpreted to suggest a deficiency in the temporal processing of visual information (Stein, 2001). Such deficits are often related to specific difficulties in the magnocellular visual pathway. The magnocellular pathway is responsible for operations of the transient visual channel, which provides short, previsual responses to stimuli that are low in spatial frequency and move rapidly. In contrast, the parvocellular visual pathway is related to operations of the sustained visual channel, which provides a longer duration response to slow-moving stimuli that have high spatial frequency. In reading and other visual tasks, these two systems mutually inhibit one another. Various findings have suggested that individuals with reading difficulties have ineffective transient system inhibition that interferes with the saccadic suppression of visual information. This leads to persistence of retinal image, so that the words on a page may seem jumbled (Lovegrove, Martin, & Slaghuis, 1986; Stein, 2001).

This example illustrates some of the difficulties that arise in attempts to link these types of problems to the reading process. Although it is clear that individuals with reading disabilities differ from typically achieving individuals on measures involving the visual system, it is not clear how the magnocellular system can be involved in word recognition. The print itself is stationary, not moving. If words are jumbled when a person is scanning words, then the task would not seem to involve the perception of individual words, but groups of words as a person reads text (Iovino, Fletcher, Breitmeyer, & Foorman, 1999). The magnocellular system operates when a person is reading continuous text; the core problem in dyslexia involves the identification of words in isolation. Thus, it is difficult to see how such a theory can explain the core reading problems associated with dyslexia. Evidence for this hypothesis is decidedly mixed, with many studies finding no evidence for deficits in magnocelluar function in people with dyslexia (Amitay, Ben-Yehudah, Banai, & Ahissar, 2002; Hulme, 1988; Ramus, 2003).

More recent attempts to explain the visual processing difficulties observed in children with dyslexia relate these difficulties to the processing of the orthographic components of written language and assume that such deficits are not related to phonological decoding. Such explanations relate to the sometimes irregular relationship of the pronunciation of words and their representation in print. The relation of phonology and orthography in English is sometimes inconsistent and English spellings are commonly irregular (Rayner et al., 2002; Ziegler & Goswami, 2005). Thus, it is hypothesized that visual system deficits are related to the ability to immediately process words that cannot be sounded out automatically—a representation of the dual-route theory of reading. In this theory, words can either be accessed through a phonological route or recognized immediately through a visual route that bypasses the need for phonological processing (Castles & Coltheart, 1993; Coltheart, 2005a).

The dual-route theory is important for hypotheses about visual processing because it suggests that words can be recognized independently of phonological processing. Talcott et al. (2000) found correlations between visual motion sensitivity and orthographic processing even when variance due to phonological processing and IQ was covaried from the relationship. However, this relationship was true for all children, regardless of the presence of a disability. In addition, there was no evidence that the relationship of orthographic processing to word recognition was stronger than the relationship of phonological processing. Eden, Stern, Wood, and Wood (1995) performed similar analyses in which they observed that measures of visual processing continued to contribute independently to prediction of reading skills after IQ and phonological processing were partialed out of the relationship. However, the amount of variance accounted for was relatively small, and the methods used capitalized on independence after the most highly correlated variables had been included. Therefore, the more recent visual processing hypotheses do not provide robust explanations for the core reading problems experienced by children with dyslexia; in this respect, they resemble any older neuropsychological hypotheses based on univariate comparisons of children with and without reading difficulties. Differences between groups in neuropsychological functions were easy to observe, but difficult to relate to the reading problem (Doehring, 1978; Satz & Fletcher, 1980).

There is a role of visual processing in reading. Words are visual stimuli, and the neural network involved in the brain clearly involves processing of graphophonemic features through the occipitotemporal region (see Figure 5.3 later in the chapter, Dehaene, Cohen, Sigman, & Vinckier, 2005; S. E. Shaywitz & B. A. Shaywitz, 2005). This area of the brain is sensitive to a variety of visual features in words and eventually becomes attuned to frequently occurring patterns of letters. Perceptual learning of these combinations occurs, which supports the automaticity of word reading essential to the development of fluency. Such connections are easier in languages that have more regular relations of graphemes and phonemes, such as Italian or German, as compared with English. But much of the neuroimaging research (reviewed below) identifies a role of visual processing as part of a broader neural network that eventuates into the language system of the brain. Studies of visual and auditory processes should attempt to link more formally with theories of word recognition in an effort to more fully develop these hypotheses.

AUDITORY MODALITY

Sensory hypotheses have also been developed in the auditory modality. The most prominent was developed by Tallal and colleagues (Tallal, 2004). To summarize, in a series of studies involving children with specific language impairment, differences between these children and normal youngsters were found in the ability to assess acoustic stimuli with spectral parameters that changed rapidly in intensity. Problems in processing rapidly changing stimuli were observed for speech and non-speech stimuli, leading Tallal and associates to hypothesize that language disabilities are caused by lower-level auditory processing problems involving the perception of rapidly changing stimuli. Tallal (1980) extended these findings to children with reading disabilities by using speech and nonspeech stimuli. She found that a subgroup of children with reading disabilities performed more poorly than nondisabled children on auditory perceptual tasks, and that performance was correlated with reading ability. However, the participants were obtained from a sample of children originally identified with oral language disorders. These correlations may have been related to the complete inability of many children to read, and thus raw scores of 0 were assigned to many of these children. Nonetheless, Reed (1989) replicated the work of Tallal (1980), finding deficits on auditory stimuli that involved speech as well as nonspeech, whereas Mody, Studdert-Kennedy, and Brady (1997) did not replicate the findings for nonspeech stimuli. Questions were raised about these studies because of the criteria used for defining the children as disabled in reading, as well as the possibility that other factors could explain the differences between the groups, such as the high comorbidity of reading disabilities and ADHD. There were also concerns about the auditory stimuli.

Several more recent studies involved samples that controlled for the presence of ADHD and used well-established definitions of dyslexia. In a study by Waber et al. (2001), children with dyslexia but not ADHD were identified from a larger group of children originally referred for evaluation of learning impairments in a clinic setting. Waber et al. (2001) found a significant difference between groups of children with good reading skills and poor reading skills in their ability to discriminate speech and nonspeech stimuli but not stimuli that showed rapid changes in their acoustic parameters. Similarly, Breier, Fletcher, Foorman, and Gray (2002) used temporal-order judgment and discrimination tasks in children with dyslexia and no ADHD, dyslexia and ADHD, ADHD and no dyslexia, and typically achieving children with no ADHD. Children with dyslexia did not show a specific sensitivity to variations in inter-stimulus intervals. They also performed more poorly than children without dyslexia only on speech stimuli, but not on nonspeech stimuli. Phonological processing measures were consistently more closely related to speech stimuli than to nonspeech stimuli. The results were independent of the presence of ADHD. Like Waber et al. (2001), Breier et al. (2002) concluded that children with dyslexia may have difficulties with speech perception that correlate with reading and phonological processing ability, but found little evidence for generalized auditory processing difficulties. In a study of adults with well-defined dyslexia, Griffiths, Hill, Bailey, and Snowling (2003) compared temporal order discrimination for long and short interstimulus intervals. They found no group differences in either short or long interstimulus intervals. There were moderate correlations between the assessments of auditory thresholds and phonological processing, but only a small group of adults with dyslexia could be characterized with elevated thresholds across different auditory tasks. Thus, the association of auditory and phonological processing skills was not robust, especially since there was also a subgroup of the controls with no reading difficulty that also showed elevated auditory thresholds.

Altogether, research on lower-level auditory deficits does not provide compelling explanations of the core reading problem apparent in children with dyslexia. In this regard, they do not explain the word recognition difficulties in a parsimonious manner, nor is the weight of the evidence as strong as that associated with explanations based on phonological processing. At the same time, there is mixed evidence that problems with speech perception (as opposed to a lower-level auditory processing problem) characterize many individuals with dyslexia. For example, Joanisse, Manis, Keating, and Seidenberg (2000) reported that speech perception deficits characterized only children who were identified with WLRD in the context of an oral language disorder. In contrast, Breier et al. (2002) did find that children with WLRD exhibited significant problems with speech perception in a sample that excluded children with indications of an oral language disorder. Breier, Fletcher, Denton, and Gray (2004) demonstrated that problems with perception of speech sounds characterized kindergarten students at risk for reading difficulties. However, in an imaging study involving the discrimination of speech sounds, Breier et al. (2003) found that children with dyslexia showed weak activation of temporoparietal areas of the brain in the left hemisphere that also corresponded to areas involving phonological processing. Speech perception problems may make it more difficult to grasp the alphabetic principle, but the specificity of such deficits to WLRD is not established.

Other Hypotheses

CEREBELLAR HYPOTHESIS

There are other recent hypotheses about the nature of dyslexia. Nicolson, Fawcett, and Dean (2001) proposed a cerebellar deficit hypothesis indicating that children with dyslexia represent a group that has failed to adequately automatize various skills, a function they argue is mediated by the cerebellum. These functions include different skills involving reading, particularly those requiring rapid naming or processing of information. This hypothesis has spawned interventions that specifically attempt to remediate these cerebellum deficits by focusing on the motor system.

There is little evidence that supports this theory, especially compared with evidence for theories based on phonological processing (Ramus, 2001). In an early study, Wimmer, Mayringer, and Raberger (1999) did not find that German children with dyslexia—who are characterized primarily by fluency and spelling difficulties—differed from controls on a balancing task, provided that ADHD was controlled. In fact, ADHD was a better predictor of performance on this cerebellar task than reading status. In a subsequent study, Raberger and Wimmer (2003) replicated these findings and were also unable to identify a link between balancing and rapid naming. Kibby, Francher, Markanen, Lewandowski, and Hynd (2003) administered tests of reading and spelling, along with assessments of language functions. They also obtained MRI scans and measured the volume of the cerebellum. Although there were small but significant differences in cerebellum volumes between dyslexic and typically achieving children, which has been reported for different cerebellar structures in several studies (see Eckert et al., 2003), there was no evidence that cerebellum volumes correlated with academic or language skills in either group. Similarly, Ramus, Pidgeon, and Frith (2003a) found no evidence for time estimation deficits in individuals with dyslexia, and no evidence for causal relations of motor function and different phonological and reading skills. In a comparison of three hypotheses about dyslexia involving (1) phonological processing, (2) low-level auditory and visual deficits, and (3) cerebellar functions, Ramus et al. (2003b) found the strongest support for phonological deficits, which often occurred in the absence of any sensory or motor disorder. They observed the presence of sensory and motor disorders in certain individuals, but were not able to link these with a reading problem. Similarly, Savage et al. (2005) found that measures of motor balance (and speech perception) did not contribute unique variance to reading and spelling outcomes if phonological processing was in the regression model. Savage (2004) reviewed theories of automaticity in dyslexia. In this review, strong evidence was found for relations of naming speed and reading fluency. However, the evidence for deficits in motor automaticity was inconsistent, with the reviewer concluding that there was much clearer evidence for language-based rather than motor-based deficits in automaticity. Ramus (2001, 2003) acknowledged that sensorimotor deficits were seen in people with dyslexia, but observed that their role in explaining the reading problems was limited.

PERIPHERAL VISION HYPOTHESIS

Similar problems have been observed in a variety of efforts to link problems with peripheral vision to dyslexia. Such hypotheses typically lead either to optometric training exercises or to interventions involving colored lenses and/or overlays. None of these hypotheses has much support in terms of the overlying theory or the efficacy of the interventions. Kriss and Evans (2005) did not find differences in the incidence of visual distortions between a sample of children with dyslexia and controls. In a critical review of colored lenses, for example, Solan and Richman (1990) found little scientific support for the underlying theory or the efficacy of different interventions, with several studies suggesting that colored lenses and filters improve reading speeds slightly in all people regardless of reading status (Iovino et al., 1999; Kriss & Evans, 2005). To reiterate, there is little evidence that interventions that do not require reading are effective for children who have reading difficulties.

It is true that dyslexia is more than a reading disability and that children with dyslexia differ from normal children on a variety of dimensions. However, these differences do not explain the reading problem. They could be related to the nature of the underlying neurobiological problems that appear to be at the root of dyslexia, but the basis for these differences has yet to receive adequate exploration (Eden & Zeffiro, 1998). It is also likely that the tests used to measure these deficits have surplus variance and/or are sensitive to comorbid conditions associated with WLRD (e.g., attention) (Doehring, 1978; Satz & Fletcher, 1980).

Subtypes of Dyslexia

In an effort to explain the variability in LDs, it has been commonly hypothesized that a number of *subtypes* exist that can be identified on the basis of how people perform on measures of cognitive–linguistic, perceptual span, and other skills (see reviews by Hooper & Willis, 1989; Rourke, 1985). The argument for the existence of subtypes in the population with LDs was based on the practical observation that even though children with LDs may appear similar with respect to their reading deficits (i.e., word recognition deficits), they may differ significantly in the development of other skills that may be correlated with basic reading development (Lyon, 1983). Thus, even within well-defined samples of children with dyslexia, there is large within-sample variance on some skills. This observation may explain, in part, why such children have been reported to differ from controls on so many variables unrelated to reading (Doehring, 1978).

The literature on subtyping dyslexia and other reading disabilities is voluminous, comprising more than 100 classification studies since 1963 (Hooper & Willis, 1989). Much of this research preceded recognition of the important link of word recognition and phonological processing, and the homogeneity in LDs that emerges from a classification based on academic skill deficits. Thus, much of the research involves children identified with LDs; although the deficits are predominantly WLRDs, the samples are very heterogeneous and this research is not reviewed here. We focus on two approaches that clearly involve WLRD and are related to a theory of reading, one involving subtypes based on component skills in word recognition (Castles & Coltheart, 1993) and the other representing an empirical search for cognitive subtypes based on the phonological limitation hypothesis (Morris et al., 1998). There are other prominent subtype hypotheses that involve distinctions of rate and accuracy of word/text reading (Lovett, 1987) and distinctions based on phonological awareness and rapid naming (Wolf & Bowers, 1999). Because these represent efforts to highlight the role of fluency, they are reviewed in Chapter 6.

Surface versus Phonological Dyslexia

The first subtyping approach is derived from the dual-route framework of reading (Coltheart, 2005a) and is based on a distinction between surface and phonological dyslexia in the acquired alexia literature (Castles & Coltheart, 1993; Coltheart, 2005b). To reiterate, the dual-route theory stipulates that the reading system comprises a sublexical system in which phonological rules relate graphemes to phonemes and a visual-orthographic system in which meaning is directly addressed. If the impairment is primarily in the sublexical system, the problem is considered *phonological dyslexia* and represents the common view of WLRD as a disorder caused by impairments in phonological processing. If the lexical system is the primary locus of impairment, the disorder is termed *surface dyslexia* and represents a problem that will be manifested with the orthographic component level of reading. The model thus predicts that people with phonological dyslexia are expected to exhibit poorer reading of pseudowords than exception words. In contrast, people with surface dyslexia are expected to exhibit better reading of pseudowords than exception words.

Findings related to this subtyping hypothesis question whether children with reading problems can be reliably characterized with surface dyslexia. Although a study by Murphy and Pollatsek (1994) reported no evidence for a subtype of surface dyslexia, Manis, Seidenberg, Doi, McBride-Chang, and Peterson (1996) and Stanovich, Siegel, and Gottardo (1997) did find some support for this hypothesis in younger children. In Manis et al. (1996) children with dyslexia had difficulties in reading both exception words and pseudowords, and the group identified with surface dyslexia performed similarly to controls matched on reading level. The researchers argued that the results were consistent with a connectionist model of word recognition (Foorman, 1994; Seidenberg & McClelland, 1989), in which reading any kind of word invokes patterns of activation that are distributed over orthographic, phonological, and semantic representations. Pronouncing pseudowords and exception words does not reflect separate routes of word recognition, but simply involves differential weighting of the connections. This observation was supported by Griffiths and Snowling (2002), who found that measures of phonological processing contributed unique variance to pseudoword reading, including phonological awareness and verbal short-term memory skills. The only unique predictor of exception word reading was an assessment of reading experience, consistent with the view that orthographic processing has a significant experiential component. They then argued that the decoding deficit that characterizes dyslexia stems from poorly specified phonological representations, whereas the exception word problem is primarily influenced by exposure to print.

In another study, Stanovich et al. (1997) also found that most children with WLRD experienced problems with both phonological and orthographic components of word recognition, leading Stanovich (2000) to suggest that surface dyslexia represented an unstable subtype with a transient delay in the development of word recognition skills. In contrast, phonological dyslexia represented a long-term deficit in the acquisition of word reading skills. This is consistent with Griffiths and Snowling (2002), who also suggested that the differences between surface and phonological dyslexia were essentially a matter of severity. Moreover, surface dyslexia appears mostly in younger children. Zabell and Everatt (2002) reported that adults with characteristics suggesting phonological or surface dyslexia were not significantly different on a variety of measures involving phonological processing. Altogether, the value of this subtyping hypothesis is its reliance on a theory of word recognition; the weakness is the weak evidence for surface, or orthographic dyslexia.

Empirical Subtyping

A prominent study design in the 1970s and 1980s involved the application of multivariate classification methods in an effort to identify subtypes of LDs (Hooper & Willis, 1989; Rourke, 1985). A subsequent study (Morris et al., 1998) differed from previous empirical approaches to subtyping, in that it was based on a model emphasizing the role of phonological processing in reading disabilities (Liberman & Shankweiler, 1991; Stanovich, 1988). It also used other theories to select potential variables, including measures of rapid naming, short-term memory, vocabulary, and perceptual skills. From a methodological perspective, the sample was large and was selected on an a priori basis for a subtyping study (i.e., it was not just a sample of convenience). Multiple definitions were used to identify children with dyslexia; children with both dyslexia and math disabilities, children with isolated math disabilities, children with permutations involving ADHD, and typically achieving children were included. The application of the clustering algorithms was rigorous and followed guidelines ensuring both internal and external validity (Morris & Fletcher, 1988).

The nine resultant subtypes are portrayed in Figure 5.1. All profiles are depicted as z-scores relative to the sample mean. There are five subtypes with specific reading disabilities, two subtypes representing more pervasive impairments in language and reading, and two representing typically achieving groups of children. Six of the seven reading disability subtypes share, however, an impairment in phonological awareness skills. The five specific subtypes (see Figure 5.2) vary with respect to impairments in rapid automatized naming and verbal short-term memory. We can see a large subtype in Figure 5.2 with impairments in phonological awareness, rapid naming, and in verbal short-term memory. There are two subtypes with impairments in phonological awareness, and in verbal short-term memory, varying in lexical and spatial skills; a subtype with phonological awareness and rapid naming difficulties; and a subtype without impairment in phonological awareness, but with deficits on any measure that required rapid processing, including rapid naming. This last subtype does not include a word recognition problem or phonological impairment, but does include difficulties on measures of reading fluency and comprehension, consistent with Wolf and Bowers's (1999) double-deficit model. The five specific subtypes can be differentiated from the "garden variety" subtypes on the basis of their vocabulary development. Children with specific subtypes of reading disabilities have vocabulary levels that are in the average range; children with more pervasive disturbances of reading and language have vocabulary levels that are in the low average range.

Altogether, these results are consistent with the phonological processing hypothesis advanced earlier in this chapter, as well as with Wolf and Bowers's (1999) double-deficit model. The results are also consistent with Stanovich's (1988) phonological-core variable-difference model. This model postulates that phonological processing is at the core of all WLRD. But reading disabilities are often more than just phonological processing problems. Children may have problems outside the phonological domain that do not contribute to the word recognition difficulties, such as impairments in vocabulary that would interfere with comprehension. More pervasive disturbances of language would lead to a garden variety form of reading disability, and the pattern could include fine motor and visual–perceptual problems that are demonstrably unrelated to word recognition.

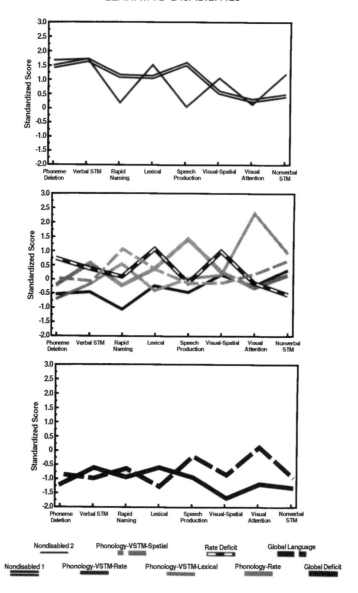

FIGURE 5.1. Z-scores for nine subtypes produced by cluster analysis of eight variables. The two subtypes in the upper panel are typically achieving. The subtypes in the lower panel are lower in overall level of function. The five subtypes in the middle panel show specific subtypes of reading disability (Morris et al., 1998). V, verbal; STM, short-term memory. From Lyon, Fletcher, and Barnes (2003a, p. 550). Copyright 2003 by The Guilford Press. Reprinted by permission.

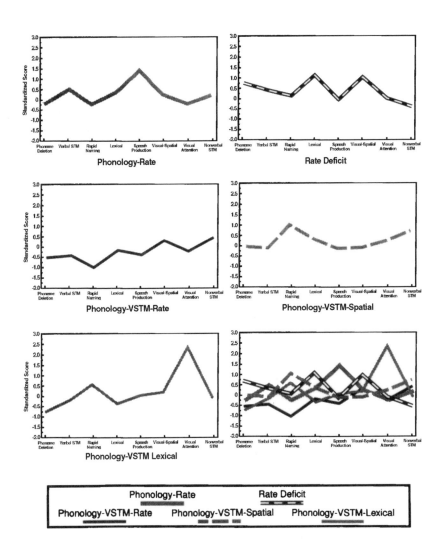

FIGURE 5.2. Z-scores for the five subtypes of children with specific reading disability subtypes plotted separately for each subtype (Morris et al., 1998). V, verbal; STM, short-term memory. From Lyon, Fletcher, and Barnes (2003a, p. 551). Copyright 2003 by The Guilford Press. Reprinted by permission.

A Definition of Dyslexia

The evolution of "dyslexia" from a vague and general term to a syn-onym for WLRD provides an example of how definitions of LDs can move from approaches based on exclusionary criteria that mostly indi-cate what LDs are not (Rutter, 1982) to inclusionary definitions that fo-cus on a key set of marker variables that lead directly to identification. As an example of an exclusionary approach, consider the definition of dyslexia formulated by the World Federation of Neurology in 1968 as summarized in Critchley (1970): "A disorder manifested by difficulties in learning to read despite conventional instruction, adequate intelli-gence, and socio-economic opportunity. It is dependent upon fundamen-tal cognitive disabilities, which are frequently of constitutional origin" (p. 11).

In contrast, consider the following definition of dyslexia, which was developed in 1994 (Lyon, 1995) and then revised by the research com-mittee of the International Dyslexia Association to take advantage of the rapid progress in research that had occurred over the ensuing decade (Lyon et al., 2003b):

> Dyslexia is a specific learning disability that is neurobiological in origin. It is characterized by difficulties with accurate and/or fluent word recog-nition and by poor spelling and decoding abilities. These difficulties typ-ically result from a deficit in the phonological component of language that is often unexpected in relation to other cognitive abilities and the provision of effective classroom instruction. Secondary consequences may include problems in reading comprehension and reduced reading experience that can impede growth of vocabulary and background knowledge. (p. 1)

Building on the research on academic skill deficits and their cogni-tive correlates, this definition indicates that dyslexia is manifested by variable difficulties with different forms of language, often including, in addition to problems with word reading, a conspicuous problem with acquiring proficiency in spelling and writing. Word-reading and spelling problems are the primary academic skill deficits in dyslexia. Although the definition emphasizes accuracy, it also explicitly notes that fluency of decoding is also involved. Reading comprehension problems are com-mon, reflecting the word decoding problems. Based on research re-viewed below, this definition identifies dyslexia as a WLRD proximally caused by core cognitive processes involving phonological processing problems and identifies both neurobiological and environmental factors as causes of WLRD. The definition is inclusionary because it specifies that people can be identified with dyslexia when they show problems with decoding single words accurately and fluently, and spell poorly. It is a model for definitions in other domains of LDs, which have not progressed to a point where such definitions are possible.

EPIDEMIOLOGY

Prevalence

The prevalence of dyslexia has been estimated to be as high as 17.4% in the school-age population (S. E. Shaywitz, 2004). However, reading disabilities in general have historically generated prevalence estimates of at least 10–15% in the school-age population (Benton & Pearl, 1978). These estimates are in the context of reports from the National Center for Educational Statistics (NCES; 2003) indicating that more than 35% of children in grade 4 read below the basic level of proficiency. Of course, as reading disabilities appear to be dimensional, prevalence depends on where the cutoff point is set, and criterion-related estimates of prevalence are not available. No prevalence estimates are available that incorporate RTI in the definition.

Dyslexia is the most common form of LD. Lerner (1989) reported that 80–90% of all children served in special education programs had problems with reading, and Kavale and Reese (1992) found that more than 90% of children in Iowa with the LD label were identified for reading difficulties. Both studies indicated that most children who have reading problems experience difficulty with word-level skills. Similarly, Leach, Scarborough, and Rescorla (2003) reported that about 80% of an elementary school sample selected because of reading problems had difficulties involving the accuracy of word reading; the remaining 20% had difficulties primarily at the level of listening comprehension. Thus, most children who are served in special education programs for LDs likely have WLRD as part of their disability (Lyon, 1995).

Gender Ratio

Although dyslexia has always been reported to be more common in males than females, several studies indicate that the gender ratio between individuals with dyslexia is not different from the gender ratio within the population as a whole (DeFries & Gillis, 1991; Flynn & Rahbar, 1994; S. E. Shaywitz, B. A. Shaywitz, Fletcher, & Escobar, 1990; Wood & Felton, 1994). Previous estimates indicating male preponderance tended to be based on clinic and school settings that were subject to referral bias. Boys are more likely to display externalizing behaviors that lead to referral, and the hyperactive-impulsive form of ADHD does appear to be more common in boys than girls (Barkley, 1997; S. E. Shaywitz et al., 1990).

More recent analyses of different epidemiological studies have questioned whether the prevalence of dyslexia is similar in boys and girls (Rutter et al., 2004), but estimated the proportions at about 1.5–2:1 in favor of males, much lower than the 3–4:1 ratio reported by earlier studies. Rutter et al. (2004) reanalyzed data from four independent epidemiological studies that permitted estimates of the gender rate for reading disability. The authors reported that, across these studies, the gender ratio ranged from about 1.4–2.7:1. They also included findings from additional studies in the United Kingdom and the United States that reported ratios of about 2:1. At the lower end, these rates are not really different from those indicated in S. E. Shaywitz et al. (1990) and Flynn and Rahbar (1994), in which a ratio of about 1.4:1 was reported.

Altogether, these studies established that there is a tendency toward male preponderance in dyslexia, but not at the magnitude suggested by clinic samples. A major question is why such differences are significant. Genetic studies have not obtained evidence suggesting that the traits associated with WLRD are sex-linked (Plomin & Kovas, 2005). Indeed, the only reliable explanatory variable identified for male preponderance has been issues related to ascertainment (Donovan & Cross, 2002). Why do schools and clinic samples commonly report higher identification rates for males than in epidemiological studies, with corresponding underidentification of girls as poor readers, if some form of ascertainment bias is not involved? Few studies find evidence of gender-based phenotypic differences in the expression of WLRD, with most studies finding very small effects of gender (Flynn & Rahbar, 1993; Canning, Orr, & Rourke, 1980).

We are not arguing that gender is not important, especially given the evidence for gender-based differences in brain structure and function (Lambe, 1999), and are certainly not suggesting that gender should not be isolated as an explanatory variable in studies of dyslexia. However, the effects appear small at best and the major importance of a gender difference, which would be a genetic link, has not been identified. In a sense, reports of male preponderance simply indicate that the distribution of reading skills is different in males and females and beg the question of whether distributions should be pooled in estimating prevalence.

DEVELOPMENTAL COURSE

Dyslexia in particular, and reading disabilities in general, reflect persistent deficits rather than a developmental lag in linguistic and reading skills (Francis et al., 1996; S. E. Shaywitz et al., 1999). Longitudinal studies show that, of children identified as reading disabled in grade 3, more than 70% maintain this status through grade 12 (Figure 3.4; S. E. Shaywitz, 2004). Studies of adults with WLRD find that the word reading difficulties persist and that the core cognitive correlates in the domain of phonological processing also persist (Bruck, 1987; Cirino, Israelian, Morris, & Morris, 2005; Ransby & Swanson, 2003). These data indicate a pessimistic outcome for youngsters with WLRD, especially because many have been identified and served in special education. Altogether, the developmental course of WLRDs is poor and such difficulties represent chronic problems for the student. These findings highlight the importance of organizing identification around instruction.

NEUROBIOLOGICAL FACTORS

The hypothesis that LDs are "unexpected" stems in part from the belief that if children who experience low achievement due to factors such as economic disadvantage and inadequate instruction are excluded from the LD category, the cause in those who have low achievement not due to the exclusions must be intrinsic to the children.

As we have noted in our review of the history of LDs (Chapter 2), the intrinsic nature of LDs was inferred initially from the linguistic and behavioral characteristics of adults with documented brain injury. As the field progressed, definitions of LDs continued to attribute them to intrinsic (brain) rather than extrinsic (e.g., environmental, instructional) causes, even though there was no objective way to adequately assess the presence of putative brain damage or dysfunction. This problem was constantly dismissed as a matter that technology would eventually resolve! This conviction was reinforced by the common nonspecific association of indirect indices of neurological dysfunction with LDs, including perceptual-motor problems (i.e., difficulty in copying geometric figures), paraclassical or "soft" neurological signs (e.g., gross motor clumsiness, fine motor incoordination), and anomalies on electrophysiological measures (Dykman et al., 1971; Taylor & Fletcher, 1983). Even at the time, the lack of specificity of these observations to either LDs or neurological integrity was widely acknowledged (Rutter, 1982; Satz & Fletcher, 1980).

Over the past two decades, the quality of the evidence has improved. It is now possible to clearly support the hypothesis that LDs in general, and dyslexia in particular, have a locus in neurobiological factors. But the evidence also suggests that causal models in which neurobiological deficits produce a child with dyslexia are simplistic and do not take into account the complex interplay of the brain and environment in development. In this section, we review studies of (1) brain structure, (2) brain function, and (3) genetics. Most of these studies explicitly identified children as reading disabled on the basis of word recognition and phonological processing abilities, so they tend to be specific to dyslexia. There is relatively little research on neurobiological factors involving LDs other than dyslexia.

Brain Structure

Research on brain structure involves either postmortem studies or the use of imaging techniques such as computed cerebral tomography (CT) and anatomical magnetic resonance imaging (aMRI). As CT did not provide particularly useful information and is regarded as having poorer resolution than aMRI, we do not discuss CT. Reviews of literature on this subject can be found in Hynd and Semrud-Clikeman (1989).

Postmortem Studies

There are a few postmortem evaluations of the brain anatomy of adults with a history of dyslexia. These cases are rare, as dyslexia is not regarded as lethal. These studies, largely by a group led by Galaburda (1993), have involved a total of 10 brains accumulated over several years. The findings indicated that individuals with dyslexia are characterized by differences in the size of specific brain structures (e.g., planum temporale) and the presence of specific neuroanatomical anomalies (Filipek, 1996; Galaburda, 1993; S. E. Shaywitz et al., 2000).

Evaluations of cortical structures in adults with a history of reading problems as children have found that the planum temporale, a structure on the plane of the temporal lobe, is symmetrical in size in the left versus right hemisphere (Galaburda, Sherman, Rosen, Aboitiz, & Geschwind, 1985; Humphreys, Kaufmann, & Galaburda, 1990). In postmortem studies of adults who presumably did not have reading problems, this structure is often larger in the left hemisphere than the right hemisphere (Geschwind & Levitsky, 1968). Because this area of the left hemisphere supports language function, the absence of this anatomical difference has been viewed as a partial explanation for language deficiencies that are hypothesized to result in reading problems. In addition, microscopic examination of cortical architecture showed minor focal distortions called "ectopias." Although also common in individuals with no history of dyslexia, these ectopias were more common than would be expected in individuals with a history of dyslexia. They were also more common in the left hemisphere. Microscopic examinations of subcortical structures have also shown differences relative to normative expectations, particularly in the thalamus (Livingstone, Rosen, Drislane, & Galaburda, 1991). These structures of the thalamus are widely believed to be involved in visual processing. Finally, examinations of the cerebellum in a subset of these brains (Finch, Nicolson, & Fawcett, 2002) revealed larger mean cell sizes in the medial posterior cerebellum relative to normal expectations, as well as unexpected distributions of cells in several parts of the cerebellum.

Altogether, postmortem studies have found clear evidence of anomalies at both subcortical and cortical levels in many parts of the brain. However, these studies are limited because the reading characteristics, educational histories, and important factors that influence brain organization, such as handedness, are difficult to ascertain in a postmortem study (Beaton, 2002; S. E. Shaywitz et al., 2000). It was not possible to correlate the size of the planum temporale or the frequency/location of ectopias with reading performance in a postmortem study, so it is difficult to establish the role of these findings in causing dyslexia.

Anatomical MRI Studies

Given the difficulties involved in obtaining brains for postmortem evaluation, as well as the aforementioned limitations of any postmortem study, investigators have turned to aMRI for the evaluation of potential differences in brain structure. The use of aMRI is desirable because it is noninvasive and is safe for children. The aMRI data can also be segmented and quantified, so that precise measurements of brain structure can be made. The findings can then be correlated with reading performance.

Studies have examined a variety of structures (Filipek, 1996; S. E. Shaywitz & B. A. Shaywitz, 2005). Given the interest generated by postmortem studies, these include the planum temporale and the temporal lobes. In addition, there have been some studies of the corpus callosum, which may reflect the fact that it is relatively easy to quantify. The cerebellum has also been studied.

This research has yielded mixed results. Studies of the corpus callosum have produced mixed findings, with some studies reporting differences in the size (Duara et al., 1991; Hynd et al., 1995). But other studies have not found differences in corpus callosum measures (Larsen, Hoien, Lundberg, & Ödegaard, 1990; Schultz et al., 1994). Studies that compare the planum temporale in individuals with and without dyslexia report both symmetry (Hynd, Semrud-Clikeman, Lorys, Novey, & Eliopulos, 1990; Larsen et al., 1990) and even reversals in the expected patterns of asymmetry (Hynd et al., 1990) in the groups with dyslexia. However, other studies have not found an association between symmetry of the planum temporale in dyslexia (Rumsey et al., 1997; Schultz et al., 1994). Leonard et al. (1996) correlated reading performance and asymmetry of the temporal lobes; higher degrees of asymmetry favoring the left hemisphere were found to be associated with better reading performance, regardless of whether a child was disabled in reading. However, Leonard et al. (2001) did not replicate this finding. In contrast, Hugdahl et al. (2003) found that the left planum temporale was smaller in a group of 23 children with dyslexia, as compared with 23 controls, at 10–12 years of age. The reduction in the planum temporale area correlated only within the group of children with dyslexia, showing a positive correlation with performance on a dichotic listening task.

Some studies reported differences between dyslexic and normal individuals in temporoparietal brain regions that extend beyond the planum temporale (Duara et al., 1991), but other studies did not find these differences (Hynd et al., 1990). Eckert et al. (2003) measured multiple brain areas in 19 controls and 18 children with dyslexia in grades 4–6 who were recruited from a family genetics study (Raskind et al., 2005). The assessments included measures of the posterior temporal lobe, the inferior frontal gyrus, and the cerebellum. The measurements that most significantly discriminated children with and without dyslexia involved the right anterior lobe of the cerebellum, and the pars triangularis in both hemispheres, an area involving the inferior frontal gyrus. Measures of the planum temporale did not discriminate the groups. Eckert et al. (2003) noted specifically that their study was "at least the eighth study demonstrating that individuals with dyslexia do not exhibit reversed asymmetry in the planum temporale" (p. 488). They argued that assessments of the temporal lobes were generally not sensitive to differences in brain structure between dyslexic and nondyslexic samples. In contrast, Silani et al. (2005) studied adults with dyslexia who, on average, had shown reduced activation in the left occipitotemporal lobe when reading. Focusing the assessment of brain structures on these areas, Silani et al. (2005) reported altered density of gray and white matter involving the left middle and inferior temporal gyri and the arcuate fasciculus in the left hemisphere. They related these alterations to inadequate connectivity involving areas demonstrably involved in reading, noting that the differences were replicated across samples from three different countries. In a study of individuals with a family history of dyslexia, Brambati et al. (2004) also found reductions in gray matter volume in similar areas of the brain, including the planum temporale. Brambati et al. (2004) also found cerebellum differences, as did Rae et al. (2002), but not like those found by Eckert et al. (2003), who reported that the cerebellar hemispheres were asymmetric. Rae et al. found symmetry in the cerebellum hemispheres of the individuals with dyslexia.

These samples are small and heterogeneous, which contributes to the variations in finding across studies. Comparisons across laboratories are also hampered by the use of different neuroimaging methods and data-analytic techniques, leading to difficulties in replicating these findings (Filipek, 1996; S. E. Shaywitz et al., 2000). The quantification of aMRI is a technically difficult set of procedures, often requiring manual drawing and a high degree of anatomical sophistication. These issues make analysis time-consuming, inevitably leading to small samples and the types of methodological factors that have emerged.

Controlling for variation in demographics, handedness, and IQ, all related to assessments of brain volumes, is also very important. Schultz et al. (1994) found statistically significant differences on multiple aMRI measures in children with dyslexia and age-matched controls, including the planum temporale and several left hemisphere structures. However, when subject selection variables (especially gender and handedness) were controlled for statistically, these differences disappeared, and the only reliable finding was a reduction of the size of the left temporal lobe in individuals with dyslexia. Pennington et al. (1999) used careful image acquisitions and elaborate morphometric analyses to measure multiple cortical and subcortical areas of the brain. These investigators found reductions bilaterally in the size of the insula and anterior superior cortex in individuals with dyslexia. In addition, the area of the brain posterior to the splenium of the corpus callosum—largely posterior temporal, parietal, and occipital regions—was larger in both the right and left hemispheres in individuals with dyslexia. These differences, however, were relatively small and occurred in a sample that had large differences between IQ scores of dyslexic and nondyslexic twin pairs, although the results were robust when age, gender, and IQ were statistically controlled.

Altogether, there is some convergence indicating subtle differences in several brain structures between dyslexic and nonimpaired readers, especially in left hemisphere regions supporting language. However, aMRI studies may be enhanced by new modalities for structural neuroimaging that are now available. Diffusion tensor imaging (DTI) is a structural neuroimaging method especially useful for assessing the integrity of cerebral white matter and brain connectivity. In an initial study, Klingberg et al. (2000) used DTI to evaluate the integrity of the cerebral white matter in areas known to support language in the left hemisphere. Comparisons of these measures in adults with and without a history of reading problems showed less development of white matter in those with reading problems. These results suggested reduced myelination of these language-mediating areas. In subsequent studies, Beaulieu et al. (2005) performed

DTI in 32 children, 8–12 years old, who ranged considerably in reading ability; only 4 readers were below the average range. These investigators reported significant correlations of reading ability and assessments of regional brain connectivity involving the left temporal parietal white matter. Similarly, Deutsch et al. (2005) evaluated 14 children, 7–13 years of age. The groups were divided into good and poor readers ($n = 7$ each). The researchers found small differences in the size of the left temporoparietal region that suggested less development of white matter in this region. Given the evidence from functional imaging studies suggesting that these regions are commonly impaired in individuals with reading disabilities, as well as the morphometry results in Silani et al. (2005) and Brambati et al. (2004), these findings are provocative. However, DTI studies of larger groups of children that include individuals with significant reading impairment are needed. It will be interesting in the future to begin to combine DTI structural assessments with functional neuroimaging studies of the same person.

Brain Function

Different types of *functional* neuroimaging methods are used to measure brain activation in response to visual, linguistic, and reading tasks among individuals who read skillfully and individuals with dyslexia. Converging evidence from a range of functional imaging methods used in studies of both groups indicates that a network of brain areas is involved in the ability to recognize words accurately, and that adults and children with dyslexia manifest different patterns of activation in these areas as compared with skilled readers. These areas most consistently involve the basal temporal (for occipitotemporal), temporoparietal, and inferior frontal regions, somewhat more predominantly in the left hemisphere (Eden & Zeffiro, 1998; S. E. Shaywitz & B. A. Shaywitz, 2005).

Imaging Modalities

Functional neuroimaging in dyslexia is based on four different modalities that vary in their data acquisition and their spatial and temporal resolution (Papanicolaou, 1998): positron emission tomography (PET), functional magnetic resonance imaging (fMRI), magnetic source imaging (MSI), and magnetic resonance spectroscopy (MRS). We also mention measures involving electrophysiological methods in context, but do not describe these studies in detail, as their potential for brain mapping is less well developed than that of these other methods. These modalities attempt to measure changes in the brain that occur during cognitive processing, and then to construct maps that demonstrate where (and sometimes when) in the brain these changes occurred. For example, metabolic changes reflected by glucose utilization or shifts in blood flow from one part of the brain to another occur, depending on the mental operation and the parts of the brain that are involved in the operation. These changes can be recorded by PET or fMRI. Similarly, there are neurons that make connections in order to support a particular activity. When neurons make connections, there are changes in the properties of these neurons that alter brain electrical activity. This activity can be recorded by an electroencephalogram (EEG). There are also changes that occur in the magnetic fields surrounding these electrical sources when a person performs an activity. MSI measures these changes, providing information about what brain areas produce the magnetic signals. MRS measures changes in brain chemistry, such as lactate or glutamine, in response to some type of challenge (Hunter & Wang, 2001).

Regardless of the modality, the principles of functional imaging are relatively straightforward (S. E. Shaywitz et al., 2000). As a cognitive or motor task is performed, the changes in glucose metabolism (PET), blood flow (PET and fMRI), electrical activity (EEG), magnetic activity (MSI), or brain chemistry (MRS) are recorded. The changes in brain activation are recorded and superimposed on an MRI of the brain so that the areas of the brain responsible for the activity can be identified. Methods like fMRI, MSI, and MRS involve no radiation, are noninvasive, are safe, and can be used repeatedly even in children. Imaging with PET requires administration of a radioactive isotope to measure changes in blood flow and/or glucose utilization. Since the half-life of these isotopes is short, the time course of an experiment is limited. Children are not usually participants in PET studies unless they have a medical disorder and can directly benefit from the evaluation, as exposure to radioactive isotopes is involved. This exposure even limits the number of times that older individuals can participate in a PET study (Papanicolaou, 1998).

These modalities also vary in their spatial and temporal sensitivity. Metabolic techniques like PET and fMRI assess brain activity that occurs after the cognitive activity has occurred. They do not occur in real time. In fMRI, serial magnetic resonance images are acquired so rapidly that they can be used to capture the changes in blood flow associated with cognitive activity (S. E. Shaywitz et al., 2000). Thus, spatial resolution with fMRI is excellent.

Methods such as MSI (and EEG) occur in real time and provide considerable information on the time course of neural events. The spatial resolution of the brain maps themselves is poor, but this problem is handled by coregistering the MSI brain map on an aMRI scan. Evoked potential and EEG paradigms have excellent temporal resolution, but the spatial resolution is very poor even with coregistration, and these methods are not generally used for functional neuroimaging. MRS is devoted specifically to chemical shifts and is also dependent on coregistration with aMRI for spatial resection. The chemical shifts occur in real time, but require longer acquisitions to measure the shift (Hunter & Wang, 2001).

Overview of Neural Correlates of WLRD

Previous research has used all four imaging modalities, and converging findings suggest that tasks requiring reading are associated with increased activation in a variety of areas, including the basal surface of the temporal lobe extending into the occipital region; the posterior portion of the superior and middle temporal gyri, extending into temporo-parietal areas (supramarginal and angular gyri); and the inferior frontal lobe areas, primarily in the left hemisphere (Eden & Zeffiro, 1998; Rumsey et al., 1997; S. E. Shaywitz et al., 2000). There are inconsistencies among studies with respect to the engagement of a particular area (Price & McCrory, 2005; Poeppel, 1996). However, it is apparent that a network of areas is involved in word recognition, each of which may be activated to a different degree, depending on specific task demands.

A simplified version of this network is shown in Figure 5.3, which shows four major participating areas. An area roughly corresponding to Broca's area is responsible for phonological processing involving articulatory mapping as in the pronunciation of words. Wernicke's area (which includes portions of the superior temporal and supramarginal gyri) is responsible for phonological processing involving letter–sound correspondence. The angular gyrus is a relay station that links information across modalities. The visual association cortex in the occipito-temporal region is responsible for graphemic analysis (Dehaene et al., 2005). Most of the empirical evidence that supports this model of the brain circuit that maintains reading is also consistent with studies of acquired reading difficulties secondary to brain damage (Dehaene et al., 2005) and the effects of transient interference with normal function in specific brain areas because of neurosurgical operations (Simos et al., 2000c). We deliberately do not address the many nuances and questions about involvement of more discrete brain regions, or discrepancies across tasks and samples (see Price & McCrory, 2005), to highlight the convergence in findings across modalities and labs.

PET STUDIES

PET is an older technology, and studies of adults with good reading versus those with dyslexia were initially conducted using this modality.

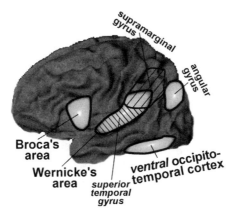

FIGURE 5.3. Simple model of a neural network for reading showing four major participating areas. An area in the frontal lobes roughly corresponding to Broca's area is responsible for articulation mapping, as in the pronunciation of words. Wernicke's area (which includes portions of the superior, middle temporal, and supramarginal gyri) is responsible for phonological processing involving letter–sound correspondence. The angular gyrus is a relay station that links information across modalities. The occipitotemporal region is responsible for graphemic analysis. Courtesy of P. G. Simos. From Fletcher, Simos, Papanicolaou, and Denton (2004, p. 265). Copyright 2004 by The Guilford Press. Reprinted by permission.

These studies found reductions in blood flow in the left temporoparietal area during performance of both reading and phonological processing tasks (Rumsey et al., 1992, 1997), but normal activation in the left inferior frontal areas among those with poor reading (Rumsey et al., 1994). Horwitz, Rumsey, and Donohue (1998) evaluated functional connectivity of the angular gyrus in adults at different levels of reading proficiency and found that the activity in the left angular gyrus occurring during a phonological task was significantly correlated with other areas involved in reading in proficiently reading adults, but not in those with dyslexia. Horowitz et al. (1998) interpreted these data as suggesting a "functional disconnection" between these areas in people with dyslexia. Other studies have also shown evidence for right hemisphere activation, which could be related to compensatory process or other nonlinguistic factors related to reading disability (Grigorenko, 2001; Wood & Grigorenko, 2001). For example, McCrory, Frith, Brunswick, and Price (2000) imaged eight adults with dyslexia and six controls, with tasks involving repetition of real words and pseudowords. The adults with dyslexia showed less activation than controls in right hemisphere regions involving superior temporal and postcentral gyri, and in the left cerebellum. They suggested that this was a compensatory pattern due to the need to shift more resources to processing of the phonetic components of the tasks, reflecting less processing of speech components that were not phonological.

A more recent PET study evaluated eight individuals with dyslexia and ten controls on conditions that involved reading words and naming pictures (McCrory, Mechelli, Frith, & Price, 2005). They found reduced activation of a left occipitotemporal area during both tasks that was independent of the degree of behavioral deficit on the activation task. McCrory et al. concluded that abnormal activation of this region is not specific to reading or to orthographic decoding, but reflects a more general impairment in the integration of phonological and visual information.

In a widely reported PET study by Paulesu et al. (2001), adults with dyslexia recruited from the United Kingdom, France, and Italy were compared with controls. Paulesu et al. (2001) showed that in people with dyslexia from the different countries, reduced activation was apparent during reading that involved the left occipitotemporal regions. This observation was important, because the phenotypic manifestations of dyslexia vary and reflect differences in the languages across these three countries, leading Paulesu et al. (2001) to suggest that phonological processing was common despite these phenotypic differences in accuracy and fluency of reading skills. Note that Silani et al. (2005) found evidence for reduced density of gray and white matter involving the middle and inferior temporal gyrus as well as the arcuate fasciculus in the left hemisphere. The latter finding was consistent with the DTI studies reviewed above, but also suggests reduced connectivity involving phonological and reading areas.

fMRI STUDIES

Studies using fMRI have also found that lack of activation of the angular gyrus is commonly observed in adults with dyslexia, but is part of a broader disruption of the temporoparietal and occipitotemporal regions of the brain. In an early fMRI study of adults, S. E. Shaywitz et al. (1998) found that adults who read well showed increased activation in temporoparietal areas (angular gyrus, Wernicke's area) and occipitotemporal areas as demands for phonological analysis increased. Adults with dyslexia did not demonstrate this pattern, but showed more activation of anterior portions of the brain (inferior frontal gyrus—areas 44, 45). In addition, the readers with dyslexia showed reversed (right greater than left) hemispheric asymmetries in activation in posterior temporal regions as compared with the group of nonimpaired readers—a finding that corresponds with previous reports of atypical patterns of hemispheric asymmetry in regional metabolism in persons with dyslexia (Rumsey et al., 1992). Pugh et al. (2000) also found evidence that the angular gyrus was poorly connected with other areas involving reading in adults with dyslexia. Studies of children using similar tasks have shown less activation of the inferior frontal area in those with dyslexia, but a similar pattern in more posterior regions of the brain (B. A. Shaywitz et al., 2002). There are many other fMRI studies on dyslexia (see Price & McCrory, 2005; S. E. Shaywitz & B. A. Shaywitz, 2005).

MSI STUDIES

MSI studies of children have revealed reliable differences in activation patterns between children with dyslexia and typically achieving children (Papanicolaou et al., 2003). For these studies, activation maps were obtained while the children completed tasks in which they listened to or read real words, or read pseudowords and had to decide whether the pseudowords rhymed (Simos, Breier, Fletcher, Bergman, & Papanicolaou, 2000a; Simos et al., 2000b). The two groups did not differ in activation patterns in the task in which they listened to words, showing the expected patterns involving predominant activation of the left hemisphere. However, on both the word recognition tasks, striking differences emerged in the activation patterns of the group with dyslexia and the typically achieving group (see Figure 5.4). In the typically achieving children, there was a characteristic pattern in which the occipital areas of the brain that support primary visual processing were initially activated (not shown in Figures 5.3 or 5.4). Then the occipitotemporal regions in both hemispheres were activated, followed by simultaneous activation of three areas predominantly in the *left* temporoparietal region (including the angular gyrus, middle temporal gyrus, and superior temporal gyrus). The frontal regions would be activated if pronunciation of the word was required. In the children with dyslexia, the same pattern and time course were apparent, but the temporoparietal areas of the *right* hemisphere were activated. On the whole, the findings are similar to those from the PET and fMRI studies, but the differences between the two groups are more strikingly lateralized.

Intervention: Imaging Studies

The relation of neuroimaging changes and response to an intervention has been evaluated in nine recent studies involving MRS, fMRI and MSI (Aylward et al., 2003; Eden et al., 2004; Richards et al., 2000, 2002, 2005; Simos et al., 2002a, 2005, in press; Temple et al., 2003). In the Richards et al. (2000) study, MRS was used to evaluate metabolic

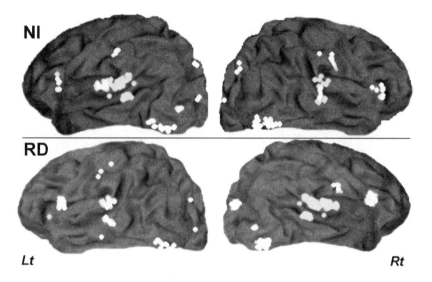

NI

RD

Lt   *Rt*

FIGURE 5.4. MSI scans from a disabled reader (lower set of images) and a nonimpaired reader (upper set of images) during a printed word recognition task in an MSI study. Note the clear preponderance of activity sources in left (Lt) temporo-parietal cortices in the proficient child and in homotopic right hemisphere (Rt) areas in the poor reader. Data from Simos et al. (2000b). Courtesy of P. G. Simos. From Fletcher, Simos, Papanicolaou, and Denton (2004, p. 271). Copyright 2004 by The Guilford Press. Reprinted by permission.

processes before and after a 3-week, 30-hour intervention focusing on phonological processing, word decoding, reading comprehension, and listening comprehension. Children received an MRS examination of the left anterior quadrant of the brain—known to be related to language processing—before and after the intervention. Prior to intervention, the MRS scans revealed a higher metabolic rate of lactate in this quadrant when children with dyslexia completed a task requiring them to decide whether words and nonwords rhymed. After the training program, lactate metabolism did not differentiate children with dyslexia from controls on the reading task. Although the investigators argued that the training program was responsible for the change in lactate metabolism, other reviewers (Gayan & Olson, 2001) have questioned the strength of these findings, largely focusing on the statistical analysis of the results.

In a subsequent study, Richards et al. (2002) recruited an additional sample of 10 children with dyslexia and age-matched controls in the 9–12 year age range. These children received 28 hours of intervention focusing on the alphabetic principle, as well as additional training on morphological awareness (Berninger et al., 2003b). This study also found significant changes in lactate activation before and after intervention, particularly in relation to the intervention that included morphological treatment.

In a third study, Simos et al. (2002a) employed MSI before and after children with severe dyslexia participated in an intense phonologically based intervention. These children ranged in age from 7 to 17 years and had very severe word recognition difficulties: Six of eight children read at the 3rd percentile or below, with the other two children reading at the 13th and 18th percentiles. The children received intervention for 2 hours a day, 5 days a week, over an 8-week period, for about 80 hours of intensive phonologically based instruction per child. Before intervention, the eight children with dyslexia uniformly displayed the aberrant pattern of activation in the right hemisphere that has been reliably identified with MSI. After intervention, the children's word-reading accuracy scores improved into the average range. In addition, in each case, there was significant activation of neural circuits in the left hemisphere commonly associated with proficient word-reading ability. There was also a tendency for reduction in right hemisphere activity. Figure 5.5 provides a

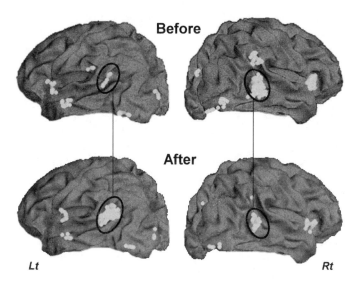

FIGURE 5.5. Activation maps from a poor reader before and after intervention. Note the dramatic increase in left temporoparietal activation associated with the significant improvement in phonological decoding and word recognition ability. Data from Simos et al. (2002a). Courtesy P. G. Simos. From Fletcher, Simos, Papanicolaou, and Denton (2004, p. 273). Copyright 2004 by The Guilford Press. Reprinted by permission.

representative example of the changes before and after intervention. These studies are intriguing and do imply a far greater role for instruction in establishing the neural networks that support reading development, an observation consistent with several additional studies.

Aylward et al. (2003) evaluated changes in response to reading intervention in 10 children with reading difficulties (averaging about 11.5 years of age) and 11 age-matched controls. The children with reading difficulties were less severely impaired than those in the Simos et al. (2002a) study, with the basis for selection a discrepancy in reading relative to verbal ability as indexed by an IQ test. The participants engaged in a 3-week intervention addressing the application of phonological and morphological strategies to word recognition. On average, the children with reading difficulties showed about one-half standard deviation improvement in word recognition ability (from a word reading quotient of about 87 to 93). They were imaged before and after the instructional period with fMRI, using a phoneme sound matching task and a morpheme mapping task. At baseline and as compared with nonimpaired readers, the children with reading difficulties showed much less activation, which varied with the tasks, of areas in the left hemisphere. After intervention, comparisons with the controls were no longer statistically significant, with the authors concluding that the brain activation patterns were normalized as opposed to indicating a compensatory pattern. The areas of the brain that changed were different from those found by Simos et al. (2002a), but the tasks and interventions were also different, and the poor readers in the Aylward et al. test were less impaired. In imaging research, slight differences in participant and task conditions can produce significant variations in activation patterns. What is similar in the studies of Simos et al. (2002a) and Aylward et al. (2003) is that the activated brain areas were largely in language areas of the left hemisphere and have been associated with the neural network supporting different aspects of word recognition. Moreover, neither study indicated compensatory patterns.

More recent studies have shown predominantly normalizing changes in brain function, but have also revealed compensatory changes largely in samples different from the first four studies. Simos et al. (2005) used MSI to assess changes in brain function in a subset of the students who received intervention in an intervention study by Mathes et al. (2005), which is described below as an example of multitiered intervention. Students at risk and not at risk for reading difficulties were imaged at the end of kindergarten (Simos et al., 2002b) and again at the end of first grade. Comparisons of spatiotemporal profiles of brain activation obtained during performance on letter–sound and pseudoword naming tasks showed clear differences at the end of kindergarten between low-risk and high-risk students. In general, the at-risk students showed early development of neurophysiological processes that reflected much greater activity in the temporoparietal areas of the right hemisphere relative to controls, essentially a bilateral pattern of activation in these regions. At the end of first grade, the at-risk group was subdivided into those who responded and those who did not respond adequately to first-grade reading instruction. The at-risk students who responded well to instruction showed essentially the same pattern as at baseline in the degree of regional activation. However, the timing of activation shifted toward a pattern like that of the not-at-risk students. The students who did not respond adequately to intervention showed patterns like those described above that are typically seen in older students with severe reading difficulties, with much greater activation of the temporoparietal areas in the right hemisphere. These patterns are depicted in Figure 5.6 for the three groups.

In a third MSI study, Simos et al. (in press) performed neuroimaging of a small group of students who had not developed adequate word recognition and fluency skills in the Mathes et al. (2005) study. These students received a 16-week intervention that involved intense training in phonological decoding based on the Phono-Graphix program (McGuiness, McGuiness, & McGuiness, 1996) for the first 8 weeks (2 hours per day) with 1 hour per day of intervention involving fluency using Read Naturally (Ihnot, 2000) for the subsequent 8 weeks. For the imaging study, 15 students provided suitable imaging data before intervention and at each 8-week interval. The intervention indicated significant improvement in word recognition, fluency, and comprehension, although individual responses to intervention were highly variable (Denton, Fletcher, Anthony, & Francis, in press). In the imaging component, the changes in brain activity after intervention were primarily normalizing and consisted of increased duration (and degree) of neural activity in the left temporoparietal region and a change in the relative timing of activity in both temporoparietal and frontal regions. In particular, the onset of activity in bilateral temporal parietal regions preceded the onset of frontal activity. These changes were apparent in individual scans involving 12 of the 15 participants. There was also some evidence for compensatory activation involving the right temporoparietal and frontal regions in about half of the participants. When participants were asked to read real words, similar changes were noted, with the most notable changes involving the duration and timing of regional activity. There was increased neurophysiological activity in the posterior portion of the middle temporal gyrus bilaterally, and decreased latency of activity in the middle temporal gyrus of the left hemisphere and in the occipitotemporal region of the right hemisphere. Correlational analysis suggested that improved read-

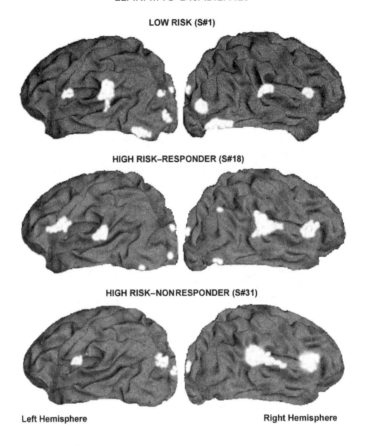

FIGURE 5.6. Activation maps from students who at the end of first grade were at low risk for reading problems; at high risk and responded to intervention; and at high risk but did not respond to intervention. Note the difference in activation involving the left temporoparietal area. From Simos et al. (2005). Copyright 2005 by the American Psychological Association. Reprinted by permission.

ing performance was generally predicted by earlier onset activity in the right occipital regions, increased duration of engagement of the left middle temporal gyrus, and prolonged onset latency of activity in the prefrontal region.

Eden et al. (2004) conducted fMRI evaluations of brain activity during tasks requiring manipulation of sounds in language before and after a phonologically based intervention involving adults with a history of developmental dyslexia. Half the adults with dyslexia received intervention for 8 weeks based on the Lindamood–Bell method. In addition to significant improvement in phonological processing and reading ability, the fMRI study showed increased activation of the inferior parietal area of the left hemisphere, interparietal sulcus, and fusiform gyrus. There were also changes in the right hemisphere. The major changes primarily represented normalization of brain processing, but some compensatory patterns were also observed.

Temple et al. (2003) conducted fMRI on 20 children who underwent intervention using the Fast ForWord method, which does not involve significant amounts of reading. There was significant improvement in reading and language skills in the children (but see below for other studies that have not demonstrated efficacy using this method). On a rhyming task, fMRI showed increased activation in the left hemisphere temporoparietal and inferior frontal region, thus representing normalizing processes. There were also improvements in other brain areas involving the right hemisphere that likely represent compensatory processes.

B. A. Shaywitz et al. (2004) performed fMRI on the students who received intervention in Blachman et al. (2004) study, with comparison groups of students in New Haven, Connecticut, who were either typical achievers or students with reading problems who received standard interventions from the school. This study required students to fly from Syracuse, New York, to New Haven because logistical factors precluded imaging the community controls from Syracuse. The results showed that prior to the intervention, students with reading difficulties exhibited much less activation of brain areas in the left hemisphere commonly associated with reading difficulties. After the intervention, students who received the experimental intervention showed greater activation of bilateral inferior frontal gyri, the left superior temporal sulcus, the occipitotemporal region of the brain involving the middle and inferior temporal gyri, and the interior aspect of the middle occipital gyrus, as well as other regions. B. A. Shaywitz et al. (2004) interpreted these results as showing normalization of left occipitotemporal regions associated with efficiency in reading, but noted compensatory changes involving the right frontal region.

Genetic Factors

Reading problems run in families and occur across family generations, which is the basis for genetic studies of reading disability and ability. This observation stems from the earliest studies of dyslexia (e.g., Hinshelwood, 1917). The risk in the offspring of a parent with a reading disability is eight times higher than in the general population (Pennington & Olson, 2005). Studies of the heritability of dyslexia and other reading disabilities show that the familiality is almost entirely genetic after adolescence, but the variability in reading disability shows both genetic and nonshared environmental influences (Petrill et al., 2006a). These studies, reviewed by Grigorenko (2001), Fisher and DeFries (2002), Pennington and Olson (2005), and Plomin and Kovas (2005), show a long history of investigations at multiple levels. As Grigorenko (2001) summarized, three areas of research converge in demonstrating that dyslexia has a heritable component. These areas involve both twin and family studies of individuals, along with linkage studies examining the role of specific genes that congregate within families that have significant heritability.

Family Aggregation

As reviewed by Grigorenko (2001) and Olson, Forsberg, Gayan, and DeFries (1999), 25–60% of the parents of children who have reading problems also display reading difficulties. The rate is higher in fathers (46%) than in mothers (33%). Children who have parents with reading difficulties are at much higher risk relative to the general population. The rates range from about 30 to 60%, depending on the method of ascertainment. If ascertainment depends on the parent's or school's identifying a child as having dyslexia, the rate is closer to 30%. If the child and parent are actually evaluated by research instruments, the rate is significantly higher.

Twin Studies

The limitation of family studies is that environments are also inherited. Studies of biologically related family members living together confound genetic and environmental influences. Twin studies can be used to address this issue by examining the concordance of dyslexia, as well as the covariance of reading achievement in general. As monozygotic twins have the same genotype, the presence of genetic influences lead to the expectation that concordance rates would be much higher in monozygotic twins than in dizygotic twins, who share only 50% of the same genotype. If shared family environmental influences are implicated, the concordance of monozygotic and dizygotic twins should be equal. Shared environmental influences account for differences between families and could include socioeconomic status, parent reading practices, and so on. Environmental influences could also be nonshared, representing factors that are not genetic and account for differences within families, such as differences in teachers and instructional practices. In general, concordance rates are quite high for monozygotic twins (almost always above 80%) relative to dizygotic twins (rarely above 50%). Therefore, differences in concordance presumably relate to genetic effects.

Beyond concordance, other studies have employed statistical methods that help separate the variance in reading skills according to genetic and both shared and nonshared environmental influences and environmental factors (DeFries & Fulker, 1985), showing that 50–75% of the variance in reading achievement can be attributed to genetic factors. Studies of reading-related processes also show significant genetic influences and varying amounts of shared and nonshared environmental influences. In addition, all of these studies show that the environment exercises significant influence on reading skills, although the contribution of genetic factors is greater. In general, genetic influences explain most of the familiality of reading disabilities and nonshared environmental factors influence lack of familiality, depending on the age of the child.

Linkage Studies

The final line of evidence comes from linkage studies that attempt to identify specific genes related to dyslexia. These studies tend to focus on families that have an unusually high number of members with dyslexia, but range in sample size, methods of analysis, and definition of the phenotype. In a comprehensive meta-analysis, Grigorenko (2005) identified 26 published reports that provide assessments of genetic linkages with "dyslexia." These reports encompassed multiple samples of extended families and twin pairs in eight countries around the world. Based on the review, Grigorenko (2005) identified eight reported susceptibility loci for dyslexia, including sites on chromosomes 1, 2, 3, 6, 11, 15, and 18. The most commonly identified locus was on chromosome 6p, which has been addressed in 14 studies. Grigorenko found that despite some nonconfirmations, there was strong evidence that this locus is involved in dyslexia and specifically for phenotypes identified with assessments of phonological decoding, orthographic coding, single-word reading, and phonemic awareness. There was no evidence that phenotypes defined by rapid naming and spelling were related to this site. Grigorenko (2005) also observed strong evidence for three loci that had been studied less frequently involving sites on chromosomes 1p, 2p, and 3cen. The findings from these studies were robust, but it is always possible that nonreplications will emerge in the future that will reduce the significance of these findings. One frequently studied site on chromosome 15q did not show a robust signal despite the fact that it is the second most studied locus. Similarly, a locus on chromosome 6q did not appear robust across studies. Evaluations of 11p and 18p were hampered by the presence of only two studies per site, with neither site showing strong evidence for a linkage at this point in time.

Grigorenko noted that the approach taken to the meta-analysis was conservative and that for some loci, the number of studies was small. A major problem for the meta-analysis was the attempt to compare across different methods for defining the phenotype, an area of controversy for genetic studies of reading disabilities; does phenotypic variance reflect genetic variance and how much of this variance is due to the phenotype or to measurement error in the tests used to assess the phenotype. The tendency to equate the phenotype to specific tests makes this distinction especially difficult. Nonetheless, the findings replicated across studies for chromosomes 1p, 2p, 3cen, and 6p despite this variation in samples, methods of analysis, countries of origin, and definitions of the phenotype. There were also variations due to whether the definition of dyslexia treats the probands as a group (category) or as a dimensional phenotype.

These molecular genetic studies also provide strong evidence for the heritability of reading difficulties and help explain why reading problems have always been known to run in families. Multiple genes may appear to be involved, particularly if the phenotypic assessment involves decoding or phonological processing. Raskind et al. (2005) suggested that the fluency of phonological decoding had a locus on chromosome 2q that represented a major gene defect, whereas accuracy of phonological decoding represented a polygenic deficit involving multiple genes. More research on the influence of phenotypic variability needs to be completed.

It is important to recognize that genetic factors do not account for all the variability in reading outcomes. Although Byrne et al. (2002) found relatively small to essentially no contributions of the environment for word reading, phonological awareness, and rapid naming measures, most studies do find nonshared environmental contributions, and some find shared environmental influences. This does not mean that some reading problems are inherited and others are due to environmental causes. Rather, the genetic risk interacts with environmental risk to produce a disability in reading; the estimates of heritability are averages across large samples. Shared environmental factors include the language and literacy environment in which the child develops. The tendencies of parents with dyslexia to read less frequently to their children and to have fewer books in the home may contribute to the outcomes of parents and their children (Wadsworth et al., 2000). Another major factor is the quality of reading instruction, which may be shared or nonshared depending on whether siblings are taught by the same teacher, receive similar interventions, and so on. These may vary at different phases in development (Byrne et al., 2002).

Family history of poor reading may give rise to limited environment–instructional interactions in the home (Olson et al., 1999; Pennington &

Olson, 2005). In a specific test of this hypothesis, Petrill et al. (2006a), examined sibling similarity in quantitative genetic model estimates from several assessments of reading in 272 school-age sibling pairs. The pairs were recruited from families involving monozygotic twins, dizygotic twins, and unrelated adopted siblings. Across different measures of word reading and related cognitive skills, Petrill et al. (2006a) found that shared environmental influences were significant, accounting for about a third to a half of the variance in word recognition and phonological awareness. Other tasks, such as rapid naming, were largely influenced by genetic factors. Of particular interest was the evidence that the estimates of environmental contributions were similar in models derived just from twins versus those that involved adopted siblings.

In an integrative review of genetic research on LDs, Plomin and Kovas (2005) characterized quantitative genetic research on children with LDs as indicating that the effects of the relevant genes are largely general and not specific to different kinds of LDs. They noted that the genes that had been associated with problems in language, reading, and mathematics are essentially the same genetic constellations that account for normal variation in these domains. In addition, genetic constellations that affect one language or academic domain also seem to affect other components of the disability. Finally, the genetic impacts are not independent, so that the genetic organizations that are associated with one particular learning disability also affect other learning disabilities. Plomin and Kovas (2005) emphasized large studies such as those from the Colorado group (Pennington & Olson, 2005) and the Twins Early Development Study (TEDS), a study of about 7,500 pairs of twins from the United Kingdom. Summarizing across studies, Plomin and Kovas observed heritability of about 0.6 for reading disability and ability and noted similar findings for analyses based on discrete groups (e.g., dyslexic versus nondyslexic) as well as studies that analyze reading as a continuous distribution. They noted that "when a gene is found that is associated with a learning disability, the same gene can be expected to be associated with variation in the normal range of ability" (p. 600). Plomin and Kovas also noted the absence of evidence for single-gene defects, stating that "it is generally accepted that genetic influence on common disorders is caused by multiple genes of small effect size rather than a single gene of major effect size" (p. 600). The researchers observed high heritability across a variety of different domains of reading abilities. When examining correlations across different domains of language, reading, and math, Plomin and Kovas found that the domains were often highly correlated, but also observed that the correlations were not perfect, which indicates that there are specific as well as general genes involved in the heritability across these domains. They concluded by noting that "definitive proof of importance of general genes will come from molecular genetic research that identifies DNA associated with learning disabilities and abilities" (p. 613). They also specifically observed the absence of evidence for a sex-linked component to the heritability of reading problems.

SUMMARY: FROM ACADEMIC SKILL DEFICITS TO NEUROBIOLOGICAL FACTORS

It is possible to define the most common form of LD, dyslexia, using inclusionary criteria. These criteria focus on the relationship of word recognition and spelling (academic skills deficits) and phonological processing (core cognitive processes). Differentiations are made relative to mental deficiency and to sensory disorders. No other exclusions seem essential, given the absence of evidence that word recognition problems vary according to putative causes. Although neurobiological studies consistently identify factors involving brain function and heritability, it is apparent that neurobiological and environmental factors interact to produce the phenotypes associated with dyslexia. This is especially apparent in the intervention-imaging studies, which imply that the neural systems that mediate the development of reading skills are malleable and dependent on experience in order to develop. We have provided only a brief review of the many functional neuroimaging studies of WLRD, deliberately highlighting the convergence across studies, but many questions remain. In a conservative summary, Price and McCrory (2005) concluded that

> functional neuroimaging studies to date have not yet established the components of reading that show reliable differences in dyslexic readers, or indeed determined which of these differences may be causal to the reading impairment in dyslexia. However, a pattern is beginning to emerge, with increased prefrontal activation and decreased occipital-temporal activation now observed over several studies. This pattern suggests that dyslexic readers largely activate the same neural system as skilled readers, but show subtle differences in how the components of this system are engaged. (p. 496)

Across modalities, these findings do suggest that in children with WLRD, or dyslexia, the functional connections between brain areas account for differences in brain activation, as opposed to specific or general dysfunction of any single brain area. Genetic studies show high heritability of word reading skills with Pennington and Olson (2005) summarizing large twin studies in the United Kingdom and Colorado as indicating that about two-thirds of individual differences in reading are attributable to genetic factors and about one-fifth to shared environmental factors. The influence of shared environmental factors is larger in young children (Petrill et al., 2006a, 2006b). Genes that influence reading may have an impact on reading and instructional practices implemented early in development, reflecting genetically driven interactions with the environment that increase estimates of heritability. Also, many of the twin and sibling studies are restricted in the range of education and SES levels of the participants, which limits generalization to reading outcomes in economically disadvantaged populations. These estimates do not mean, however, that reading achievement in poverty is due to genetic factors or that genetic factors constrain the effects of intervention, particularly in younger children (Pennington & Olson, 2005).

The phonological processing hypothesis provides a robust explanation of the word reading difficulties characteristic of dyslexia, but dyslexia is more than just a reading disability. Many children with dyslexia have problems in other areas, such as math (or ADHD). Impairments in other components of the reading process, particularly fluency, are difficult to explain solely on the basis of phonological processing, although the failure to develop word recognition ability is the most parsimonious explanation of the fluency and comprehension problems. There are hypotheses based on other factors that differentiate children with reading disabilities (not always well defined as dyslexic) from typically achieving children, but these hypotheses do not provide strong explanations of the core reading problem. The impact of this research, and the coherent explanation of dyslexia that has emerged, are best judged by the impact of the research on the treatment of WLRD, which we address in the rest of this chapter.

WORD RECOGNITION INTERVENTIONS

Reading disabilities have a deleterious effect on educational, social, and occupational well-being. Thus, a substantial amount of research on the development of reading-related skills during the preschool period, early identification and prevention of reading failure in kindergarten and the early grades, and remediation of reading problems in later elementary and middle school grades has taken place in the last decade. We begin with research on children who struggle because of word recognition difficulties. This research, and the specific teaching methods and approaches that have been studied, are described here in relation to (1) early identification and intervention studies to prevent reading failure at classroom and tutorial levels and (2) reading remediation studies for older students. Whenever possible, we begin with a well-known commercial program and then discuss specific methods derived from research. Many evidence-based reviews of specific programs can be found on the Florida Center for Reading Research website (www.fcrr.org).

The primary focus of this review is on studies that reflect academic therapies, which are the only consistently proven methods for helping students with LDs. The history of intervention is replete with interventions derived from theories of auditory and visual processing, theories based on hypothesized brain deficits, and even odder theories (diet, exercise). Many of these programs can be dismissed simply because they do not require students to read. For example, the Fast ForWord programs provide a set of computer games that slow and magnify the acoustic changes within normal speech, but do not have a reading component (Scientific Learning Corporation, 1999). A recent randomized study of the effectiveness of these programs indicated that although some aspects of students' language skills improved, actual reading skills were not significantly enhanced (Rouse & Kreuger, 2004; see also Pokorni, Worthington, & Jamison, 2004). As discussed in the next section, if there is one cardinal intervention principle for students with LDs, it is that training in motor, visual, neural, or cognitive processes without academic content does not lead to better academic outcomes.

Empirical Syntheses

There is considerable evidence supporting the use of specific instructional procedures addressing word recognition difficulties in poor readers. This research parallels studies demonstrating at a classroom level the importance of explicit instruction in the alphabetic principle as a component of any reading program. The National Reading Panel (NRP, 2000) conducted a meta-analysis of 96 studies designed to improve phonemic awareness skills. The analysis yielded effect sizes that were in the large range immediately after intervention (0.86) and remained strong over the long term (0.73). There was evidence of generalization to reading and spelling in the moderate range (0.53–0.59). The NRP found that phonemic awareness instruction was most effective when it included a letter component, when instruction focused on one or two types of phonemic manipulations as opposed to multiple types, and when students were taught in small groups. Programs lasting less than 20 hours were typically more effective than longer programs, with single sessions lasting about 25 minutes. There was little difference in effectiveness between classroom teachers and computers.

Similar findings were apparent in the NRP meta-analysis of data derived from studies of the effectiveness of phonics instruction on a variety of reading outcomes, most often word recognition. Seventy-five studies were screened, and 38 were retained for meta-analysis. The overall effect size of phonics instruction was in the moderate range (0.44). Programs that included phonics instruction were more effective than comparisons that provided either implicit or no phonics instruction. Programs in which phonics was taught "systematically" were more effective than programs that taught less systematically. Phonics instruction was effective in individual tutorial programs (0.57), small-group programs (0.42), and whole-class programs (0.39). It was much more effective when introduced in kindergarten (0.56) or first grade (0.54), as compared with grades 2–6 (0.27). Phonics instruction was more effective in kindergarten (0.58) and grade 1 (0.74) for students at risk for reading problems. It tended to be less effective for students who were defined with LDs in reading (0.32) and had a negligible effect size in low-achieving readers in grades 2–6. As suspected, word recognition skills were most significantly affected in younger students (effect size = 0.60–0.67), with effects on spelling (0.67) and reading comprehension (0.51). Again, gains were smaller in all domains after grade 1.

At this point in the development of reading interventions, the issue is not whether to provide phonics instruction; rather, the question is how to integrate phonics instruction with instruction in other components central to learning to read. Individuals who argue that the solution to reading difficulties is simply to introduce more phonics instruction in the classroom, without incorporating instruction in other critical reading skills (e.g., fluency, vocabulary, comprehension), are not attending to the NRP findings or the converging scientific evidence. This is true for programs that attempt to enhance the reading abilities of all students in the classroom, as well as programs that attempt to enhance reading in students with LDs.

Prevention of Reading Disabilities

Prevention programs typically include assessments to identify students with difficulties in acquiring foundational skills in word recognition and fluency and target interventions to address specific deficits. Some of these programs also address academic needs in the area of vocabulary and comprehension. Studies designed to assess the capability of specific approaches to prevent reading disabilities have accumulated in recent years because of the increased ability to predict which students will develop such difficulties as they enter and proceed through school (Foorman et al., 2004). Thus, these studies largely target students who are at risk for reading difficulties because of early phonological processing and/or word recognition difficulties. In this section, we distinguish studies that attempt to intervene at a classroom level from those that attempt to identify students who are at risk and pull them out for intervention. We review only studies that begin in kindergarten or grade 1, but note that preschool interventions are also demonstrably effective (Lonigan, 2003).

Classroom Studies

Classroom studies either attempt to introduce new comprehensive reading programs into the classroom with an accompanying emphasis on professional development, or offer a classroom-level intervention that the teacher provides or directs. It is well known that introducing reading curricula into the classroom, with professional development linked explicitly to the curriculum, typically results in improved reading scores for the classroom as a whole, as well as accelerating reading development in students who are at risk for reading difficulties (Snow et al., 1998). We present three examples involving (1) Direct Instruction, (2) the University of Texas–Houston classroom intervention study, and (3) Peer Assisted Learning Strategies.

DIRECT INSTRUCTION

We use the term "Direct Instruction" to refer to the method of intervention developed by Engelmann and colleagues (e.g., Engelmann, Becker, Hanner, & Johnson, 1978). Direct Instruction programs include an extensive professional development component that helps teachers understand the rationale for this approach to reading instruction, lesson plans, methods for error correction, and grouping strategies. The curriculum extends beyond phonics into fluency and comprehension. Direct Instruction lessons are typically fast paced and follow a prescribed lesson plan. The lessons usually last 35–45 minutes and contain 12–20 tasks. These methods are based on task analytic and behavior management systems, but line up with the emphasis on phonological processing and word recognition. The programs include opportunities for practice using individualized workbooks that match the content in the group lesson.

Adams and Engelmann (1996) provided a review of research based on this particular reading methodology. They reported that effect sizes from studies comparing Direct Instruction programs with contrast groups receiving standard practice yielded large effect sizes that generally exceeded 0.75. Adams and Carnine (2003) provided a comprehensive synthesis of approximately 300 studies involving reading that utilized Direct Instruction methods; 17 were research studies that met very specific inclusion and exclusion criteria, including the presence of a comparison group, pretest scores, and the ability to isolate Direct Instruction as the primary reading methodology. The average effect size for these studies that specifically included students with LDs was 0.93, which is in the large range. This was comparable to the effect sizes reported by Adams and Engelmann (1996) for students in general education classrooms (0.82) and in all special education categories (0.84). Disaggregating the results showed that the effect sizes tended to be larger for secondary/adult groups (1.37) relative to elementary groups (0.73). Gains were apparent on criterion-referenced measures (1.14) as well as norm-referenced tests (0.77). Quasi-experimental studies yielded an average effect size of 0.90, and experimental studies that included a randomized controlled experiment (RCE) yielded an average effect size of 0.95, supporting findings reported by the NRP (2000). For studies that lasted up to 1 year, the average effect size was 1.08, relative to studies that persisted for more than 1 year (0.77).

One limitation of the Adams and Carnine (2003) study is that it did not compare effect sizes within domains of reading. Often the outcome measures are reading composites, and it would be useful to know more about differences in the impact of Direct Instruction programs on word recognition, reading fluency, and comprehension. In a more recent study, Carlson and Francis (2002) carried out a 4-year RCE of a version of Direct Instruction through a program (Rodeo Institute for Teacher Excellence; RITE) that involved schoolwide implementation of a Direct Instruction model. The evaluation involved 20 schools that implemented the RITE Program and 20 demographically comparable comparison schools. The RITE program included implementation of a Direct Instruction curriculum and extensive professional development through an institute providing teachers with professional development in the model as well as classroom management and on-site coaching. Results revealed that the overall program was successful in increasing the reading abilities of students in the targeted schools relative to comparison schools. The effect sizes in both word recognition and reading comprehension were in the large range. Those students who were exposed to the program early and spent more years in the program outperformed all other students, including those within the target schools. Thus, students who began in kindergarten and were assessed for the final time in grade 3 had the best outcomes. There were direct links of professional development for teachers to improvements in teaching skills, fidelity of implementation, and student performance. The number of students who read at levels of word recognition and reading comprehension that met considered consensual benchmarks was reduced over time in both domains.

Direct Instruction programs have been widely criticized despite the significant evidence base indicating effectiveness. The criticisms include

the possibility that the results of Direct Instruction programs do not extend to comprehension skills and begin to fade in upper elementary
grades. Others suggest that the scripting of programs deprofessionalizes
teachers. Another concern is the behavioral component of Direct Instruction programs, which some have suggested impairs critical thinking. Although there is evidence in some early studies that the effects begin to fade, this is a characteristic of many of the types of schools in
which programs like Direct Instruction are implemented. It also reflects
the use of norm-referenced achievement tests that represent comparisons
against age-based cohorts that are cross-sectional samples. Thus, the
drop in scores is not really a decline, but a reduction in the rate of accel-
eration. The concerns about scripting, deprofessionalization of teachers,
and the impact on critical thinking do not appear to be supported by objective evidence. Using a scope and sequence does not eliminate the need
for teacher judgment and skill, content expertise, and the ability to assess and monitor student progress. More research is needed to evaluate
the apparent decline in effect sizes, a problem apparent in many intervention studies.

FOORMAN AND COLLEAGUES

Foorman et al. (1998) contrasted the effects of reading curriculums that
varied in the explicitness of instruction in word recognition for at-risk
students receiving Title I services in eight schools in grades 1–2. The students were taught by one of three approaches: (1) explicit code—a basal
curriculum (Open Court Reading, 1995), which provided explicit instruction in word recognition, along with instruction in comprehension
strategies; (2) embedded code—a phonics program (Hiebert, Colt, Catto,
& Gury, 1992), which emphasized the learning of phonics concepts
within the context of whole words; and (c) implicit code—a curriculum
that stressed contextual reading; responses to literature; writing, spelling, and phonics in context; and integration of reading, writing, listening, and speaking, with no decontextualized instruction in phonics. All
students received the same amount of time in the respective programs,
with comparable student–teacher ratios. The teachers received professional development and support for implementing each of the approaches. These approaches were compared to standard instruction.

   Growth curve analyses were conducted on measures of phonological awareness, word reading, and spelling administered at four time
points between September and April. Figure 5.7 shows an example of
the results using a word-reading task administered four times during the
school year. Across a variety of literacy outcomes, students in the explicit
code group improved at a faster rate than students who received implicit

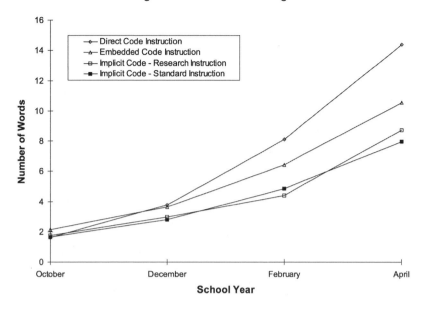

FIGURE 5.7. Growth in word reading raw scores at four time points during the school year by curriculum. Students who participated in the direct (explicit) code condition showed more rapid growth and higher end-of-year performance. From Foorman, Francis, Fletcher, Schatschneider, and Mehta (1998, p. 46). Copyright 1998 by the American Psychological Association. Reprinted by permission.

code instruction, and had significantly higher April scores in word reading, phonological processing, and spelling. The means for students in the embedded phonics condition were between those of the other two groups. A significantly higher percentage of students in the implicit and embedded code groups than in the explicit instruction group showed little improvement in word reading over the year. In addition, Foorman et al. (1998) found that the relation between phonological analysis and word reading was stronger for explicit code students than for implicit code students, suggesting that the effects of explicit instruction on word reading stemmed from its effects on phonological awareness.

PEER-ASSISTED LEARNING STRATEGIES

An alternative and cost-effective classroom-level intervention has been developed based on collaborative learning (Jenkins & O'Connor, 2003). Collaborative learning refers to a set of practices involving small-group instruction and students working together in learning activities. Such activities emerge from a number of the models reviewed above, often integrating cognitive, behavioral, and constructivist principles. As a set of practices, cooperative learning has a large empirical base that provides strong support for its use at a classroom level (Jenkins & O'Connor, 2003). This is partly because such practices facilitate classroom management and differentiated instruction by their focus on smaller groups within the classroom.

In the reading area, the most well-developed form of collaborative learning intervention is represented by Peer-Assisted Learning Strategies (PALS), most fully elaborated in a systematic research program involving more than 30 studies over the past 20 years by a research group at Vanderbilt University led by Doug and Lynn Fuchs (Fuchs & Fuchs, 2000, 2005). PALS is a classroom-level intervention in which students who have stronger academic skills are typically paired with students with weaker academic skills for about 30 minutes of instruction three to five times per week. Often the instruction efforts are divided into those that involve word recognition and decoding skills and other strategies involving comprehension. There is an extensive literature on the efficacy of PALS, which has been developed for reading and math and used in research from kindergarten into secondary school (Fuchs & Fuchs, 2000, 2005). We provide examples of studies in which PALS was implemented in different formats in kindergarten and grade 1, noting that the research base extends beyond grade 1.

In a kindergarten study, Fuchs et al. (2001a) compared three groups of students; the first group received phonemic awareness instruction based on the Ladders to Literacy program (O'Connor, Notari-Syverson, & Vadasy, 1998), and this was the only instruction provided for this group. A second group received instruction in both phonemic awareness based on Ladders to Literacy and beginning word recognition skills; the third group was a classroom comparison group that received neither of these interventions. The decoding instruction was based on PALS. The results indicated that the two treatment groups did not differ on phonological awareness skills at the end of kindergarten, but exceeded levels apparent in the comparison group that received standard instruction. On decoding and spelling tests, students who also received the decoding component of PALS exceeded the group that received only phonological awareness instruction, whose performance was comparable to the comparison group.

A second study utilized the same comparison groups with different students, but focused on non-Title 1 schools. Thus, Fuchs and Fuchs (2005) compared three kindergarten groups: (1) that received PALS with and without phonological awareness training, (2) that received only phonological awareness training, and (3) that received neither intervention. The two intervention groups were generally comparable on a variety of phonological awareness, reading, and spelling measures, but performed at higher levels than the comparison group. There was little evidence that the phonological awareness training added to the value of PALS, which emphasized decoding skills. These studies demonstrate that classroom-level interventions that involve the teaching of word recognition skills are not enhanced when phonological awareness instruction is added. They also attest to the power of classroom-level interventions that result in more differentiated instruction in the classroom.

In other intervention studies involving first-grade PALS, Fuchs and Fuchs (2005) reported evidence that PALS improved not only word recognition skills, but also reading fluency and comprehension. Mathes, Howard, Allen, and Fuchs (1998) found that first-grade PALS improved reading skills in both low- and average-performing first-graders, documenting that PALS is not detrimental to high achievers. In summarizing the results of several studies involving PALS in first grade, Denton and Mathes (2003) found that PALS resulted in 69–82% of the poorest readers in the classroom progressing to the average range by the end of the intervention, based on an admittedly arbitrary criterion of word reading above the 25th percentile. Nonetheless, extrapolating this reduction to the total school population indicates that PALS potentially reduces the population base rate for reading difficulties from 25 to 5–6%, results that are similar to those reported by Foorman et al. (1998).

Tutorial Studies

In the next section, we review studies that are largely independent of classroom-level interventions. These studies typically utilize a tutoring model in which at-risk students are pulled out of the classroom for additional instruction. Although initial studies focused on individualized tutoring, more recent implementations utilize small groups of three to five students. We begin with a widely available program and then examine specific studies of tutoring.

READING RECOVERY

A popular early intervention program for first-grade students reading in the lower 20% of their classes is Reading Recovery (RR) (Clay, 1993). This intervention provides daily, individual 30-minute lessons to students in first grade who are identified as being at risk on the basis of a survey of reading skills. A complete RR program includes 20 weeks of lessons, although the actual duration of the program varies from student to student. The RR program stresses that basic decoding and phonics skills should be taught in the context of authentic reading and writing activities and emphasizes teaching students to employ multiple strategies (use of context clues, word attack, etc.) to identify words, rather than focusing on only one strategy, such as "sounding out" words. The RR teacher is responsible for selecting text for each individual student such that the student will be challenged, but not frustrated, and can be successful with teacher support. A major emphasis is on the teacher's observational skills and judgment.

Shanahan and Barr (1995) provided a comprehensive review of the effectiveness studies conducted to date with RR, reporting that the program does result in substantial gains in reading for approximately 70% of participating students. However, they noted that many of the studies reviewed were methodologically deficient. A recent meta-analysis also found that RR was effective for many grade 1 students (D'Agostino & Murphy, 2004). This study disaggregated RR outcomes by whether the outcomes involved standardized achievement tests or the Observation Survey, an assessment developed by Clay (2002), that is specific to the RR curriculum. It also separated results for students who successfully completed RR (i.e., met program criteria and were discontinued) versus those who were unsuccessful or left the program before receiving 20 lessons (i.e., were not discontinued) and according to the methodological rigor of the studies. When the comparison group was composed of low-achieving students, average effect sizes on standardized achievement tests for all discontinued and not discontinued students were in the small range (0.32), and higher for discontinued (0.48) than not discontinued (−0.34) students. This finding was consistent with that of Elbaum, Vaughn, Hughes, and Moody (2000), who reported that RR was less effective for students with more severe reading problems. D'Agostino and Murphy (2004) found that analyses based on just the more rigorous studies included in their meta-analysis, in which evaluation groups were more comparable on pretests, showed smaller, but significant effect sizes on standardized measures. Disaggregation according to whether the student was discontinued or not was not possible. Effect sizes were much larger for the Observation Survey measures, but these assessments are tailored to the curriculum and also have severely skewed distributions at the beginning and end of grade 1, which suggests that the Observation Survey should not be analyzed as a continuous variable in program evaluation studies (Denton, Ciancio, & Fletcher, 2006).

Concerns about the efficacy of RR revolve around two issues: (1) whether RR is successful with the lowest-performing students and (2) whether RR is cost-effective. In terms of the first concern, RR has typically targeted students who perform in the lowest 20% of their classes. The actual performance level of participants varies from school to school. Although the research from the developers of RR continues to indicate efficacy for about 70% of the students in the program, its reported effects are much weaker when students who do not meet the program's exit criteria are included in the analyses of outcomes. It should also be noted that much of the research reported by the developers of RR has not been scrutinized by rigorous peer review prior to publication.

In a review by Elbaum et al. (2000), it was found that gains for the poorest readers were often minimal, which Elbaum et al. suggested may be related to the need for more explicit instruction in decoding. Several studies support this observation. Iversen and Tunmer (1993) compared the reading growth of students enrolled in the standard RR program with students enrolled in a modified RR program supplemented with explicit instruction in the alphabetic principle. Although both RR groups significantly outperformed control students on a variety of reading measures, students in the modified RR program progressed significantly faster than those in the standard program. Tunmer, Chapman, and Prochnow (2003) noted that in New Zealand, which, as its country of origin, has significant implementation of RR, there remains a large gap in reading skills between economically advantaged and economically disadvantaged students. In one study, Chapman, Tunmer, and Prochnow (2001) followed students who were placed in RR programs, observing that many experienced severe difficulties in phonological awareness and decoding skills before entering the program. Participation in RR did not reduce these difficulties, which they attributed to the absence of attention to explicit instruction in the alphabetic principle. More recently, Tunmer et al. (2003) modified an RR program in New Zealand to include phonological awareness and explicit phonics instruction, implementing it with economically disadvantaged minority students. Comparing the modified program in seven schools with a historical control cohort from the same schools revealed that students who received the modified program scored higher than the historical controls on all phonological awareness and reading measures, including standardized measures of reading achievement and measures like those employed in RR. These gains persisted through grade 2. There was evidence that the modified program reduced the achievement gap characteristic of economically disadvantaged students in New Zealand.

The second issue with RR involves its cost-effectiveness (Hiebert, 1994). The professional development component is expensive and, because RR requires one-on-one tutoring, many schools find it difficult to implement on a long-term basis. The question, however, is whether any reading intervention in elementary schools needs to be provided on a 1:1 basis. In their meta-analysis, Elbaum et al. (2000) found that larger groupings of three students to one teacher were just as effective as 1:1 groupings across a range of interventions. Vaughn et al. (2003b) system-

atically manipulated group size in order to compare interventions delivered 1:1, 3:1, and 10:1. Across a variety of reading assessments involving word recognition, fluency, and comprehension, outcomes were
comparable for 1:3 and 1:1 interventions, and both of these were better
than interventions in group sizes of 10:1. These findings support conclusions reached by the NRP (2000). More recently, Iversen, Tunmer, and
Chapman (2005) developed a version of RR for small groups, observing
no differences in outcomes for students taught in 1:1 and 1:2 formats.

OTHER TUTORIAL STUDIES

Torgesen and Colleagues. Torgesen et al. (1999b) evaluated the
long-term effects of a prevention study that began in kindergarten and
followed students through grade 4, with intervention through grade 2.
Students were identified for the study in the first semester of kindergarten, based on scores on tests of letter name knowledge and phonological
awareness. The 180 students in the final sample were randomly assigned
to four treatment conditions: (1) phonological awareness training plus
synthetic phonics (PASP) instruction embedded within real-word reading
and spelling activities (embedded phonics); (2) phonics instruction embedded with real-word reading and spelling activities; (3) a regular kin-
dergarten/classroom support group receiving individual instruction to
support the goals of the regular classroom program; and (4) a best practices control group. Students in each treatment condition were provided
with 80 minutes of one-on-one instruction each week during kindergarten and grade 1. Results revealed that the PASP program was associated
with significantly higher gains in alphabetic reading skills (decoding)
and spelling than the embedded phonics and the classroom support
treatments. Students in the embedded phonics and classroom support intervention groups outperformed the best practices group. Students in all
three treatment groups performed equally well on measures of single-
word reading, indicating that enhanced preventative instruction is beneficial, no matter what the training format. At the end of the grade 2, students who received the most explicit instruction in the alphabetic principle had much stronger word reading skills than students in all the other
groups. In addition, students who received the most explicit instruction
showed the lowest retention rate (9%), with retention rates in the other
three conditions ranging from 25% (implicit phonics), 30% (classroom
support condition), and 41% (no treatment comparison group). As a
group, students in the most explicit condition demonstrated word-level
reading skills that were in the middle of the average range. However, in
this same group, 24% of the students were still well below average levels
in these skills, based on a criterion of word reading above the 25th per-

centile. Extrapolated to the entire population, this would lead to an overall failure rate of 2.4% in the population from which these students were selected. This figure, of course, is far below the approximate 20% figure reported for students commonly assumed to be at risk for reading disabilities and the 37% of grade 4 students performing below basic level in reading on the National Assessment of Educational Progress (NAEP; NCES, 2003).

Torgesen (2004) presented preliminary data from a new generation of prevention studies. In introducing preventative instruction to grade 1 students at risk for reading difficulties, the provision of PASP in groups of three to five students for 45 minutes a day (about 30 weeks) led to significant improvement, with only 8% of the at-risk individuals performing below the average range as defined by word recognition skills (below the 26th percentile at the end of grade 1). This suggests a population failure rate of 1.6%. These results persisted through grade 2, although outcomes were slightly poorer for comprehension than for word recognition, with a comprehension test suggesting that 4.1% were reading below average levels.

Blachman and Colleagues. In a series of studies, Blachman (1997; Blachman, Ball, Black, & Tangel, 1994) exposed 84 low-income, inner-city kindergarten students to 11 weeks of instruction. One teacher instructed a small group of four to five students in several aspects of phonological awareness and letter sound knowledge for 15–20 minutes per day, four days a week. The students completed 41 15–20–minute lessons, for a total of 10–13 hours of instruction. At the end of the 11 weeks, students receiving the phonological treatment significantly outperformed control students on tasks assessing the reading of phonetically regular words and related tasks. A follow-up study conducted in February and May of grade 1 showed that these gains were maintained if the curriculum contained the same emphasis on phonological skill development and on the relation of these skills to decoding, word recognition, and textual reading.

Vellutino and Colleagues. Vellutino et al. (1996) identified students who had scores below the 15th percentile in real-word and pseudoword reading skills at the beginning of the second semester of grade 1. These students were in schools that were selected because of the high probability of the students having strong literacy backgrounds. The schools were largely middle class and above, and the sample was predominantly Caucasian. These students received 30 minutes of daily individualized tutoring. Approximately half of this tutorial was devoted to explicit code-based activities, as well as word recognition and writing activities, and the other half was devoted to activities involving the use of decoding and other strategies for word recognition and comprehension in text reading. At the end of only one semester of remediation, approximately 70% of the students were reading within the average or above average range based on national norms. These results translated to a reading failure rate, based on those reading below the 26th percentile in word recognition skills, of approximately 1.5–3% of the overall population, depending on whether severely impaired and moderately impaired readers were both included in the tally (3%), or only severely impaired readers (1.5%) were included. Further, students who responded well to remediation, and "caught up" to their normal reading peers, generally maintained these performance levels once the intervention was discontinued. In a follow-up evaluation, Vellutino et al. (2003) reported on outcomes through grade 4, exploring differences in students according to the amount of progress made in the intervention. Poor readers who were most difficult to remediate performed well below the normal readers, as well as below the poor readers who were readily remediated, on kindergarten, grade 1, and grade 3 tests evaluating phonological abilities. They did not differ on semantic, syntactic, and visual measures, although all tutored groups tended to perform below the normal readers on these measures as well as on most of the phonological measures.

Vellutino et al. (2003) found that although most students maintained their gains, a significant number did not maintain their progress, especially those who were the most difficult to remediate. The investigators suggested that these students may not have received the type of individualized, comprehensive, and integrated approach to reading instruction they needed to consolidate their initial gains and become functionally independent readers after tutoring was discontinued.

Berninger and Colleagues. In a series of studies, Berninger and her colleagues evaluated a variety of interventions and training methods for students in grades 1–2 at risk for reading difficulties. The interventions often manipulated relations between written and spoken words (Berninger et al., 1999); different components of reading, such as combinations of word recognition and comprehension training (Berninger et al., 2003b); or various combinations of phonological and orthographic awareness training (Berninger et al., 1999). Many of the interventions were done over very short periods of time, but always included highly structured lesson plans. In general, Berninger and her colleagues reported that interventions that expanded the unit of analysis at a sublexical level to include orthographic and morphological relations were generally more effective than those that involved only phonological relations. In addition, interventions that were more integrative and involved more components of reading, such as both word recognition and comprehension training, were more effective than those that involved only one component of reading.

In other studies, Berninger and her colleagues made comparisons of RTI based on assessments of growth, much like those done by Vellutino et al. (2003). Berninger et al. (2002a) compared faster and slower responders based on an assessment of growth curves in response to intervention. They found that students who responded faster in first grade maintained their gains in second grade and tended to have higher levels of initial reading ability and Verbal IQ. Similar findings were reported by Stage et al. (2003). Slower responders had more difficulties in the language area—particularly on measures of phonological and orthographic awareness, rapid naming, and verbal reasoning skills. In the responder groups, there were subsets of fast responders who consistently showed better development of word recognition than reading comprehension ability. Slower-responding students made reliable gains with continued tutoring, but needed longer durations of instruction.

Altogether, these studies provided a rich research base demonstrating the efficacy of early intervention studies. The next section discusses a new generation of studies that attempts to build upon this research base by layering classroom-based interventions and small-group instruction.

Multitiered Intervention Studies

The examples of prevention research reviewed to this point involve *either* classroom intervention or tutorial intervention. As both approaches demonstrate efficacy, why not evaluate the effects of layering classroom and tutorial interventions (O'Connor, 2000; Vaughn, Linan-Thompson, & Hickman, 2003b)? Such implementations must involve a determination of who needs tutoring, that is, which students do not respond to classroom level intervention. In this section, nine recent studies involving multitiered classroom (Tier I) and tutorial (Tier II) interventions are reviewed (see Vaughn, Wanzek, Woodruff, & Linan-Thompson, in press, for another review).

Three studies involved approximately one semester of intervention in either kindergarten (Al Otaiba, 2000) or grade 1 (Berninger et al., 2000; Vadasy, Sanders, Peyton, & Jenkins, 2002). In each of these studies, the intervention was followed by a second intervention. Although Vadasy et al. (2002) did not find evidence for additional benefits of the second intervention, Berninger et al. (2000) and Al Otaiba (2000) found that the second level of intervention led to significant gains.

Other studies used longer time frames in kindergarten and/or grade 1. O'Connor, Fulmer, Harty, and Bell (2001) evaluated a multitiered intervention program for students in grade 1 who were identified as being at risk. In Tier I, classroom teachers were provided with professional development addressing differentiated reading instruction geared toward low-achieving students. In the second tier, supplemental small-group reading instruction was provided for about 30 minutes per day, three times per week. The content varied, depending on needs for word recognition and fluency. At the end of grade 2, comparisons with a group that did not receive the tiered interventions showed higher levels of performance on word recognition, fluency, and comprehension in the tutored students.

In an earlier study, O'Connor (2000) evaluated the effects of multitiered intervention in kindergarten. Fifty-nine students representing the lowest 40% of kindergarteners were identified as being at risk on an assessment battery involving vocabulary, memory, letter identification, rapid naming, and phonological awareness measures. The intervention focused on the provision of professional development to kindergarten teachers, with an emphasis on differentiated instruction in the classroom. In addition, students who seemed to struggle received 1:1 tutoring. The study found that 28% of students who received both levels of intervention continued to struggle. The provision of additional intervention involving small-group 1:1 intensive interventions substantially reduced the number of students who continued to struggle at the end of grade 1. Following these students into grade 2 revealed, however, that the tutored students tended to lose ground in comparison with students who were not at risk.

O'Connor, Fulmer, Harty, and Bell (2005) reported on a study of 103 kindergarteners and 103 first-graders who received three layers of intervention. The first layer consisted of professional development in reading instruction for kindergarten and first-grade teachers. The kindergartners subsequently received an additional intervention providing small-group instruction for students who were struggling. Depending on rate of progress, students continued in the second layer through second and third grade. Using historical controls, O' Connor et al. (2005) found a significant reduction in the rate of placement in special education, which was 15% prior to the study; after 4 years of participation, the rate of placement dropped to about 12% if just one layer (professional development) was provided and to about 8% if the second layer was added.

Simmons, Kame'enui, Stoolmiller, Coyne, and Harn (2003) summarized a kindergarten–grade 1 intervention program that also layered classroom and supplemental interventions. This study began in kindergarten, identifying 113 students who performed in the bottom 25% of all students in seven schools. Identification was based on a curriculum-based assessment of letter naming and initial sound fluency. The at-risk kindergarteners were assigned to one of three interventions. All interventions provided 30-minute, small-group, pull-out supplements to typical kindergarten instruction. One intervention (Code) provided 30 minutes of both strategic and systematic instruction in the alphabetic principle, phonological awareness and decoding instruction, as well as practice and application through handwriting, spelling, and related tasks. The second program (Code/Comprehension emphasis) provided two 15-minute segments involving (1) phonological and alphabetical skills and (2) vocabulary and comprehension activities. The third intervention addressed a comparison group that received 30 minutes of instruction emphasizing phonological awareness and decoding skills derived from a commercial program. Results revealed that the Code emphasis group obtained higher scores in word recognition relative to the Code/Comprehension emphasis or the commercial program groups.

In first grade, students who scored at or above a specified fluency benchmark of naming 20 letter sounds per minute on a nonsense word fluency measure received either the monitoring condition or a maintenance intervention. The maintenance intervention involved 30 minutes of instruction focused on decoding, word recognition, and connected text reading. Findings revealed an interaction of entry-level skills and whether the student benefited from the maintenance program. Students who entered with higher scores on nonsense word fluency performed comparably whether they received the maintenance or the monitoring condition. Students whose scores met the fall benchmark but were at the low end of the score continuum revealed lower rates of growth on an oral reading fluency measure. A third group of students, who received kindergarten intervention but did not respond strongly, continued small-group instruction in first grade. Three conclusions can be drawn from these findings: (1) students who responded strongly to kindergarten intervention and scored well above fall benchmarks did not require further intervention to reach end of first-grade benchmarks; (2) students who received kindergarten intervention and barely reached fall benchmarks required additional intervention to maintain adequate growth; and (3) students who did not respond strongly to kindergarten and fell far below fall first-grade benchmarks required extensive intervention in first grade. These latter results support the adjustment of instruction according to student needs and show that certain forms of kindergarten instruction led to improved reading in at-risk students in first grade (Coyne, Kame'enui, Simmons, & Harn, 2004).

Vaughn et al. (2003a, 2003b) provided a multitiered intervention that began with kindergarten students in six schools. In this study, kindergarten teachers were provided with professional development and in-class support. Students identified as being at risk were randomly assigned to supplemental small group intervention (i.e., multitiered intervention) or to only the enhanced classroom intervention. Interestingly, in addition to generic professional development, the classroom implementations included support through kindergarten PALS. The interventions included an emphasis on phonological awareness and beginning decoding as well as elements of the Direct Instruction model, including error correction, explicit instruction, and purposeful examples. The lesson plan was sequenced, and progress was monitored in all at-risk students. The intervention involved approximately 50 daily sessions over 13 weeks and supplemented the Tier I instruction. Results revealed that at-risk students who received multitiered intervention performed at significantly higher levels than historical control students on measures involving word recognition, fluency, and comprehension. In addition, students who received multitiered intervention outperformed students who were at risk and received enhanced classroom instruction, although the effect sizes were smaller relative to historical controls.

Mathes et al. (2005) evaluated the effectiveness of two small-group pull-out interventions in grade 1 relative to enhanced classroom instruction alone in a sample of 292 students who were identified as being at risk for reading difficulties. These students represented the bottom 20% of students in terms of early reading development in about 30 classrooms in six non-Title I schools. All identified students received enhanced classroom reading instruction, representing the district's professional development program with enhanced materials and the use of assessments to inform instruction. The two pull-out interventions, provided to randomly assigned subgroups of the at-risk students who also received enhanced classroom instruction, were constructed to reflect different philosophies in early reading intervention. One approach (Proactive Reading) was modeled on Direct Instruction principles. It consisted of 120 fully articulated lessons designed in five strands targeting phonological awareness, alphabetic decoding, orthographic knowledge, fluency development in decodable text, and comprehension strategies. The other intervention (Responsive Reading) also involved explicit instruction in the alphabetic principle, as well as fluency and comprehension strategy instruction. There was no predetermined scope and sequence. Rather, teachers were provided with guidelines consisting of a sequence of useful phonic elements and a list of high-frequency words and designed lessons to respond to student needs reflected in daily assessments and observations. In contrast to those in Proactive Reading, students in Responsive Reading read text leveled for difficulty but not explicitly phonetically decodable. A typical lesson would involve fluency work (repeated reading with modeling) and assessment of one student in the group for the first 8–10 minutes, 10–12 minutes of explicit instruction in phonemic awareness and phonics, and supported reading and writing for the remaining 20 minutes. Both interventions were provided in small groups of three students to one teacher for about 40 minutes each day for about 8 months.

The results revealed that all three groups obtained scores that were in the average range at the end of the year on measures of word recognition, fluency, comprehension, and spelling. The two groups that received pull-out intervention generally did not differ from one another, but had higher outcomes involving phonological awareness, word reading, and oral reading fluency than the group that received only enhanced classroom instruction. Figure 5.8 provides an example of the overall pattern of results, comparing in one cohort growth in reading fluency on a CBM probe administered every 3 weeks for the three at-risk groups and a comparison group that was not at risk. It is apparent that the two groups that received the pull-out interventions had greater growth than the group that received only enhanced classroom instruction. Note that the two pull-out groups had average fluency rates close to the end of first grade benchmark of 60 words per minute, and the demographically comparable not at-risk group had rates close to the second-grade bench-

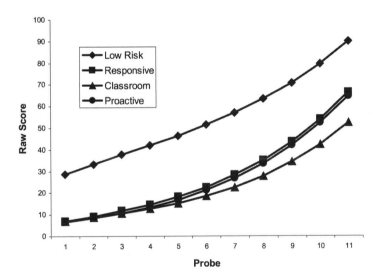

FIGURE 5.8. Growth in reading fluency based on curriculum-based assessments every 3 weeks for students in grade 1 who were (1) identified as being at low risk for reading problems, (2) participated in one of two small-group interventions (responsive, proactive), or (3) received only enhanced general education classroom intervention. The groups that received the small-group interventions showed faster rates of growth and higher end-of-year performance as compared with the at-risk group that received only enhanced classroom instruction. From Mathes et al. (2005, p. 169). Copyright 2005 by the International Reading Association. Reprinted by permission.

mark. Based on a criterion of the 30th percentile in word recognition skills, about 16% of the group that stayed in the classroom did not achieve in the average range at the end of the year, which translates to 3% of the schools' first-grade populations. Less than 10% of students who received the two pull-out interventions failed to achieve in the average range, representing population rates that were under 1.5%. These results demonstrate that pull-out intervention has a value-added impact relative to classroom instruction alone, even instruction of generally high quality. It is important to recognize that the participating classroom teachers had been provided with an aggressive professional development program targeting reading instruction by their school district, and that these students received the beneficial effects of the professional development, screening, and progress monitoring provided by the researchers.

McMaster, Fuchs, Fuchs, and Compton (2005) randomly assigned 33 first-grade teachers, half in high-poverty schools and half in middle-class schools, to validated classroom treatment with PALS (22 teachers) or to their standard practice (11 control classrooms). The researchers monitored student response to whole-class instruction weekly for 7 weeks. On the basis of the students' level of performance, combined with the amount of improvement they showed over the 7-week period, results revealed that the use of PALS reduced the proportion of inadequate responders from 28 to 15%. The students who failed to demonstrate adequate response to PALS were then randomly assigned to three secondary service conditions: (1) none (i.e., continue in classroom PALS without modification), (2) classroom adaptations to PALS (i.e., received a modified form of classroom PALS), or (3) one-to-one adult tutoring. Adult tutoring involved three weekly sessions that combined a strong focus on word-level instruction with story-reading practice and self-regulation. Results showed that adult tutoring was more effective than the other two secondary conditions, further reducing unresponsiveness to 2–5%, depending on how unresponsiveness was calculated (McMaster et al., 2005).

Vellutino et al. (2006) provided intervention to children identified as being at risk for reading problems upon kindergarten entry. The intervention involved instruction in emergent literacy skills, including print concepts, letter identification, letter–sound correspondence, phonological awareness, guided reading, and story comprehension. The intervention was provided in small groups of two to three children per teacher for about 30 minutes twice weekly. A comparison group of kindergarten children was included that received no intervention in kindergarten. At the end of the kindergarten year, the intervention group had substantially higher scores on a variety of literacy outcomes. In first grade, children were again screened for reading problems. Those who continued to struggle were randomly assigned to pull-out interventions that involved either an emphasis on teaching the alphabetic principle or a guided reading intervention. Both interventions involved a range of literacy-related activities, but differed in their emphasis. At the end of first grade, there were no differences between the two groups that received the small-group instruction. In a follow-up at the end of third grade, 84% of the students who had received intervention in only kindergarten or both kindergarten and first grade were performing in the average range on a variety of literacy measures. This translates to an inadequate response rate across the schools of 3.2% (assuming a risk designation of the bottom 20% of the population).

Summary: Prevention Studies

The classroom and tutorial studies reviewed in this section show that early intervention may reduce the number of students who are at risk for reading difficulties, including those who might eventually be characterized with LDs in reading as well as those who are economically disadvantaged and may be poorly prepared to read. Intervention studies that address the bottom 10–25% of the student population may reduce the number of at-risk students to rates that approximate 2–6% (Denton & Mathes, 2003; Torgesen, 2000). In examining these programs, it is clear that both classroom and small-group tutorial programs are effective (i.e., successful intervention programs do not require 1:1 tutoring). In addition, the most effective programs were comprehensive, integrated programs that emphasized instruction in the alphabetic principle, teaching for meaning, and opportunities for practice. As these components differentially impact word recognition, comprehension, and fluency, respectively, such findings are not surprising.

Of particular interest were the results of studies that attempted to layer classroom and tutorial interventions. When this layering occurred, such as in the provision of tutorial instruction for at-risk students from classrooms with an intervention emphasizing PALS, or where the core reading program was apparently strong, the number of at-risk students appears to go below 2% in some studies. Moreover, outcome studies show that these changes are effective through grade 5 and that domains involving word recognition, fluency, and comprehension are impacted.

Reading Remediation Studies

Empirical Syntheses

Although it is difficult to bring students with WLRD up to grade level if the intervention begins after grade 2, remedial studies tend to yield effect sizes that are comparable to those of early intervention studies. The problem is that the student's access to print is so delayed that a year of reading experience—essential to building fluency—has been missed (Torgesen et al., 2001). In a comprehensive meta-analysis of intervention studies for students identified broadly as learning disabled, Swanson (1999) grouped intervention studies into four instructional models: those providing only direct instruction, those providing only strategy instruction, those providing both direct instruction and strategy instruction, and those providing interventions that could not be categorized as either direct instruction or strategy instruction. A variety of interventions were placed in each of those domains. Direct instruction included interventions that involved breaking tasks into smaller steps, administering probes, use of feedback and diagrams, modeling of skills and behaviors, and related interventions. In contrast, strategy instruction included attempts at student collaboration, teacher modeling, reminders to use strategies, multiprocessing instructions, dialogue, and other interventions related to the attempt to teach students strategies. Overall, the results indicated that interventions that provided both direct instruction and strategy instruction were more effective than those that involved only direct instruction or strategy instruction. The studies that included strategy instruction resulted in larger effect sizes than those that did not (0.84 vs. 0.67); methods that included direct instruction had larger effect sizes than those that did not (0.82 vs. 0.66). Combining direct instruction and strategy instruction yielded larger effect sizes (0.84) versus either direct instruction alone (0.68) or strategy instruction alone (0.72). Note that these effects are in the moderate-to-large range, showing that remedial reading interventions across a variety of different methods improve reading outcomes. These effects were observed in word recognition, comprehension, and fluency. There are many examples of remedial reading programs. In the next section, we begin with commonly utilized programs and then move to highlight some of the more recent studies.

Multisensory Methods

Historically prominent remediation approaches used with disabled readers have been characterized as multisensory in nature, were provided in an individualized fashion, and were used to develop spelling and writing skills as well as reading skills. An early example of this type of method was the Fernald approach (Fernald, 1943), which incorporated principles of language experience and whole-word (not whole-language) instruction in the teaching format. In essence, the reading material to be learned was provided by the students through the dictation of their own stories. Fernald (1943) argued that this type of approach could help to overcome the negative feelings that many students have because of their prolonged difficulties in learning to read. From these stories, the students selected words they wished to learn and worked directly on them, repeatedly saying and tracing the words until they could be written from memory. Words that were mastered were kept in a file, and these words were used to generate additional reading material. The Fernald approach emphasized learning words as wholes and discouraged teaching students how to "sound out" new words. Given what is now known about the importance of decoding skills in the learning-to-read process, it is not surprising that the Fernald method was not substantiated by research evidence (Myers, 1978).

Other programs considered "multisensory" were derived from the early work of Samuel and June Orton under the general rubric of "Orton–Gillingham" approaches. Early versions of these programs emphasized the need for instruction to all sensory modalities. These approaches required the student to learn associations between letters and sounds. Students were taught to see a letter (visual), hear its sound (auditory), say its sound (auditory), trace the letter (tactile), and write the letter (kinesthetic). Words mastered were eventually inserted into sentences and passages to promote text reading and reading comprehension. There was an emphasis on understanding the structure of language and sounding out words.

These early efforts were reformulated by Anna Gillingham and Betsy Stillman in the 1960s and have continued to evolve. Many of the remedial approaches reviewed in this chapter, including approaches used in research by Blachman, Berninger, Wolf, and others that emphasize the importance of explicitly and systematically teaching students about the structure of language reflect the influence of these earlier remedial approaches (Moats & Farrell, 1999). Similarly, commercial programs such as the Lindamood Sequencing Program for Reading, Spelling, and Speech (Lindamood & Lindamood, 1998) and Phono-Grafix (McGuiness et al., 1996) reflect the influence of Orton–Gillingham instruction. In response to the students of interest, these programs initially focused primarily on word recognition, but have expanded to incorporate activities related to reading fluency and comprehension, writing, and oral language development under the rubric of multisensory structured language education.

As outlined in Birsh (1999), the content of multisensory structured language instruction involves six components: (1) phonology and phonological awareness, (2) sound–symbol association, (3) syllable instruction, (4) morphology, (5) syntax; and (6) semantics. This content is embedded in five principles of instruction: (1) simultaneous, multisensory teaching to all learning modalities (visual, auditory, kinesthetic) to enhance memory and learning; (2) systematic and cumulative organization of material; (3) direct teaching through continued teacher–student inter-action; (4) diagnostic teaching involving continued assessment of individual needs; and (5) both synthetic (putting parts of language together to form a whole) and analytic (presenting the whole and breaking it down into constituent parts) instruction. With the exception of the multisensory component, which remains controversial, principles 2–5 characterize many effective approaches to reading remediation for students with word recognition and fluency difficulties, along with the focus on explicit teaching of the structure of language.

Older versions represented as Orton–Gillingham approaches have received little research support (Hallahan, Kauffman, & Lloyd, 1996), and more recent versions are just beginning to be rigorously evaluated. The NRP found only four studies with adequate methodological quality that involved variations of older multisensory Orton–Gillingham programs. Two of these programs yielded positive effect sizes and two did not. For example, Oakland, Black, Stanford, Nussbaum, and Balise (1998) implemented the Dyslexia Training Program, an adaptation of the widely employed Alphabetic Phonics program developed at the Texas Scottish Rite Hospital, for 2 years of daily instruction in small groups. In relation to a comparison group of students who were served in "regular practice" classrooms, effect sizes associated with the Dyslexia Training Program were not regarded as significant (NRP, 2000). Two years of instruction resulted in changes from about the 3rd percentile of word recognition ability to the 10th percentile.

In another study, students with identified reading disabilities in grades 2 and 3 who were provided services in public school special education resource rooms received one of two programs in which phonics was taught explicitly, one of which was an alphabetic (synthetic) phonics program based on an Orton–Gillingham model and the other an analytic phonics method (Recipe for Reading). Students in these two groups were compared with a group that received an intervention involving teaching sight-word recognition skill (Foorman et al., 1997). Although there was a clear tendency for students who received the alphabetic phonics program to show better gains in phonological analysis and word-reading skills at the end of 1 year of intervention, these differences were not apparent when verbal intelligence scores—higher in this group—were controlled in the analysis. Foorman et al. (1997) also noted that the size of the instructional groups was too large to promote adequate implementation of any of the programs.

There is efficacy data from less rigorous evaluation studies that support these types of programs, and more rigorous studies are emerging. Studies that compare instruction with and without the traditional multisensory components do not indicate differences in outcomes (Clark &

Uhry, 1995; Moats & Farrell, 1999). Wise, Ring, and Olson (1999) also did not find that a multisensory articulatory component, as in the Lindamood program, was a necessary component of their own intervention. The strength of these programs likely involves the intense, systematic approach to instruction, the link with specific types of struggling readers, and possibly the explicit attention to the structure of language. Although there is limited evidence for the efficacy of programs under the multisensory rubric, other programs, reviewed below, that are similar in content and structure do show positive effects.

Lovett and Colleagues

The longest continuing program on reading remediation research is directed by Maureen Lovett at The Hospital for Sick Children in Toronto. In the initial phase of this research, children with severe reading disabilities were randomly assigned to either an intervention that is a modification of Reading Mastery, a Direct Instruction program, called Phonological Analysis and Blending/Direct Instruction (PHAB/DI), or to a program with a metacognitive focus that teaches word recognition through the application of different strategies called Word Identification Strategy Training (WIST). Both programs recognize the importance of decoding instruction that helps children break apart words and the importance of instruction that maximizes transfer of learning. The PHAB/DI program emphasizes letter sound units, and the WIST program focuses on larger subsyllable units. In the initial evaluations, both programs were more effective than an active comparison group (classroom survival skills) on standardized and experimental measures (Lovett, Warren-Chaplin, Ransby, & Borden, 1990). These programs resulted in different patterns of transfer of learning, thus showing treatment-specific effects. For example, PHAB/DI was associated with stronger results specifically on phonological decoding, such as with pseudowords; the WIST program resulted in generalization to regular and exception words in English. As Lovett, Barron, and Benson. (2003) observed, these programs did not normalize reading skills, and 35 hours of instruction did not seem to be adequate. However, the students in these interventions were largely in upper elementary and middle school classes when they began the intervention and entered with very severe reading difficulties, often below the 5th percentile.

Lovett et al. (2000a) conducted an RCE in which PHAB/DI and WIST were combined and compared with longer-term intervention with PHAB/DI or WIST alone and to an active control condition. The study provided about 70 hours of instruction in different sequences that involved going from PHAB/DI to WIST, WIST to PHAB/DI, or either intervention alone for the same amount of overall instructional time. Generalized treatment effects on standardized measures of word identification, passage comprehension, and phonological decoding were demonstrated for all four reading instruction sequences. Results showed that the combination of PHAB/DI and WIST, in either order, was more effective than either intervention alone on measures of nonword reading, letter sound knowledge, and different word identification measures. Thus, 35 hours of instruction in PHAB/DI combined with 35 hours of instruction in either WIST or RAVE-O (Retrieval, Automaticity, Vocabulary elaboration, and Enrichment with language-Orthography) was more effective than 70 hours of PHAB/DI or WIST—the latter interventions more effective than teaching math and study skills.

These studies occurred in special research classrooms where children were referred for reading difficulties. Subsequent research has employed these programs in school settings. A combined program (PHAB/DI and WIST) is now called the "PHAST" (phonological and strategy training) Track Reading Program. In an ongoing study in which the PHAST Track Reading Program was implemented in community schools in Toronto, initial data showed that the students who received these interventions made substantial gains on standardized and experimental measures, achieving on average about two-thirds of the program gains achieved in the laboratory-based interventions. There was considerable variability in the response to the community-based interventions, which may reflect differences in the fidelity and the vitality of implementation.

Morris, Lovett, and Wolf

The PHAST Track Reading program has also been employed in recent multisite intervention studies involving collaboration by Lovett's group, Wolf's group in Boston, and Morris at Georgia State University (Morris et al., 2006). In the initial 5 years, a group of students received different combinations of the interventions in schools in Toronto, Atlanta, and Boston. The samples were carefully constructed to control for variations in socioeconomic status (SES), ethnicity, and intellectual levels, all involving students in second and third grade. Half the children at each site and in each group were from lower SES backgrounds, and within lower and middle SES levels, half were white or African American. Four treatment groups were compared. One group received the original PHAST Track Reading Program (decoding and word identification focus). The second group received a combination of PHAB/DI and Wolf's RAVE-O program (Wolf, Miller, & Donnelly, 2002), which is described in Chapter 6 in the section on fluency interventions. These two programs, which combined direct instruction methods emphasizing the alphabetic principle with different forms of language focus and strategy instruction, were compared against two comparison groups, one that was taught Direct Instruction math and study skills and one that received PHAB/DI along with study skills training. Results showed that students who received either combined condition achieved higher levels of word recognition and comprehension ability than students who received only PHAB/DI; all three groups performed at higher levels than the math comparison group. This intervention, which involved approximately 70 hours of instruction, resulted in changes of about 0.5 standard deviations. Approximately 50% of students who received the two combined interventions showed word recognition ability that approximated the average range. This study revealed that these multidimensional programs yielded a gain for children with lower IQs equivalent to that for those with higher IQs at entry, and a benefit for children from lower SES environments equal to that for those from more advantaged circumstances.

Olson and Colleagues

Olson and Wise (2006) summarized a series of computer-based remedial studies for students with significant reading problems defined on the basis of difficulties with decoding skills. These students were generally identified with disabilities in grades 2–5 and had word recognition scores that were in the lower 10% of their classmates. In their initial studies, Olson and Wise (1992) pulled students from regular reading or language arts classes to read interesting instructional-level stories on a computer during approximately 28 half-hour sessions over a semester. Decoding support for targeted words in the stories was available in various forms through the use of synthetic speech. The group that received computer-based instruction showed significantly better gains in phonological decoding skills and word recognition than a randomly assigned control group of poor readers who remained in their regular remedial reading or language arts classes. However, the gains in the computer-trained group were much less dramatic in poor readers with the lowest scores on measures of phoneme awareness.

In a study of 200 students randomly assigned to two conditions, Wise et al. (2000) developed a longer computer-based *Phonological* intervention. This program had a main focus on phonological awareness and decoding in 50–60 half-hour sessions over a semester taught in small groups (usually 3:1). One-third of the intervention time was in computer-based and small-group interactive instruction in phonological and articulatory awareness—based, in part, on a program developed by Lindamood and Lindamood (1998). Another third of the intervention time was spent on practice in the phonological decoding of nonwords and in building nonwords and words spoken by the computer. The final third of the intervention included reading instructional-level stories on the computer with decoding assistance when requested for difficult words, answering occasional multiple-choice comprehension questions, and reviewing targeted words at the end of the session.

The second condition was *Accurate Reading in Context,* an intervention that also spent a third of its time in small-group interaction and having interactive discussions regarding use of comprehension strategies (Palinscar & Brown, 1985), to balance with the highly motivating small-group phonological awareness activities in the Phonological condition. The remaining two-thirds of the Accurate Reading intervention involved reading stories independently on the computer, as described for the Phonological condition. The main purpose of this second intervention was to compare the benefits of the Phonological condition with benefits from Accurate Reading practice with stories without explicit phonological instruction.

When compared with the Accurate Reading in Context group at the end of intervention, the Phonological group in the Wise et al. (2000) study made three times more improvement in phonological awareness and two times more improvement in the phonological decoding of nonwords. However, the results for standard score gains in word reading depended on the grade/reading levels of the poor readers, and on whether the measure of word reading was time limited or unlimited. Combined across grades 2–5, those in the *Phonological* condition showed significantly greater standard score gains on two untimed measures of word reading, but this main effect was qualified by a significant interaction with their grade/reading level: Phonologically trained poor readers in grades 2–3 showed substantially greater gains in untimed word reading, but there was no significant advantage for phonologically trained students in grades 4–5, in spite of their superior phonological skills. An *opposite* treatment main effect was found for an experimental measure of time-limited word reading. The Phonological group actually had significantly smaller gains, and this treatment difference tended to be larger for the poor readers in grades 4–5, where growth in rapid and accurate word reading was clearly better in the group that spent most of its time accurately reading stories on the computer. This result is consistent with those of other studies, reviewed later in Chapter 6 on fluency, that showed significant fluency gains from text-reading practice (e.g., Stahl, 2004).

The Wise et al. (2000) study included follow-up tests 1 and 2 years after the end of intervention. Although the Phonological group's advantages in phonological skills did remain significant 1 and 2 years after intervention, there were no significant differential training-group main effects or interactions for any of the reading or spelling measures at follow-up tests. Wise et al. (2000) hypothesized that better long-term transfer to reading from improved phonological skills might be attained from longer and more intensive intervention to "automatize" phonological skills and from continued support for the application of those skills in reading.

Olson and Wise (2006) concluded that there is still little evidence that older poor readers experienced specific long-term benefits than can be specifically attributed to a heavy emphasis on sublexical phonological intervention as provided in many interventions (e.g., Lindamood & Lindamood, 1998). With that controversial conclusion, they cited Torgesen et al. (2001), noting that this study resulted in similar reading gains for two conditions that, like those in Wise et al. (2000), were quite different in their emphasis on explicit phonological intervention. Although the Torgesen et al. (2001) Embedded Phonics intervention did include a sublexical component, these results parallel those in the earlier section "Prevention of Reading Disabilities" showing that the addition of phonological awareness training to the decoding component of PALS (which has a sublexical component) has no value-added impact on reading outcomes. Mathes et al. (2005) also found comparable gains for two reading interventions that varied the amount of phonological awareness and sublexical phonics intervention. Berninger et al. (2003b) found that interventions that combined word recognition training with a significant sublexical component and reflective reading comprehension improved word recognition skills more than in a group that only received practice in reading skills or in a group that received only intervention in word recognition. Outcomes for word recognition in the group that simply practiced reading skills was not different from a fourth group that received only reading comprehension instruction. However, all three intervention groups showed higher reading comprehension scores relative to the comparison group that simply practiced reading. The Colorado interventions provide the most extreme distinctions, but keep in mind that the computer reading condition provided pronunciations as targeted words were highlighted, so implicit learning of their print–speech relations was supported (Foorman, 1994).

Blachman and Colleagues

The emphasis on interventions that combine different components that include explicit instruction in the alphabetic principle and different aspects of strategy instruction can be found in other older and more recent interventions. Blachman et al. (2004) reported the results of a reading intervention as compared with standard practice intervention in a sample of second- and third-graders with poor word recognition ability. The intervention involved 8 months of individualized tutoring (average of 105 hours) in a program that emphasized explicit instruction in phonological and orthographic connections in words as well as text-based reading. Each lesson was built around a five-step core that included (1) review of sound–symbol associations, (2) practice in word building to develop new decoding skills, (3) review of previously learned regular words and high-frequency sight words, (4) oral reading of stories, and (5) writing words and sentences from earlier components of the lesson. Each lesson also included activities that involved additional reading of narrative and expository text to enhance fluency, comprehension, and engagement, along with other writing activities and games.

Figure 5.9 shows representative pre–post changes on measures of word reading accuracy, comprehension, and fluency of text reading. Across multiple outcomes, students who received the intervention had greater gains in word recognition, fluency, comprehension, and spelling than students who received their interventions through the schools. These gains were maintained in a 1-year follow-up. These students generally began the intervention with word recognition skills that approximated the 10th–12th percentile; at the end of the intervention their scores approximated the 23rd percentile in word recognition, with higher scores in spelling, slightly lower scores on measures of reading fluency, and comparable scores on comprehension. The effect sizes were generally in the moderate-to-large range across reading domains, rang-

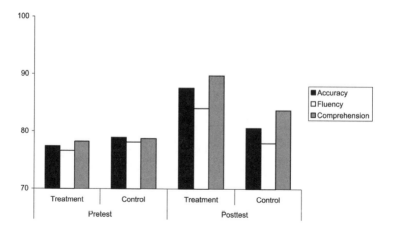

FIGURE 5.9. Pre–postintervention results for treated and control subjects on the accuracy, rate, and comprehension measures of the Gray Oral Reading Test (GORT). Clear differences in treatment and controls are apparent. Data from Blachman et al. (2004).

ing on standardized tests from 0.55 for reading comprehension to 1.69 for word recognition.

Torgesen and Colleagues

Other intervention studies parallel these results, generally showing that the nature of the program is less important than its comprehensiveness and intensity. In a highly visible study, Torgesen et al. (2001) enrolled students reading below the third percentile in word recognition ability in grades 3–5 in an intense 8-week program in which the students received 2 hours of instruction per day, 5 days per week (about 67 hours over the 8-week period). The interventions involved either the well-known Lindamood–Bell Auditory Discrimination In-Depth program or a program called "Embedded Phonics" developed for this study. Both interventions incorporated intervention principles that have been found to be effective for students with significant reading difficulties. These included ample opportunities for structured practice of new skills, the cuing of appropriate strategies in context, and explicit instruction in the alphabetic principle. A time-by-activity analysis showed that the Lindamood–Bell program involved about 85% time in instruction in phonological decoding, about 10% in sight word instruction, and 5% time in reading and writing connected text. The Embedded Phonics program, in contrast, involved about 20% instructional time in phonological decoding, 30% in sight word instruction, and 50% in reading or writing connected text.

There was little difference in the relative efficacy of the two interventions, so Figure 5.10 collapses across the two interventions. As depicted in Figure 5.10, the results showed significant improvement of about one standard deviation in word recognition, slightly less than one standard deviation in comprehension, and little change in fluency. The gains in word recognition and comprehension persisted for 2 years past the intervention (Figure 5.10). About 70% of the students who received one of these interventions were able to read in the average range, defined as word recognition scores above the 25th percentile, after the intervention and, most remarkably, 40% exited special education. Disappointing, however, was the absence of changes in fluency. In explaining the absence of improvement in fluency, Torgesen et al. (2001) suggested that reading rate was limited because the number of words in grade-level passages that the students could read "on sight" was much smaller than the number that could be read by average readers. Thus, when comparing fluency rates on stories that were at the student's instructional level, there were no rate differences. However, grade-level passages reduced the fluency differences because there were too many words the students did not have as part of their sight word vocabulary. There is a strong re-

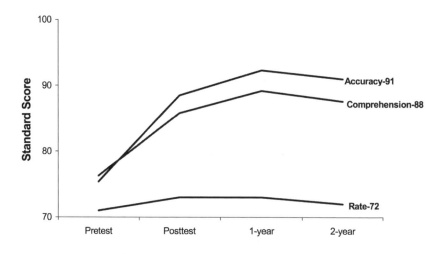

FIGURE 5.10. Growth in accuracy, rate, and comprehension scores from the GORT collapsed across treatment at pretest, posttest, and 1- and 2-year follow-ups. There is more growth in the accuracy of word reading and in comprehension as compared with reading fluency. Data from Torgesen et al. (2001).

lationship between reading fluency and practice, so that if students are not able to access print for 3–5 years, it would be very difficult to close this gap. Torgesen (2002) estimated that students in the interventions would have to read for 8 hours per day for a year in order to close the gap created by the delay in the students' access to print.

Torgesen (2004) reported preliminary data that represented another attempt to evaluate a cohort similar in age and decoding impairment. In this study, students with severe reading difficulties in grades 3–5 received an intense phonologically based intervention, or an intervention that included a fluency-oriented component addressing repeated reading of words and passages. Initial results did not show differences between the two interventions. Although both interventions led to significant improvement in word-reading accuracy and in comprehension, little change in norm-referenced fluency scores was apparent, paralleling the findings of Torgesen et al. (2001).

Berninger and Colleagues

Berninger et al. (2003a) identified 20 students in grades 4–6 who were participating in a family genetics study. These students read one standard deviation below their Verbal IQs on one of several different measures. The selection criteria resulted in a sample that tended to be much higher in Verbal IQ than other samples, with the students also tending to have higher reading scores at baseline. These students were randomly assigned to an intervention involving about 28 hours of either extensive phonological awareness intervention or intervention in morphological awareness. The phonological intervention emphasized word building through phonological analysis and synthesis, whereas the morphological treatment emphasized word building and generation with larger units of words. Each student received intervention in groups of 10 over a 3-week period. Results showed gains of about a half standard deviation in word recognition for both conditions as compared with pretreatment scores. It should be noted that this sample had much higher language proficiency scores and few students with attention problems, or compared with those in other remedial studies reviewed in this chapter.

Summary: Remedial Studies

Remedial studies show that foundational skills can be improved in students with LDs in reading, typically characterized by word recognition difficulties. The effects are most apparent in word recognition, but also show transfer to comprehension. Fluency gains are often smaller, but vary across studies and may reflect the age and the severity of reading difficulties of the students addressed by the study. For example, Blachman et al. (2004) obtained stronger gains in fluency than Torgesen et al. (2001), but most of the students were younger and their difficulties less severe than those in Torgesen et al. (2001). Wise et al. (2000) also found age-related changes in fluency gains. A variety of approaches are associated with improvement, including commercial programs that were incorporated in different studies (Lindamood–Bell, Phono-Graphix), research-based approaches (PHAB/DI, RAVE-O, PHAST, PASP), and programs that were not reviewed (Spell-Read; Rashotte, MacPhee, & Torgesen, 2001; see Florida Center for Reading Research, 2005, 2006). It is clear that the program is less important than how it is delivered, with the most impressive gains associated with more intensity and an explicit and systematic delivery (Torgesen et al., 2001). There are also associations with the length of instruction; many hours are required to accelerate reading development in older students (grade 2 and beyond). To reiterate a critical finding, programs that are explicit, oriented to academic content, teach to mastery, provide scaffolding and emotional support, and monitor progress are particularly effective. Outcomes are specific to the content of instruction, so that more comprehensive programs are emerging. Future development of remedial programs must involve more

attention to reading fluency, which seems least responsive to intervention (see Chapter 6).

CONCLUSIONS

This extensive review of research on WLRD, or dyslexia, illustrates the
research advances that have been made over the past 30 years around
the world in understanding dyslexia. What is especially impressive about
the research is not only the growth within domains of inquiry, such as
cognitive processing, brain function, genetics, and intervention, but also
the integration across domains. It is clear that research across different
areas involving children and adults with dyslexia is linked and is beginning to produce an integrated, coherent view of dyslexia. The starting
point for any coherent theory is a classification that is reliable and valid,
and that yields identification criteria indicating the presence or absence
of the class of interest. In this respect, dyslexia is unique among LDs in
terms of generating definitions that are inclusionary and that clearly
specify how to go about identifying people with dyslexia. This research
shows that the primary academic skill deficits that lead to identification
of dyslexia involve problems with the accuracy and fluency of decoding
skills, and spelling. Cognitive research identifies reliable correlates and
predictors of these marker variables, the most robust involving phonological awareness. Additional cognitive processes involve rapid naming
of letters and digits as well as working memory for phonological material. Dyslexia has reliable neurobiological correlates, with a burgeoning
evidence base on the neural correlates of word recognition and dyslexia.
There is also substantial research identifying specific genetic markers of
dyslexia that involve several different genes. Intervention studies have
shown that dyslexia can be remediated when it is identified later in development. Most impressive are the results of studies that simply attempt to immunize all children against dyslexia and to prevent it from
becoming a disability. Although prevalence estimates remain high, and
will always depend on the criteria used to designate a reading problem,
there is reason for optimism in terms of actually reducing the number of
students who have intractable reading problems and who require long-
term remediation. A key for all research efforts is to focus on clearly defined phenotypes, which for dyslexia we suggest should stem from the
assessment of academic skill deficits.

To achieve these goals, it is imperative that the concept of response
to instruction be incorporated into definitions of dyslexia and other
LDs. In the absence of a definition that includes response to instruction,
prevalence assessments will remain difficult. It is noteworthy that other

medical disorders that are essentially dimensional, such as obesity and hypertension, are defined in relation to intervention outcome. Imagine specifying criteria for obesity or hypertension in the absence of studies indicating at what point treatment is indicated in order to reduce risks for strokes, heart attacks, and diabetes (Ellis, 1984; Shaywitz, 2004). As we turn to other domains of LDs, the reader should notice the contrast in the degree to which research and practice have developed for WLRD versus other domains of LDs.

CHAPTER 6

Reading Disabilities

Fluency

The question of whether a subgroup of reading disability can be characterized specifically by difficulties in reading fluency is not adequately studied, but it seems likely that this is this case. Wolf and Bowers (1999) and Lovett, Steinbach, and Frijters (2000b) have provided evidence for a "rate deficit" group that does not have problems in the phonological domain, but often has difficulties with comprehension because of fluency difficulties. Morris et al. (1998) found a rate deficit subtype that, although not phonologically impaired, did show difficulty on any task that required speeded processing. As Wolf and Bowers hypothesized, this subtype also had difficulties with reading fluency and comprehension, but not word recognition. Wimmer and Mayringer (2002) also showed that German speakers could be identified with fluency problems and no apparent difficulties with decoding or spelling. The primary issue is not so much whether a specific reading fluency subgroup can be identified, but whether the primary correlate is phonological processing and whether such LDs are really independent of a WLRD. In this chapter, we review evidence primarily on academic skill deficits, core cognitive processes, and interventions pertaining to reading fluency disability. There are few data on epidemiology, developmental course, or neurobiological correlates that pertain specifically to this form of LD.

ACADEMIC SKILL DEFICITS

The primary core academic skill deficit characterizing people with specific reading fluency problems is reading speed, which is a proxy for the automaticity of word and text reading. Contemporary views of fluency conceptualize it as more than just an outgrowth of word recognition skills. For example, the NRP (2000, p. 3-5) defined fluency as "the ability to read a text quickly, accurately, and with proper expression." Meyer (2000, p. 15) defined fluency as the "ability to read connected text rapidly, smoothly, effortlessly, and automatically with little conscious attention to decoding." The importance of fluency, however, extends beyond the development of word recognition skills and involves the concept of automaticity (Logan, 1997). When decoding is an automatic process, oral reading of text is effortless and requires little conscious attention, thereby permitting more resources to be allocated to higher-order processing of the meaning of the text (Wolf et al., 2003). Moreover, it seems possible for a person to develop fluency difficulties despite accurate word recognition because of difficulties with attention, executive functions, and other skills that influence the efficient allocation of resources (Denckla & Cutting, 1999). Fluent readers can perform multiple tasks simultaneously, likely because of the efficient use of cognitive resources that reflect the operation of these skills. Most definitions of fluency also include an emphasis on prosody, or the ability to read with correct expression, intonation, and phrasing. We do not discuss this component of fluency, inasmuch as in poor readers its lack is not usually regarded as a disability and would be secondary to the problem with automaticity.

The measurement of fluency is less daunting than measurement of reading comprehension (see Chapter 7). Excluding prosody, the latent construct is automaticity of word and text reading, so that fluency essentially boils down to the reading rate (adjusted for accuracy), and sometimes with concern for prosody. As we discussed in Chapter 4, fluency can be assessed by the amount of time needed to accurately read single words, a list of words, short passages, or longer texts. These measures tend to be highly correlated. Jenkins, Fuchs, van den Broek, Espin, and Deno (2003) found that fluency in reading words on a list and in a passage were both sensitive to reading impairments in WLRD. Moreover, identifying individuals with rate deficits is no more difficult than identifying people with word recognition difficulties. It presently involves a decision about cut-points on a dimension. As we already discussed, the problems will emerge when efforts are made to create a subgroup of inaccurate word readers, who always have fluency problems, and compare them with a subgroup primarily impaired in fluency.

Subtype Hypotheses

The critical question for a fluency disability is similar to that identified for reading comprehension in Chapter 7: whether people with difficulties associated with accuracy of word recognition can be differentiated from those impaired primarily in the speed of either word decoding or text reading. In reading comprehension, few would dispute that there are poor readers whose primary breakdown is either at the level of comprehension or the accuracy and fluency of word recognition and text reading. Fluency itself is a process that is dissociable from word recognition and comprehension. However, all three processes are highly correlated, especially in younger children or in those who have reading difficulties. Part of the definitional problem is that people with isolated difficulties in fluency have not been studied as frequently as those with problems involving decoding or comprehension. However, there are subtyping studies that (1) separate poor readers who are inaccurate word readers from those whose problem is with the automaticity of word reading or the fluency with text reading, or (2) separate poor readers according to patterns of impairment on assessments of phonological awareness and rapid naming, which are essentially proxies for word reading accuracy and text reading fluency. We review these studies in the next section, as they help set the stage for understanding the core cognitive correlates of reading fluency.

Rate versus Accuracy

Lovett (1987; Lovett et al., 2000b) proposed two subtypes of reading disability, based on the hypothesis that word recognition develops in three successive phases. The three phases are related to response accuracy in identifying printed words, automatic recognition without the need to "sound out" words, followed by developmentally appropriate maximum speed as components of the reading process become consolidated in memory. Children who fail at the first phase are "accuracy disabled"; those who achieve age-appropriate word recognition but are markedly deficient in the second or third phase are "rate disabled."

The strength of the Lovett subtype research program is its extensive external validation. In a study of the two subtypes (rate disabled vs. accuracy disabled) and a normal sample matched on word recognition ability to the rate-disabled group, children in the accuracy-disabled group were deficient in a wide array of oral and written language areas external to the specific reading behaviors used to identify subtype members; the rate-disabled group's deficiencies were more restricted to deficient connected-text reading and spelling (Lovett, 1987). Reading comprehension was impaired on all measures for the accuracy-disabled group and was highly correlated with word recognition skill, but the rate-disabled group was impaired on only some comprehension measures. Additional subtype–treatment interaction studies (Lovett, Ransby,

Hardwick, & Johns, 1989; Lovett et al., 2000b) found some differences between the accuracy- and rate-disabled groups on contextual reading, whereas word recognition improved for both groups.

Double-Deficit Model

Recent research continues to emphasize the importance of the basic distinction between accuracy and rate, but uses cognitive proxies for this relation. In the model developed by Wolf and associates (Wolf & Bowers, 1999; Wolf et al., 2003), the authors propose that although phonological processing contributes considerably to word recognition deficits, accurate and fluent reading of text is also a critical academic skill. Children may demonstrate fluency deficits that are somewhat independent of problems with phonological processing. When isolated deficits in fluency occur, the most reliable correlate occurs on tasks that require rapid naming of letters and digits. Thus Wolf and associates have postulated a "double-deficit model" of subtypes.

This model specifies essentially three subtypes: one characterized by deficits in both phonological processing and rapid naming; another with impairments only in phonological processing; and a third with impairments only in rapid automatized naming. Wolf and associates (Wolf & Bowers, 1999; Wolf et al., 2003) have summarized evidence that supports the external validity of this subtyping scheme, which is reviewed in the next section.

As a subtyping hypothesis, there are several issues posed by the double-deficit framework (Vellutino et al., 2004). The most significant is whether the phonological awareness and rapid naming deficits are really independent within the double-deficit group. It may be that within this group, both deficits are driven by the severe problem with phonological processing that characterizes this group (Compton, DeFries, & Olson, 2001; Schatschneider, Carlson, Francis, Foorman, & Fletcher, 2002). It is well known that serial-letter-processing accounts of word recognition are not viable (Gough, 1984). Moreover, some studies find that controlling for prior experience eliminates the unique contribution of rapid naming, but not phonological processing, to word-reading outcomes (Wagner et al., 1997). This is an odd contrast with heritability studies, which find little evidence for environmental influences on rapid naming (Petrill et al., 2006a, 2006b). Finally, there are inherent methodological problems identified by Schatschneider et al. (2002) and Compton et al. (2001) that involve difficulties in defining single- versus double-deficit typologies. When both phonological processing and rapid naming are impaired, a child is more severely impaired in both dimensions, which makes it difficult to match single- and double-deficit-impaired children.

Children with double deficits tend to have more severe problems in either phonology or rapid naming as well as in reading, as compared with children with a single deficit. Not surprisingly, given the measurement issues, Spector (2005) found that such subtypes were unstable over the course of a year; only about half of a sample of children identified at the beginning of grade 1 as belonging to classifications based on single and double deficits in phonological awareness and rapid naming maintained group membership at the end of the year.

CORE COGNITIVE PROCESSES

The core cognitive processes correlated with reading fluency include word recognition, rapid naming, speeded processing, executive functions, and orthographic processing. It is obvious that people with word recognition problems will have problems with fluency and comprehension. As these skills are really markers of a WLRD, we do not further discuss them (see Chapter 5). The importance of the link between word reading accuracy and fluency is that in defining specific fluency difficulties, the accuracy of word reading must be ensured.

The core process that has received most attention in the rate deficit group involves rapid automatized naming, which is where the involvement of speeded processing and other cognitive skills tends to emerge. Fluency is also likely related to the ability to process increasingly large sublexical units of words, which some consider an orthographic process. A major question is the link between tasks that mimic the reading process, such as rapid naming of letters laid out left-to-right like text, and linguistic capabilities that support orthographic processing, and whether rapid naming is a proxy for any form of speeded processing.

Rapid Automatized Naming

Three lines of evidence support the relation of naming speed as a separate contribution to reading difficulties. First, naming-speed tasks, especially the ability to name letters rapidly, consistently contribute independently to variance in reading achievement beyond what can be attributed to phonological awareness ability. This finding is apparent not only in studies that attempt to predict longitudinal outcomes (Schatschneider et al., 2002; Wolf & Bowers, 1999), but also in studies that look at the relation of different latent variables through confirmatory factor analysis (McBride-Chang & Manis, 1996; Wagner et al., 1994).

Second, subtyping studies compared children who have deficits in both phonological awareness and rapid naming with children who have only a single deficit (Lovett et al., 2000b; Wolf & Bowers, 1999). These studies show that children with double deficits have more severe reading difficulties than children who have only single deficits. Moreover, the naming-speed group, unlike the double-deficit or phonological deficit group, does not appear to be significantly impaired in phonological processing or decoding (Wimmer & Mayringer, 2002). However, these studies are subject to the methodological problems identified above. Moreover some investigators do not identify all the subtypes predicted by the classification (Waber, Forbes, Wolff, & Weiler, 2004).

Finally, the cluster analysis study of Morris et al. (1998) found evidence for a subtype with impairment in both phonological awareness and naming speed, as well as subtypes with impairment in only phonological awareness or speed of processing. The subtype with double deficits was more impaired in reading than subtypes impaired in only one domain. Moreover, the subtype with rate impairment was not impaired in phonological awareness or in the accuracy of word recognition—just in fluency and comprehension. At the same time, the rate-deficit subtype occurred with low frequency, representing less than 10% of a large group of children with reading disabilities.

Is Rapid Naming Just a Phonological Task?

Despite the preceding evidence, researchers argue as to whether rapid naming contributes to reading achievement independently of its phonological component (Vellutino et al., 2004; Vukovic & Siegel, 2006). Any task that requires retrieval of information with an articulatory component has to involve phonological processing. As rapid-naming tasks are moderately correlated with phonological awareness measures, this appears to be a reasonable conclusion. In this interpretation, naming speed is essentially a measure of how rapidly an individual can access phonologically based codes. Nonetheless, naming speed and phonological processing are dissociable, just as word recognition and fluency are dissociable (see Chapter 5).

Rapid Naming and Other Cognitive Processes

The alternative view is that measures of naming speed involve nonphonological processes that are also related to reading (Wolf & Bowers, 1999). To complete rapid naming tasks, a variety of cognitive processes may be implicated, including executive functions that involve response inhibition and set shifting and lexical processes that permit retrieval and naming (Denckla & Cutting, 1999; Wolf et al., 2003). These processes, of course, are also involved in fluent reading of text, begging the question of what rapid naming tests actually measure. Wolf et al. (2003, p. 361) noted that "the components of naming speed represent a mini-version or subset of the components of reading."

It is significant that naming speed is not the most predictive component of rapid letter naming. In a component analysis of rapid-naming tasks, both Neuhaus, Foorman, Francis, and Carlson (2001) and Wolf and Obregon (1992) found that the pause time between stimuli, which is when these other cognitive processes should be operating, was most strongly associated with reading difficulties. Of course, the interstimulus interval is when other cognitive processes, involving attention and executive functions, and lexical retrieval would be operating if a person was reading a passage out loud. Clark, Hulme, and Snowling (2005) found that rapid naming of letters and digits accounted for unique variance in exception word reading when phonological skills were controlled. However, in evaluating the different components of naming, neither the average item duration nor the average pause duration uniquely predicted reading ability. Rather, the number of pauses in naming was the unique predictor. Thus, deficits of rapid naming were interpreted as "top-down" or strategic factors that reflect differences in reading practice and experience. This is consistent with findings of Schatschneider et al. (2004), who suggested that rapid letter naming predicted reading because it was a simple assessment of reading ability, noting that only letter and digit naming—not color and object naming—seemed to predict reading ability.

Rapid Naming and Speeded Processing

The final issue involves the specificity of rapid-naming deficits to reading difficulties. In reviewing research on rapid automatized naming, some investigators found evidence for deficiencies on any task involving speeded and/or serial processing (e.g., Waber et al., 2001; Wolff, 1993). Catts, Gillispie, Leonard, Kail, and Miller (2002b) found that some poor readers have a general deficit in speeded processing that accounts for their rapid-naming deficits. Speed of processing also uniquely predicted reading outcomes, with Catts et al. suggesting that such measures represented an "extraphonological" influence in some children's reading difficulties. Waber, Wolff, Forbes, and Weiler (2000) demonstrated that unlike phonological awareness tasks, rapid naming measures do not differentiate children who have learning difficulties in other areas. Children with ADHD often show difficulties on measures of rapid automatized naming (Tannock, Martinussen, & Frijters, 2000). However, Semrud-Clikeman, Guy, Griffin, and Hynd (2000) found that children with reading problems had slower naming speeds than children with ADHD and no reading problems. Based on these types of data, Waber et al. (2001) argued that these difficulties reflect common brain-based problems with timing or rapid processing that occur across many learning impairments.

Studies of children with brain injury provide evidence that the accuracy and speed of word recognition can and should be differentiated, but also contribute to concerns about the specificity of these difficulties to reading. Barnes, Dennis, and Wilkinson (1999) matched children with traumatic brain injury on their word-decoding accuracy. Comparisons of reading rate and naming speed showed that fluency was worse in children with traumatic brain injury, paralleling observations of non-brain-injured children with rate deficits (Waber et al., 2001; Wolf & Bowers, 1999). Moreover, fluency is related to reading comprehension scores in both populations (Barnes et al., 1999; Morris et al., 1998).

Many of the issues involved in determining the link of rapid naming to reading reflect differences in the use of nomenclature. We have been careful to differentiate components of reading that involve accuracy, fluency, and comprehension, reserving the term *dyslexia* for difficulties that specifically involve the accuracy of word recognition skills. Other researchers (e.g., Wolf & Bowers, 1999) tend to use the term *dyslexia* to refer to any form of reading difficulty, often describing a "variety of dyslexias." Thus, in their thorough review of the link of dyslexia and rapid naming, Vukovic and Siegel (2006) did not find evidence that rapid naming constituted a specific core cognitive process in dyslexia. However, dyslexia was defined as WLRD with a core phonological deficit. The link of rapid naming and word recognition is relatively weak and difficult to differentiate from phonological processing. If the reading component is a fluency assessment, rapid naming of letters clearly accounts for unique variance in proficiency even if the assessment is based on the reading of lists of words and pseudowords as fast as possible. If, in contrast, the outcome was fluency of word recognition, rapid naming accounted for most of the unique variability in outcomes (Petrill et al., 2006b; Schatschneider et al., 2004). The subtype identified by Morris et al. (1998) that had difficulties with speeded processing was not impaired in word recognition or phonological processing and should not be labeled with *dyslexia*.

Although it is possible to differentiate accuracy and rate components on measures of phonological awareness and rapid naming, more research needs to be done to establish the significance of a subgroup specific to reading fluency. It is clear, however, that fluency must be considered independently of accuracy in evaluating the outcomes of reading intervention studies. Studies of older children show that accuracy may

improve in children with severe reading difficulties without corresponding improvements in fluency (Torgesen et al., 2001).

Orthographic Processing and Cross-Linguistic Studies

Orthographic Mapping

Another major correlate of developing fluent and automatic word and
text reading likely involves the capacity to process increasingly large
units of words (Foorman, 1994). As we discussed in Chapter 5, the visual
association areas in the occipitotemporal regions of the brain may become very specialized for the fast mapping of orthographic relations. As
the child becomes able to instantaneously recognize increasingly larger
units of words, word recognition becomes automatized, which allows
more efficient allocation of resources to comprehension processes.

Reading can be thought of as matching the orthographic units that
are present in text to their phonological representations in speech. With
phonological recoding, children can access many relations of the orthographic units they see with the sounds of words that exist in the spoken
language (Foorman, 1994; Ziegler & Goswami, 2005). As reading develops, children learn more about the orthographic patterns and become
able to process increasingly large units of words, recognizing many
words by sight. The origin of this development, however, is in the phonological code that indicates the relation of sound to print (Lukatela &
Turvey, 1998).

Cross-Linguistic Studies

The issue of phonological–orthographic mapping is especially important
for understanding how reading develops in different languages. English
is a language characterized by often arbitrary relations of sound and
print, particularly because many orthographic units have multiple pronunciations. Other languages have much more transparent relations of
phonology and orthography. For example, German, Italian, and Spanish
are languages in which the pronunciation of words is fairly reliably sig-
naled by how the word appears in print. The question is whether these
differences in the relation of phonology and orthography are related to
the development of reading and whether reading problems are different
by virtue of this variation.

A review of the cross-linguistic research is beyond the scope of this
book (see Caravolas, 2005; Seymour, 2005; Ziegler & Goswami, 2005).
Seymour (2005) summarized a series of studies comparing the early development of reading across several different European languages. He

found that the complexity of syllables and the depth of the orthographies influenced how rapidly children learned to read. In languages that had deep and inconsistent orthographic structures in which the syllabic structure was also complicated, such as English and Danish, reading developed most slowly. In contrast, reading developed much faster in a language like Italian or Spanish that has a relatively transparent orthography and simple syllabic structures. Thus, learning to read is affected by the complexity of the orthographic relations in print when children begin to read. Ziegler and Goswami (2005) identified three factors that influenced reading development across languages: (1) the availability of phonological units that can be explicitly accessed before reading; (2) the consistency of orthographic units, which may have multiple pronunciations, and phonological units, which may have multiple spellings; and (3) the size of the orthographic unit that is available within the written language system, which they termed the "granularity problem." They developed the "psycholinguistic grain size" theory to help explain differences in lexical organization and processing strategies that would characterize skilled reading across different language orthographies.

Even in languages like Chinese, children are sensitive to the phonological components that are expressed in Chinese logograms and attend to the regularity by which the phonological component of the Chinese logograms affects pronunciation (Hanley, 2005). Although English readers have strong phonological awareness skills, Chinese readers tend to have better syllable and morpheme awareness (Tan, Spinks, Eden, Perfetti, & Siok, 2005). However, all of these linguistic skills are operating at a sublexical unit with variations that reflect, in part, the relation of the phonological and orthographic units.

Reading Problems in Other Countries

In examining differences in the manifestations of reading problems across different languages, phonological skills still seem to drive the acquisition of word recognition and fluency (Caravolas, 2005; Wimmer & Mayringer, 2002). However, in orthographies where the relation of phonological and orthographic units is more inconsistent, such as in English, many more readers who are inaccurate will emerge. Pseudoword reading is especially difficult. Thus, Aro and Wimmer (2003) compared pseudoword reading controlled for letter patterns, onsets, and rimes in German, Dutch, English, Swedish, French, Spanish, and Finnish speakers in grades 1–4. Only English was associated with a low rate of accuracy (about 90%) by the end of grade 1. In German poor readers, difficulties with pseudoword reading were less common; poor reading was often characterized by fluency and spelling problems when the primary correlate was phonological processing. However, some German poor readers had poor fluency with adequate spelling and had more difficulties with rapid naming (Wimmer & Mayringer, 2002). In a longitudinal study, Wimmer, Mayringer, and Landerl (2000) composed German speaking groups based on the double-deficit model and compared their reading and spelling development 3 years later. They reported that phonological awareness deficits earlier in development were weakly linked with phonological decoding, but more strongly related to spelling and foreign word reading. In contrast, naming speed was related to reading fluency, spelling, and foreign word reading. They suggested that when reading was taught with synthetic phonics methods in a language with a more regular relation of phonology and orthography, the acquisition of reading was less affected in earlier phases by phonological processing than in later phases that build up orthographic relations of words.

In contrast, Ziegler, Perry, Ma-Wyatt, Ladner, and Schulte-Karne (2003) found that patterns of reading strengths and weaknesses were similar in German and English speakers: Both groups of children showed more difficulties in reading pseudowords than real words and had slow reading speeds. In a study of Dutch children (de Jong & van der Leij, 2003), phonological awareness and rapid naming tasks were administered in kindergarten, grade 1, and grade 6. Rapid naming discriminated good and poor readers through grade 6; phonological awareness deficits diminished by grade 6. This finding may have reflected a ceiling effect because, in a second study, poor Dutch readers struggled with phonological processing if task demands were increased. Caravolas, Volin, and Hulme (2005) found that phonological awareness was a unique predictor of reading in Czech- and English-speaking children and that good and poor readers in both languages had similar phoneme awareness difficulties. In another review, Goswami (2002) argued that the core deficit in WLRD in studies across several countries and languages involves phonology and that the manifestation of this difficulty varies depending on the orthography of the language.

Much of this research on orthographic processing continues to focus on dyslexia and attends less to children who manifest primary problems with fluency. It would be interesting to follow Wimmer and Mayringer (2002) and look for poor readers in regular and irregular orthographies who vary in spelling ability and examine the correlates of poor reading fluency. Another interesting question is whether performance on a rapid-naming task is somehow more closely associated with the capacity for orthographic than phonological processing, which was implied by Wimmer et al. (2000) and others (see Wolf et al., 2003). Manis, Doi, and Bhader (2000) found that rapid naming accounted for significant variability in reading even when phonological awareness and vocabulary were controlled. The unique contribution of rapid naming was stronger for orthographic processing; phonological awareness was more closely related to pseudoword reading. Other studies that address the relation of rapid naming and orthographic processing have found that both phonological and orthographic processing are related to rapid naming performance, questioning whether the rapid naming component is specific to orthographic processing (e.g., Bear & Barone, 1991; Holland, McIntosh, & Huffman, 2004). Although it has been suggested that these findings reflect a relation of rapid naming tasks and fluency to some sort of timing mechanism that is independent of phonological processing (Bowers & Wolf, 1993), the evidence for this hypothesis is weak, given that rapid naming tests are essentially proxies for reading fluency assessments.

NEUROBIOLOGICAL FACTORS

Brain Structure and Function

Studies of brain injury in adults have not isolated fluency deficits as a specific type of alexia. There are also no structural or functional neuroimaging studies of a subgroup of LDs with isolated fluency difficulties. A study using regional cerebral blood flow assessments of hemodynamic changes in brain activation found that rapid naming tasks involving objects and objects blended with colors activated the parietal lobes. Color naming did not result in reliable changes in brain activation (Wiig et al., 2002). Misra, Katzir, Wolf, and Poldrack (2004) used fMRI to assess brain activation in response to naming tasks for objects and letters. They found that the network typically implicated in word reading was activated (see Figure 5.3), with some differences when the letter and color tasks were used. Moreover, there was additional activation of areas involving eye movements and attention, which would be expected in a task requiring serial processing of stimuli.

In their neuroimaging study of response to a phonologically mediated intervention with children identified with decoding problems (Blachman et al., 2004), B. A. Shaywitz et al. (2004) observed significant changes in the occipitotemporal regions of the brain that they related to improvements in fluency based on the view that this ventral visual region is important for rapid processing of letter patterns. Similarly, when poor decoders received an intervention emphasizing both decoding and fluency (Denton et al., in press), Simos et al. (in press) found normalization of latency of responses in this region specifically on a task designed to assess the fluency of word reading. Such changes were less apparent on a pseudoword decoding task that resulted in more change in the temporoparietal regions.

Altogether, there are emerging studies of rapid naming and reading fluency that involved skilled adults and children with WLRD. We could not identify neuroimaging studies specifically addressing children who are impaired in fluency. These studies tend to support the view that rapid-naming tasks are proxies for the reading of connected text, given the similarities in the areas of the brain that are activated in reading.

Genetic Factors

Although there are no genetically sensitive studies of a fluency subgroup, there is evidence for common and separate heritability of the accuracy and fluency of word-reading skills when treated as dimensions. Davis et al. (2001) found that rapid naming measures had significant heritability even when reading measures were included in the model. In a study of 800 twin pairs, Compton et al. (2001) found evidence of a common set of genes for phonological processing, rapid naming, and reading in affected twins. This group also showed evidence for genetic influences that were specifically involved in the relation of rapid naming and reading. In contrast, a control group of unaffected twins also revealed common genetic influences for phonology, rapid naming, and reading, but no evidence of an independent relation of rapid naming and reading. There was little evidence of shared environmental influences in the affected group, which included children 8–18 years of age. In a similar sample of mostly older children, Tiu, Wadsworth, Olson, and DeFries (2004) found that measures of phonological processing and rapid-naming skills both made significant genetic contributions to reading. In a study of younger twin pairs, Petrill et al. (2006a) found significant heritability of rapid naming of letters that was not explained by phonological measures and that generally had a smaller relation with the environment than phonological measures. These findings support the hypothesis that naming speed is etiologically distinct from phonological awareness. In this respect, Raskind et al. (2005) compared the heritability of component skills involving accuracy and fluency of pseudoword reading. Using a variety of genetic association methods and a genome-wide scan, the researchers found evidence for involvement of chromosome 2 for fluency, but not accuracy, of pseudoword decoding. There was also clear evidence for shared genetic etiology for these two correlated processes.

SUMMARY: FROM ACADEMIC SKILL DEFICITS TO NEUROBIOLOGICAL FACTORS

Reading fluency is an important reading skill that is correlated with, but also independent of, word recognition. The core cognitive correlates involve rapid naming, orthographic processing, and other cognitive skills that regulate attention, inhibitory processing, and lexical retrieval. A major issue concerns what is actually measured by rapid-naming tests and whether they are proxies for text-reading fluency. Although there is disagreement about whether rapid naming reduces strictly to the domain of phonological processing, most of the evidence suggests independence, particularly if the criterion is a fluency measure. The neuroimaging and genetics studies show clear evidence for independence of phonological processing and rapid naming. A limitation of research in English-speaking countries is the reliance on one language, with research on other languages more strongly suggesting that children can have specific difficulties involving fluency. The research base addressing children with specific fluency difficulties is sparse, as the next section on treatment will show. Neurobiological studies are emerging and are most interesting in suggesting the possibility of different genetic mechanisms for phonological awareness/decoding and naming speed/fluency.

READING FLUENCY INTERVENTIONS

In contrast to studies that target either the prevention or remediation of students identified with word recognition difficulties, there are few examples of interventions that are specific for students who have problems primarily in reading fluency. It is likely that interventions that address fluency deficits could be applied to these students if they were identified as a separate subgroup. But most attempts to intervene in the fluency area usually involve students who began with problems with word recognition, and typically attempt to include both word recognition and fluency components in the intervention. The most frequently studied interventions involve different ways of encouraging students to practice reading, such as by repeated reading or guided oral reading, and simply trying to increase the amount of time a student spends in independent reading.

Empirical Syntheses

The NRP (2000) reviewed classroom and tutorial studies addressing intervention studies involving fluency. The panel identified 16 studies that included 398 students who were poor readers and 281 students who were good readers. The NRP found comparable, moderate effect sizes (around 0.50) for both poor readers and average readers. Although a variety of intervention programs were examined, the only domains in which they could be characterized as effective involved repeated reading and other guided-reading oral interventions. In general, these types of interventions involved repeated oral readings with a model or with a peer or parent. They did not necessarily focus on students who were poor readers.

Kuhn and Stahl (2003) followed the NRP report on fluency with a review of a broader range of studies. These authors expanded the NRP report by including studies that involved repeated reading, assisted reading in clinical settings, and approaches to fluency development that involved the entire classroom. This synthesis did not compute effect sizes, but we include it here because it was a follow-up to the NRP report.

In evaluating this literature, Kuhn and Stahl confirmed the NRP finding that practice-based interventions for fluency were efficacious. However, gains were generally lower in students with reading difficulties. Approaches that involved some form of assistance, such as reading with a model or listening during reading, appeared more effective than approaches that did not involve assistance, such as silent sustained reading. These findings suggest that teacher guidance and monitoring is a critical component of fluency instruction. Kuhn and Stahl noted that little evidence supported simple repeated reading of passages and stories; time spent in oral reading of connected text, as opposed to repetition, may be responsible for the effect of repeated reading on fluency and comprehension.

In an empirical synthesis of interventions addressing students with LDs, Chard, Vaughn, and Tyler (2002) found 24 published and unpublished studies that reported specific findings involving fluency. These studies included repeated reading, both with and without a model, and sustained silent reading, and evaluated issues involving the number of repetitions, text difficulty, and the extent of improvement. Chard et al. (2002) found 21 studies that addressed whether repeatedly reading text resulted in improved reading fluency in students defined with LDs. These studies yielded an average effect size in the moderate range (0.68). In 14 studies, almost all single cases involving modeling by an adult, all studies were associated with positive effect sizes in the small-to-large range. Peer modeling was also associated with small-to-moderate effect sizes. Modeling with an audiotape or computer in four small studies showed small-to-moderate effects. A variety of factors influenced effect size estimates, including the amount of text, text difficulty, number of repetitions, types of feedback, and criteria for repeated reading. Like the NRP, Chard et al. concluded that more research is needed, reflecting the lack of attention to fluency development. At the same time, it is apparent that an emphasis on fluency building as part of either classroom or tutorial interventions is essential to improving performance in this domain.

Interventions for Struggling Readers

As Torgesen et al. (2001) graphically demonstrated, a common finding in remedial approaches for reading in students with word recognition deficiencies is improvement in word reading and comprehension, but little change in fluency. Although early intervention will help address some of these difficulties for many students, the reduced efficacy of many remedial approaches may be due to persistent word recognition difficulties that could have been reduced through earlier intervention. For example, early intervention programs do seem to impact fluency as well as word recognition (Torgesen, 2002). This finding may well reflect the earlier access to print afforded by early intervention and more rapid development of decoding skills that promotes the opportunity to read and acquire the repeated exposures to words that facilitates rapid processing at a larger orthographic level. Nonetheless, remedial studies may continue to produce students who respond to instruction in the alphabetic principle, but continue to have fluency difficulties. In turn, many of these students may be unable to comprehend primarily because their slow reading rate places too many demands on their ability to process what they have read. In addition, students who are not fluent do not enjoy reading, so they are less likely to read, which contributes to the failure to build sight word vocabulary, a key to the development of accurate and fluent reading skills.

Read Naturally

A commercial program specifically targeting fluency is Read Naturally (Ihnot, 2000). In Read Naturally, students read nonfiction passages designed for students in grades 1–8. Students practice oral reading of short, interesting passages (i.e., repeated reading), read with a videotape at a challenging pace, and time and graph their reading rates (e.g., words correct per minute) so they are constantly aware of their progress. A comprehension component involves discussion of passages with the teacher and answering questions about what they have read. There is little research on Read Naturally. Hasbrouck, Ihnot, and Rogers (1999) reported cases that had benefited from Read Naturally, but these were not controlled evaluations. In their study of inadequate responders, Denton et al. (in press) found that 8 weeks of instruction (1 hour per day) based on Read Naturally led to significant improvement in reading fluency skills, but little improvement in decoding or comprehension abilities. More research on the effectiveness of this approach to reading fluency would be useful.

Fluency-Oriented Reading Instruction

Stahl, Huebach, and Cramond (1997) developed fluency-oriented reading instruction, a classroom approach to facilitate automatic word recognition and fluency with three components: (1) a redesign of the basal reading lesson to include specific components involving fluency; (2) a period involving free reading in school; and (3) a component involving reading at home. The redesign of the basal reader largely involved an attempt to introduce differentiated instruction by dividing students into two groups based on their reading levels, with modifications of fluency instruction based on the amount of assistance needed. The school and home components were designed to increase the amount of time spent reading connected text.

An initial evaluation of the program (four teachers, two schools, eventually expanded to ten teachers and three schools) showed positive results. On average, students gained about 2 years in overall reading growth on an informal inventory. Of particular importance was the finding that over the 2-year period, even struggling readers improved in fluency, with only 2 of about 105 students reading below second-grade level by the end of the year. Reading practice clearly improved fluency in this study.

Stahl (2004) summarized the initial findings from a larger-scale attempt to evaluate fluency-oriented reading instruction that included control groups. The first year of the study involved 9 schools and 28 classrooms across three sites and compared fluency-oriented reading instruction with a program that emphasized repeated reading of a wide range of materials. A third group served as a classroom curriculum control and was simply followed over time. Historical controls were also included and evaluated. Stahl (2004) reported that both interventions that involved fluency instruction resulted in better outcomes than the historical and curriculum controls, and there were no systematic differences between the two treatments. Results were especially dramatic for the students who were struggling readers, who also received supplementation of the fluency program using Direct Instruction principles to address decoding weaknesses (following Lovett et al., 1990). In evaluating performance relative to students who had been in the same school programs in the past (historical controls), improvements in word recognition, oral reading rate and accuracy, and comprehension were apparent. The effects on struggling readers, many of whom would likely have had LDs, were especially interesting.

A second wave of the initial study is under way to replicate and extend these initial findings. The key to both approaches may involve the scaffolding of texts to the readers' instructional level. Stahl (2004) suggested that scaffolding may explain why approaches like the two interventions improve fluency and comprehension, but approaches based on sustained silent reading (e.g., drop everything and read) do not appear to have major effects on reading improvement.

RAVE-O

Not surprisingly, fluency is emerging as a major emphasis in the remedial area, with newer efforts perhaps best characterized by the RAVE-O program developed by Wolf et al. (2002). RAVE-O stands for Retrieval, Automaticity, Vocabulary elaboration, and Enrichment with language-Orthography. It is designed to facilitate the development of automaticity in reading subskills, to facilitate fluency in decoding and comprehension processes, and to enhance interest and engagement in reading and language use in students with LDs in this area.

RAVE-O is based on a developmental model of fluency (Wolf et al., 2003) that emphasizes the multiple contributions to proficient comprehension made by the student's familiarity with common orthographic patterns, as well as the student's knowledge of a word's meaning(s), morpheme parts, and grammatical uses. A major premise is that the more a student knows about a word, the faster the student will retrieve and read it. The game-like format includes intensive work on rapid orthographic pattern recognition; building word webs; learning word retrieval and comprehension strategies; playing games with language through computer games enhanced with animation; and rapid, repeated reading of short (1-minute) mystery stories that incorporate the multiple meanings and syntactical uses of core words.

This program is typically used in conjunction with a word recognition program and is being evaluated along with the PHAST Track Reading Program by the Morris, Wolf, and Lovett research group described in Chapter 5. Morris et al. (2006) found that RAVE-O enhances word recognition, fluency, and comprehension better than instruction based only on the decoding skills programs. To date, there is no strong evidence from these studies that RAVE-O produces larger gains in fluency at the word level than a program like PHAST, which teaches strategies for generalizing from the alphabetic principle to larger sublexical units at the morphosyntactical level. This finding highlights the importance of including instruction that focuses on increasingly large sublexical units for people with decoding and fluency difficulties.

One question is whether a program like RAVE-O leads to more improvement in reading connected text, as well as comprehension, as compared with a program that emphasizes the generalization of word recognition strategies. This possibility would reflect the focus of programs like RAVE-O on fluency at the sublexical, word, and connected text levels. Previous theories of how fluency emerges focused on accurate and fluent word recognition, which is supported by the comparable word-level fluency results of programs like WIST. If RAVE-O leads to stronger gains in fluency at the connected text level and comprehension, such findings would support a more comprehensive approach to intervention at the text level of proficiency and comprehension. In addition, it would be interesting to compare the effects of programs like RAVE-O and WIST in children identified as having fluency, but not accuracy, difficulties.

Although programs like RAVE-O focus more broadly on fluency at the text level, most theories of how fluency emerges also focus on accurate and fluent word recognition, which is supported by programs like WIST. To illustrate, in a series of remedial studies specifically addressing fluency deficits (Levy, 2001), students identified with fluency difficulties received a variety of interventions. Most also had word recognition problems. These studies were specifically designed to evaluate whether transfer in fluency is mediated at the level of word recognition or at the level of text reading. In general, the studies summarized by Levy (2001) show that the reading fluency of poor readers is limited by their slow rate of processing at the level of the individual word. She found that simple practice in a "repetition of names" game led to significant gains in word recognition skills, particularly for poor readers. Words were learned best through word training study, in which the student was taught to read a list of words as fast as possible. The alternative involved having students read a story four times in succession that contained the same word. For the poor readers, transfer to improved reading speed occurred regardless of whether a similar or different story context was used. However, Levy (2001) reported that context was not an essential component of the experience and that teaching automaticity of word reading was possible for poor readers and also made them more successful. There was clear evidence for transfer across linguistic levels in context. In other studies, there appeared to be little additional benefit of highlighting shared orthographic units. However, blocking according to the orthographic unit, which has the effect of making the orthographic relation more explicit, resulted in more automaticity. These results are consistent with the premises of RAVE-O, showing that grouping words into similar orthographic patterns accelerates fluency.

Levy (2001) noted that many poor readers were very slow in generalizing across words. In one of the few studies that targeted students with specific fluency difficulties, Thaler, Ebner, Wimmer, and Landerl (2004) provided computerized training on repeated reading of 32 words over 25 days to a sample of 20 German-speaking children. Each word was designed to emphasize the onset segment and was presented up to six times per day. Although fluency for reading the trained words improved over the 5-week period, there was only a slight improvement in reading untrained words. In a different study of poor readers who spoke Dutch, de Jong and Vrielink (2004) trained grade 1 students to rapidly name serially presented letters. There was little evidence of improvement when rapid serial naming of letters was directly trained. Thus, training students on orthographic processing does not generalize strongly to new words and is difficult to achieve.

CONCLUSIONS

There is clear evidence for a dissociation of reading fluency deficits from those involving word recognition and comprehension. In addition, cognitive processes that focus on rapid naming and orthographic processing appear related to fluency deficits. Problems remain in how reading fluency deficits are defined. Another problem concerns the specificity of rapid-naming deficiencies to children with reading disabilities. There has been little work done specifically on people with difficulties in reading fluency in North America.

Fluency interventions have focused largely on procedures that lead to repeated exposures to words. This approach is likely to be maximally effective if the reading material is scaffolded to the child's instructional level in reading. To develop fluency, children need to be engaged with print as soon as they begin to read. One reason that children who learn to decode later in their development remain slow readers may be the cumulative effects of lack of experience, which prevents the development of a sight word vocabulary (Torgesen et al., 2001). Interventions based on broader views of fluency that extend beyond repeated reading are emerging, such as the RAVE-O program. As the importance of learning to process larger orthographic units becomes more fully appreciated, it seems likely that approaches to reading and spelling instruction that explicitly focus on these opportunities will be linked to fluency.

CHAPTER 7

Reading Disabilities

Comprehension

Research on children with word recognition difficulties tends to (1) compare them with children who are typically achieving and (2) not consider impairments in other areas, such as fluency, comprehension, or even math and written expression. This approach is used because the findings of studies involving word recognition do not appear to vary because of other comorbidities, at least when the reading problem and its correlates are examined. But this is not the case in research on other forms of LDs, where inclusion of children with word recognition problems may obscure the results. Thus, studies of children with specific problems in reading comprehension focus on comparisons of children with poor word recognition and poor reading comprehension skills, versus those who have good development of word recognition skills, but poor development of reading comprehension (Nation & Snowling, 1998; Oakhill, Yuill, & Parkin, 1996; Stothard & Hulme, 1996). If a study of reading comprehension contains a large number of children who decode words poorly (e.g., Perfetti, 1985; Shankweiler et al., 1999), the most likely cause of reading comprehension problems is the inability to decode. Proficient reading comprehension assumes accurate and fluent decoding.

There is good evidence that reading comprehension difficulties can occur in the absence of word recognition problems and that oral language disorders are not synonymous with WLRD (Bishop & Snowling, 2004). Catts, Adlof, Hogan, and Weisner (2005) found clear evidence that children with specific language impairments had distinct disorders, although comorbidity was apparent if the language-impaired child had phonological processing difficulties. More pertinent are studies that identify children specifically impaired in reading comprehension, but not decoding. However, the research base is much less developed for such difficulties than for LDs involving word recognition. There is little work on neurobiological correlates or developmental course, though some studies of the latter are available. Neurobiological research specific to children with LDs involving reading comprehension is also scant. There is a good body of research on remediating comprehension in children with LDs.

ACADEMIC SKILL DEFICITS

The primary academic skill deficits used for defining LDs in the reading comprehension domain are, simply put, deficits in the variety of abilities that allow the reader to abstract meaning from text. This is a complex set of processes that in many respects parallels the ability to comprehend language, and many models of reading comprehension and its development highlight the close relation of comprehension processes in reading and listening comprehension, noting also the differences in language systems by eye and by ear (Gough & Tunmer, 1986). For example, making inferences is likely based on similar processes in reading and listening comprehension, but text comprehension also requires processes that are more specific, such as sensitivity to story structure (Perfetti, Landi, & Oakhill, 2005). We return to this issue below.

Reading comprehension assumes adequate decoding ability and approaches levels of listening comprehension as decoding skills become accurate and fluent. However, as we discussed in Chapter 4, the assessment of reading comprehension is not straightforward. There is always concern about how well reading comprehension tests measure processes specific to the comprehension of written language, as opposed to other language processes that must be in place in order for reading comprehension to take place. Measures of word recognition accuracy have a relatively transparent relationship between the content of the tests and performance requirements for word reading. However, standardized reading comprehension tests differ from everyday reading contexts along several potentially important dimensions, including passage length, immediate versus delayed recall, and learning and performance requirements (Pearson, 1998; Sternberg, 1991). At this point in time, a single assessment may not be adequate, as it is difficult to determine the source of a child's comprehension difficulties based on a single measure. Exactly how to measure and define the component academic skills is a significant and understudied area (Francis et al., 2005b).

Subtypes of Poor Comprehenders

Evaluating components of reading skills has shown clear evidence for subgroups based on variations in accuracy, fluency, and listening comprehension. Based on the Simple Model of Reading (Gough & Tunmer, 1986), Aaron, Joshi, and Williams (1999) found four subgroups of poor readers whose difficulties were in the following areas: only decoding, only listening comprehension, both decoding and listening comprehension, and orthographic processing/speed. Catts, Hogan, and Fey (2003) evaluated decoding and listening comprehension in a much larger cohort that oversampled for children with oral language impairments, identifying subtypes that were stable over time involving only decoding, only listening comprehension, both decoding and listening comprehension, and a nonspecific group. Like Leach et al. (2003), Catts et al. (2003) found that even in older students (grade 4), about 70% of the poor readers in their sample, deliberately overidentified with students who had poor oral language ability, had problems involving decoding. Such findings contrast with a recent report on adolescent literacy that suggested that well over half of poor readers in middle and high school have specific problems with reading comprehension (Biancarosa & Snow, 2004), but are more consistent with Nation's (1999) estimate that poor comprehenders accounted for 15% of poor readers.

The Reading Components Model is a useful approach to subtyping, but whether it should be expanded to include fluency (Chapter 6) is unclear. Joshi and Aaron (2000) found that 48% of the variance in reading comprehension could be explained by decoding and listening comprehension, but another 10% could be explained if a rapid letter naming test was added. Such measures, as we discussed in Chapter 6, are essentially proxies for fluency (Schatschneider et al., 2004). Children in the unspecified subtype in Catts et al. (2003) were not characterized by fluency difficulties, and this group of researchers has not found much evidence suggesting a need to expand the Reading Components Model to include fluency. Nonetheless, as Joshi (2003) suggested, the Reading Components Model focuses on the primary manifestations of the reading problem and leads immediately to targeted remedial instruction. It represents a primary research strategy in studying poor comprehenders.

The issue of discrepancies between reading comprehension and listening comprehension is trickier. In Chapter 3, we pointed out that this version of an aptitude–achievement discrepancy model had the same psychometric problems as any bivariate discrepancy model. Thus, Badian (1999) found the same patterns of instability over time for this type of definition that have been described for IQ–achievement definitions of WLRD (see Chapter 3). In addition to this problem, however, a definition based only on discrepancies between listening and reading comprehension will not isolate a specific subgroup of poor comprehenders because it does not address the measurement of word recognition skills. It is not possible to define a group with specific LDs in reading comprehension without formally measuring word recognition abilities and ensuring that these skills are in the average range.

CORE COGNITIVE PROCESSES

Cognitive models of comprehension (Perfetti et al., 2005) include processes related to the surface code (decoding, accessing word meaning, and syntax), to building text-based representations (pronominal reference, deriving word meaning from context, making bridging inferences within the text), and to constructing a mental model of the situation described by the text (using general knowledge to make inferences, integrating the goals of the reader). Individual differences in comprehension could arise from failures in any of these processes or with more general cognitive processes, such as working memory operations and retrieval from long-term memory, that are involved in constructing representations of the text base and the situation model (van den Broek, Rapp, & Kendeou, 2005). The presence of a specific LD involving reading comprehension presumes that decoding is intact; research generally demonstrates that children who are good at decoding, but poor at comprehending, can decode and access meanings that are stipulated or provided by the surface code of the text (Barnes, Johnston, & Dennis, in press), so research has focused on the latter two classes of processes.

For identifying relevant cognitive processes, research addressing children with reading comprehension difficulties uses three major experimental designs in an attempt to identify core deficits underlying comprehension difficulties. One design compares age-matched children who are good at decoding but poor at comprehending with children who are good at both (chronological-age design). A second design compares children who are good at decoding/poor at comprehending with younger children matched for level of reading comprehension to the older disabled children (reading comprehension-level match design). The third design attempts to train children in skills, the lack of which is hypothesized to contribute to the reading comprehension deficits, to determine whether training actually improves reading comprehension. The findings from the three methods are consistent in identifying core cognitive correlates involving language, listening comprehension, working memory, and a variety of processes that support meaning construction such as inferencing.

Language

Children with good decoding/poor comprehending often have more basic deficits in vocabulary, morphology, and understanding of syntax that impair reading comprehension (Nation, Clarke, Marshall, & Durand, 2004; Stothard & Hulme, 1992, 1996). The language deficits of these children are typically not severe enough to classify them as speech and language impaired (Nation et al., 2004); furthermore, their phonological skills are typically not deficient (Cain & Oakhill, 1999; Nation, Adams, Bowyer-Crane, & Snowling, 1999; Oakhill, 1993). The comprehension of reading can be no stronger than the comprehension of language, a clear example being vocabulary: a child may be able to decode a word, but if he or she does not know the meaning, comprehension of the text will be impaired.

Ultimately, language development is at the heart of reading comprehension. In studies by Catts and colleagues that look specifically at language skills in poor comprehenders, and comprehension skills in children with oral language impairments, the overlap is high and problems with vocabulary and syntax are common links (Catts & Hogan, 2003). Some studies of lexical processing in poor comprehenders that control for both levels of decoding and basic language skills such as vocabulary, show that poor comprehenders have problems on a variety of measures involving semantic judgment and fluency (Nation & Snowling, 1998; Nation et al., 1999).

Listening Comprehension

Language comprehension and listening comprehension are sometimes both used to refer to receptive language skills. However, in the reading comprehension area, listening comprehension means more than just receptive language skills. It includes discourse-level processes that serve as overarching control processes that impact reading and listening comprehension. Thus, *listening comprehension* is a term that needs to be unpacked and refers to a process as hard to measure as reading comprehension. We address some of the processes underlying both reading and listening comprehension below. Just focusing on the term as it is used in the comprehension area, it is well established that difficulties in listening comprehension parallel problems with reading comprehension (Shankweiler et al., 1999; Stothard & Hulme, 1996). Most studies comparing reading and listening comprehension in normative samples show high levels of overlap. Children cannot understand written language any better than they can understand oral language. It is possible that dissociations of listening and reading comprehension occur in some cases, so that reading comprehension is better than listening comprehension. This would seem most likely in older children and adults, but there is little research demonstrating these dissociations. Regardless, any language or cognitive difficulties that hinder oral language comprehension will also affect individuals' ability to read text or even to comprehend text read to them.

Working Memory

A specific cognitive skill commonly identified as a source of difficulty in studies of poor comprehenders is working memory. Both listening and reading comprehension make demands on working memory as a storage resource in which words and sentences are held for more extended processing and integration with prior knowledge and as a mental workspace in which previous interpretations of text can be revised in relation to incoming information (Barnes et al., in press). Several studies document relations of verbal working memory and comprehension and show that working memory is impaired in poor comprehenders (Stothard & Hulme, 1992; Nation et al., 1999). Cain, Oakhill, and Lemmon (2004b) found that learning of novel vocabulary from context (i.e., incidental word learning) was impaired in poor comprehenders when the context was not adjacent to the new word; working memory capacity, but not immediate memory span, was related to the successful inferring of meanings of novel words from context. Interestingly, poor comprehenders with average vocabulary knowledge were not impaired in learning new vocabulary that was directly taught (i.e., not inferred from context), but poor comprehenders with weak vocabulary knowledge had difficulty learning novel vocabulary even with explicit instruction. Cain, Oakhill, and Bryant (2004a) found that working memory, as assessed by a sentence span test, contributed unique variance to inference making, comprehension monitoring, and story structure knowledge even when decoding ability, verbal IQ, and vocabulary were controlled. Similar patterns are seen in populations of children with brain injury, who frequently present with poor comprehension and adequate decoding (Barnes et al., in press). The consistency in findings in children with poor comprehension supports a central role of working memory as a mediator of poor reading (and listening comprehension). The relation of storage/integration and inhibitory processes in working memory to individual differences in various comprehension processes requires further study. However, even in studies that involve working memory, assessments of higher-order processes contribute unique variance to comprehension outcomes, as shown in the next section.

Higher-Order Processes

Reading comprehension cannot be explained solely on the basis of word recognition, oral language, and working memory. Even when decoding, basic language skills, and working memory are controlled, deficits in reading comprehension still arise (Cain, Oakhill, & Bryant, 2000; Cain et al., 2004a; Nation & Snowling, 1998) because of difficulties with discourse-level skills involving inferencing, comprehension monitoring, text integration, and other metacognitive skills related to comprehension that are partly, but not completely, explained by variability in working memory (Cornoldi, De Beni, & Pazzaglia, 1996; Cain et al., 2004a, 2004b).

Inferencing

A substantial body of research shows that poor comprehenders understand literal or stipulated meanings provided by the surface code of the text, but have difficulty making inferences that require interpretation or integration of text (see Oakhill, 1993). The difficulties are apparent even when working memory demands are controlled (Oakhill, 1993), in children with intact vocabulary and oral language skills (Barnes & Dennis, 1996), and even when differences in background knowledge are controlled (Barnes et al., in press). It may be that the inferencing problems do not reflect a fundamental inability to make an inference, but an inability to do so in the context of text comprehension, representing a strategic deficit. Cain and Oakhill (1999) found that prompting the poor comprehender to engage in a strategy that would support making an inference led to improved inferencing, and reducing both working memory and metacognitive demands also results in improved inferencing (Cain, Oakhill, Barnes, & Bryant, 2001; Barnes & Dennis, 2001). As we review below, the use of explicit prompts and other strategies to support inferencing in intervention studies also attests to the strategic nature of the inferencing problem (Vaughn & Klingner, 2004). However, it should be noted that although metacognitive and strategic interventions improve inferencing and reading comprehension, this is not the same as saying that comprehension strategies and metacognitive abilities are causally related to skilled and less skilled comprehension.

Prior Knowledge and Inferencing

A variety of studies have examined the role of prior knowledge in comprehension. Obviously, children and adults with better vocabulary knowledge and greater breadth and depth of general knowledge and who read more will have better reading comprehension skills that emphasize integration of new information with prior knowledge. The issue is to control for prior knowledge, especially in evaluating inferencing and related processes. To investigate the construction of a situation model in text comprehension that controls for prior knowledge, a variety of populations of poor comprehenders have been studied, including typically developing children (Barnes, Dennis, & Haefele-Kalvaitis, 1996), neurologically normal children who are poor at decoding and comprehension (Barnes & Dennis, 1996), neurologically normal children who are good at decoding with poor comprehension (Cain et al., 2001), children with spina bifida and hydrocephalus who are good decoders and poor at comprehension (Barnes et al., in press), and children with poor comprehension as a result of acquired brain injuries (Barnes & Dennis, 2001). The paradigm used across these studies controls for prior knowledge by teaching children a pretend world. They then hear or read a story that requires them to integrate knowledge of the pretend world with events depicted in the story. Inferences are evaluated that involve (1) *coherence* (i.e., necessary for maintaining story coherence and (2) *elaboration* (i.e., elaborate on objects and people in the story).

Analyzing only those inferences for which children had adequate knowledge as demonstrated by the ability to remember the needed background at the end of the task, findings across studies were similar. First, poor comprehenders took longer to master the knowledge base, so that the difficulties in acquiring knowledge were not simply a matter of experience and exposure (Barnes & Dennis, 2001). Second, older poor comprehenders performed similarly to younger, skilled comprehenders. Both groups made fewer inferences than older skilled comprehenders. Third, the sources of their difficulties with inferencing were similar (Barnes et al., in press; Cain et al., 2001). When inferences required retrieving knowledge from memory over time, the differences were larger, reflecting a larger processing burden; in contrast, when the knowledge and text necessary for an inference were cued, the differences were smaller because the processing burden was reduced. Third, elaborative inferences were easier to make than coherence inferences (Barnes et al., 1996) as measured when the processing burden was reduced, but more coherence than elaborative inferences were made in the context of story comprehension at all levels of comprehension ability. Thus, the attempt to maintain semantic coherence characterizes even poor comprehenders.

Of particular interest are the findings showing that it took longer to master the knowledge base. In a similar vein, Cain et al. (2001) reported that although good and poor comprehenders with adequate decoding skills had comparable recall of the knowledge base at the end of the experiment, one week later the poor comprehenders recalled less of the knowledge base than the good skilled comprehenders. Understanding more about the origins of this difficulty in acquiring and retaining knowledge would be an important direction to pursue. Is it related to more general language or learning difficulties, to working memory and resource allocation problems, or to other factors, such as exposure and experience.

Comprehension Monitoring

There are several metacognitive processes that are used to control and check comprehension when reading (and listening). Successful comprehension monitoring requires the reader to identify inconsistencies in the text, gaps in understanding, or the need to seek information from other parts of the text (Cataldo & Cornoldi, 1998). Nation (2005) summarized a variety of studies indicating that children who are poor comprehenders have difficulties with comprehension monitoring. Thus, it is not surprising that a focus on comprehension monitoring is a common part of strategy instruction in reading comprehension interventions.

Story Structure Sensitivity

As a final example of a higher-order process that is specific to reading comprehension, consider the child's sensitivity to the nature of the text that he or she is reading. Texts have different genres and can represent narrative stories, expository text, poems, directions, hypertext, and other genres. Each genre carries a distinct linguistic style and is often laid out in ways that vary. Understanding this variation facilitates comprehension.

In addition to effects of genre, other aspects of the structure and text provide important information that facilitates comprehension, including the title of the story, the first sentence of the paragraph, beginning and ending paragraphs, and related aspects of story structure. Children who struggle with comprehension are less aware of genre and story structure variation. They do not attend to this type of information, but do respond to efforts that attempt to teach them about text features and how attending to these features facilitates comprehension (Perfetti et al., 2005).

EPIDEMIOLOGY

Prevalence

Estimates of *specific* reading comprehension difficulties from epidemiological studies are not available. Badian (1999) defined reading comprehension difficulties using both a low achievement definition at the 25th percentile and a 1.5 standard error discrepancy definition with listening comprehension as the aptitude measure in a population of more than 1,000 children in grades 1–8. She reported an overall prevalence of 2.7% for the discrepancy definition and 9.1% for the low achievement definition—both low, given the cut-points. However, there was no control for level of word recognition ability, so the prevalence of *specific* reading comprehension difficulties could not be determined. Sample-specific studies of children who have age-appropriate word recognition skills but poor reading comprehension yield estimates that range from 5 to 10%, depending on the exclusionary criteria used to define the groups (e.g., Cornoldi et al., 1996; Stothard & Hulme, 1996). Nation (1999) estimated that 15% of poor readers had problems specific to comprehension.

The relation of reading comprehension difficulties and age is unclear, although it seems likely that specific reading comprehension problems are more apparent in older children and emerge after the initial stage of learning to read. Shankweiler et al. (1999) were able to identify only a few second- and third-graders, sampled for different types of LDs, with good word recognition and poor comprehension skills. Leach et al. (2003) found that only about 20% of a sample of children with reading problems had specific comprehension difficulties and that most of these children were identified after second grade. In contrast, Badian (1999) found that the prevalence rates for the discrepancy definition decreased slightly by eighth grade, but increased for the low achievement definition. The sample of children with impairments was small for each grade level, and the children were not identified with *specific* reading comprehension difficulties. If a child has a significant oral language disorder, it seems likely that reading comprehension problems will be identified earlier in development, but many of these children will also have poor word recognition skills (Catts, Fey, Tomblin, & Zhang, 2002a). Children with more subtle difficulties in language comprehension may be those children who are identified later in development, if at all (Nation, Clarke, & Snowling, 2002). As with any definition of LDs, incidence varies depending on decisions about cutoff points on norm-referenced tests.

Gender Ratio

Badian (1999) found male:female gender ratios of about 2.4:1 for the discrepancy definition and 1.6:1 for the low achievement definition of reading comprehension difficulties. These numbers are somewhat higher than the overall findings in Chapter 5, but this is the only study examining gender ratios for comprehension.

DEVELOPMENTAL COURSE

The developmental course of specific reading comprehension disability has not been studied. Recent studies in this area have addressed how poor comprehension early in a child's reading history may influence not only later reading comprehension, but also continued development of word-decoding skills. Although decoding and comprehension disabilities have been shown to be dissociable, children who are good at decoding but poor at comprehending may begin to fall behind in their decoding skills in the later school grades (Oakhill et al., 2003) because of diminished experience with text. As they read less and truncate their exposure to less common words (Cunningham & Stanovich, 1999), their sight word vocabularies do not keep pace with those of peers who have stronger comprehension abilities and read more frequently. Moreover, their poor ability to use semantic cues to decode less frequent words may constrain higher levels of lexical development (Nation & Snowling, 1998). This pattern has been referred to as a Matthew effect (Stanovich, 1986) and was clearly apparent in the nondiscrepant poor comprehenders in the Badian (1999) study, where prevalence increased with age.

NEUROBIOLOGICAL FACTORS

We provide only a brief discussion specific to neurobiological factors related to reading comprehension. This is largely because poor comprehenders have not been studied from either a neuroimaging or genetics perspective as a separate group. In addition, functional neuroimaging research on reading comprehension tends to focus on specific subskills, such as word recognition, working memory, or semantic processing.

Brain Structure and Function

The areas of the brain that support access to meaning and language comprehension are fairly well understood. There are no anatomical MRI studies of poor comprehenders. Individuals can sustain an injury to the brain that results in specific language (and reading) comprehension difficulties. The areas of the brain that are involved correspond closely to the areas identified in Figure 5.3 that are responsible for phonological processing and cross-modal processes in word recognition. Interestingly, patients who sustain aphasias that affect language comprehension vary in the degree to which reading comprehension is affected, but both domains are typically impaired.

In a review of neuroimaging studies involving sentence and discourse processing, Gernsbacher and Kaschak (2003) identified several studies that looked both at processing sentences and at processing at the level of discourse. For both of these general classes of tasks, the paradigms do not correspond generally to reading of authentic text. Instead, readers (or listeners) must identify anomalies or process some specific component of the discourse, such as prosody or emotion. In summarizing the results of sentence comprehension studies, Gernsbacher and Kaschak (2003, p. 102) indicated that "the processing of sentences does involve Wernicke's area (word/phonological processing), superior and middle temporal regions (phonology/lexical/semantic processing), Broca's area (production/syntactic analysis), inferior frontal gyrus (phonological/syntactic/semantic processes), middle and superior frontal regions (semantics), and the right hemisphere homologues to these regions." In summarizing discourse studies, Gernsbacher and Kaschak (2003, p. 105) noted that "the processing of discourse therefore appears to be a distributed network of brain regions. These include the areas involved in lower levels of language processing (words, sentences, etc.) as well as areas specific to discourse: right temporal and frontal regions (important for the integrative aspects of discourse processing, as well as both temporal lobes). The exact function of these regions is not yet known" (p. 105).

In another review focusing on functional imaging studies involving comprehension of written sentences, Caplan (2004) found that some processing operations at the sentential level involve similar brain areas regardless of whether language is written or spoken. Different brain regions supported different aspects of sentence processing, but there was variability in the regions that were supported. Thus, studies of fairly specific sentence and discourse characteristics tend to focus on processes that support comprehension, reflecting the fact that reading (and listening) are essentially unobservable processes that require the joint operation of multiple domains in order to abstract meaning from text (or words).

Genetic Factors

There are no studies that we could identify that specifically addressed the heritability of poor reading comprehension in individuals identified as having these disorders. As a dimension, Petrill, Deater-Deckard, Thompson, Schatschneider, and De Thorne (in press) found strong heritability of reading comprehension in a young sample of twins, as measured by the Passage Comprehension cloze procedure used in different Woodcock tests (e.g., Woodcock et al., 2001; see Chapter 4). The magnitude was similar to that observed for word recognition. In this study, letter and word recognition, phonological awareness, and oral language vocabulary showed significant shared (and nonshared) environmental influences, but reading comprehension showed only significant nonshared environmental influence. However a study of adult twins reared apart found similar heritabilities for word reading but a lower estimate for reading comprehension (Johnson, Bouchard, Segal, & Samuels, 2005).

In a first grade sample, Byrne et al. (in press) obtained a heritability estimate of .76 for Woodcock Passage Comprehension, very similar to the estimates from Petrill et al. (in press). A fluency assessment based on the TOWRE (Torgesen et al., 1999; see Chapter 4) yielded a heritability estimate of .82. The correlation of the heritability estimates was .97, indicating no significant independent genetic influences for decoding and comprehension for younger children based on this cloze procedure. In an older sample from the Colorado study, Keenan, Betjemann, Wadsworth, DeFries, and Olson (2006) created composite measures of reading comprehension and listening comprehension across several different tasks that involved varying passage lengths and response formats, including the knowledge-based inferencing task described on p. 191. These measures yielded heritability estimates of .51 for reading comprehension and .52 for listening comprehension. A decoding composite yielded a heritability estimate of .65. The correlation of the heritability estimates for decoding and reading comprehension was .85 for listening comprehension and .80 for reading comprehension. Although these estimates show strong common genetic influences, they are significantly less than 1, indicating significant independent genetic influences. These studies, along with Petrill et al. (in press) suggest greater independence for word recognition and reading comprehension among the older compared to the younger twins. These results, like those of different cognitive mechanisms, also support the Reading Components model.

Different language skills related to reading comprehension have been shown to have varying degrees of heritability across a variety of studies (Plomin & Kovas, 2005), and oral language disorders certainly have a significant heritability component (Bishop & Snowling, 2004). There is overlap in the heritability of reading and language problems, but these are also independent disorders. In particular, semantic and syntactic components of language development are heritable, commonly characteristic of children with oral language disorders, and certainly affect reading comprehension. Many of these individuals have reading comprehension deficits, but it is the heritability of the language problem that contributes to both the oral language and reading comprehension difficulties. In contrast, children whose primary problem is WLRD have language difficulties that are more specific to phonological processing and that lead to impairments in word recognition. It cannot be said that LDs that specifically involve poor reading comprehension are inherited, but it can be said that the language components of these disorders share distinct heritable features. More research on the dimension of reading comprehension that expands the assessment beyond cloze procedures (e.g., Kennan et al., 2006) is needed.

SUMMARY: FROM ACADEMIC SKILL DEFICITS TO NEUROBIOLOGICAL FACTORS

Although the comprehension-related deficits discussed above have been well documented and replicated across studies employing different procedures and criteria for group membership, questions remain concerning how to measure academic skill deficits in reading comprehension, and debate ensues about the core cognitive processes that underlie reading comprehension disability (Snow, 2002; Stanovich, 1988). Nonetheless, studies of children with WLRDs, comprehension disability, or both, children with neurodevelopmental disorders, and typically achieving children support a dissociation between these two components of reading. This work also shows that these two aspects of reading are associated with different cognitive deficits, suggesting that different forms of intervention will be necessary to remediate these two distinct forms of LDs. There is a need for neurobiological studies to focus on comprehension either as a dimension or, especially, as a category distinct from WLRD.

READING COMPREHENSION INTERVENTIONS

General Instructional Approaches

General approaches are often classified into two different types of instruction: specific skills instruction and strategy instruction (Clark & Uhry, 1995; Swanson, 1999). As the name suggests, specific skills instruction focuses on teaching skills that can be applied to texts, such as vocabulary, finding the main idea, making inferences, and finding facts. Vocabulary can be taught through either explicit instruction approaches or contextual approaches (NRP, 2000). Skills such as finding the main idea and making inferences can be taught by having children read short passages and answer questions. However, for such approaches to be effective, the teacher must provide the instruction in an explicit and systematic manner.

In contrast to specific skills instruction, strategy instruction is "viewed as [instruction in] cognitive processes requiring decision making and critical thinking" (Clark & Uhry, 1995, p. 107). Strategy instruction in reading comprehension is an outgrowth of several cognitive psychology theories and concepts, notably schemas, metacognition, and mediated learning. For example, schemas involve the idea that a reader brings certain psychological frameworks, or "mental schemas," to a text. During reading, in order for the reader to comprehend, facts must be added or adjusted to the reader's mental schema. The study of metacognition has also had considerable influence on reading comprehension research.

It has been found that "good readers who possess meta-cognitive skills in reading are aware of the purpose of reading and differentiate between task demands. They actively seek to clarify the purposes or task demands through self-questioning prior to reading the given materials . . . [and] evaluate their own comprehension of materials read" (Wong, 1991, pp. 239–240). As is true for other skill domains (e.g., memory), the teaching of metacognitive strategies is beneficial to poor comprehenders even though metacognition is not causally related to comprehension skill, but may be considered an essential part of comprehension (Perfetti et al., 2005).

Finally, the concept of cooperative learning, which involves the effects of student–teacher interactions on the student's later ability to solve problems independently, has also influenced reading comprehension theory and instruction. For example, Maria (1990) conceptualized reading instruction as an interaction between reader, text, and teacher. The reader brings decoding ability, oral vocabulary, and background knowledge to the text. The text is no longer perceived as having a single meaning for all students. Rather, meaning is constructed through this interaction. The teacher is viewed as a manager and facilitator who provides direct instruction in strategies, but who also encourages independence (Clark & Uhry, 1995).

Other intervention methods based on these types of cognitive strategies have been developed to teach reading comprehension. For example, Palinscar and Brown (1985) have developed a teaching method called "reciprocal teaching" that has been found to enhance reading comprehension skills. In addition, Pressley and his colleagues have developed interventions based on "transactional strategies" to increase reading comprehension skills that are based in part on Vygotskian concepts (Pressley, 2006). In this method of instruction, students are "provided with direct instruction in a number of comprehension strategies and are encouraged to talk about and choose a strategy for understanding what they read . . . students are provided with positive instruction when a strategy is successful" (Clark & Uhry, 1995, p. 111). Instruction also involves teacher modeling of different comprehension strategies.

Bos and Anders (1990) developed an interactive teaching model, which is similar to Pressley's (2006) transactional teaching method, that is also based on Vygotskian principles. This model incorporates six teaching–learning characteristics: (1) activating prior knowledge; (2) integrating new knowledge with old knowledge; (3) cooperative knowledge sharing and learning; (4) predicting, justifying, and confirming concepts and text meaning; (5) predicting, justifying, and confirming relationships between concepts; and (6) purposeful learning. Initially, a teacher models these strategies for the students, but gradually moves away from being an instructor to being more of a facilitator.

Although the specific skill training and strategy instruction methods have some similarities, the most effective instruction for students with reading comprehension disabilities involves explicit instruction, multiple opportunities for instruction, and carefully sequenced lessons (Clark & Uhry, 1995). Strategies based on cognitive concepts (i.e., strategy instruction) appear to be the most effective methods of intervention for reading comprehension and have provided the best results to date for improving disabled readers' comprehension.

This general observation seems true even for older poor readers. In a recent report on adolescent literacy from the Carnegie Foundation (Biancarosa & Snow, 2004), it was noted that 70% of adolescents need differentiated literacy instruction. It is not known how many of these students have problems specifically at the level of reading comprehension, and the report is probably incorrect in suggesting that poor decoding accounts for a minority of these poor readers. Indeed, Catts, Taylor, and Zhang (2006) reported that three times more adolescents in grades 8 and 10 had problems with decoding as compared with specific comprehension problems, with 6.5% having specific comprehension problems, 3.7% having specific decoding problems, and about 19% with both decoding and comprehension problems. Neither the comprehension nor the decoding problems should be minimized. Within poor eighth grade readers, Catts, Hogan, and Adlof (2005) found that about 30% had a specific listening comprehension problem, 13% had specific decoding problems, and 33% had both decoding and comprehension difficulties. By 10th grade, only 3% had specific decoding problems, but difficulties in both remained common. Decoding problems should not be minimized in older students and adults. The causes of reading difficulties are diverse and a focus on comprehension is needed, especially given the evidence below indicating that explicit instruction improves reading comprehension even in students for whom decoding and fluency is an issue.

The Carnegie report made 15 recommendations for teaching reading comprehension in adolescents (see Table 7.1), beginning with the need for "direct, explicit comprehension instruction, which is instruction in the strategies and processes that proficient readers use to understand what they read, including summarizing, keeping track of one's own understanding, and a host of other practices" (p. 4). We describe some of these practices below, but the idea that the instruction is explicit is key, given that many assume that simply reading broadly and frequently will in itself improve comprehension. However, as an earlier study of teachers whose students achieve higher and lower reading achievement scores showed, children develop better comprehension skills when instruction

TABLE 7.1. Recommendations for Enhancing Reading Comprehension from the Carnegie Report

 1. Provide explicit instruction in the strategies and processes that support comprehension.

 2. Teach comprehension in content areas.

 3. Self-directed learning should motivate students to read and write.

 4. Support collaborative learning around a variety of texts.

 5. Provide intervention in small groups for those who struggle with reading comprehension, writing, and content areas.

 6. Employ diverse texts that range in difficulty level and topics.

 7. Require intensive writing in all subject areas.

 8. Develop technology as an instructional tool.

 9. Provide assessments of student progress and program efficacy.

10. Provide extended time for literacy. In secondary schools, 2–4 hours of literacy instruction and practice in language arts and content classes is needed each day.

11. Provide ongoing professional development in literacy.

12. Evaluate student and program outcomes.

13. Create teacher teams across content areas that meet regularly.

14. Provide leadership from teachers and principals who understand reading instruction.

15. School districts should have a comprehensive, coordinated literacy plan from preschool to high school that is interdisciplinary, interdepartmental, across grade, and coordinated with outside resources and the community.

---

is explicit (Knapp, 1995, p.8): "Students do not acquire the ability to search for deeper meaning by osmosis. Teachers must structure opportunities for children to learn how to analyze and think about what they have read."

Other recommendations target both instruction and infrastructure areas. The need to involve content teachers (e.g., those who teach history, science, language arts, etc.) in explicit reading comprehension instruction is critical, as considerable time will be needed to enhance comprehension abilities in all students. Engaging older students, whose interest in schooling in general often diminishes in the face of other interests, is also very important. Recommendations for collaborative text learning, diverse texts, intensive writing, more time devoted to literacy-related activities, and ongoing monitoring of student performance represent themes readily apparent in the specific intervention examples described below and in Chapter 4. To accomplish these tasks, infrastructure changes will be needed, particularly comprehensive, district-wide literacy plans that link reading instruction across domains and grades from K to 12.

Efficacy of Reading Comprehension Instruction

Empirical Syntheses

Fortunately, there are interventions that are effective specifically in the area of reading comprehension with students who vary in the extent of impairment in word recognition, fluency, and listening comprehension. Most interventions specifically addressing reading comprehension take place at a classroom level and generally target students generically identified as being "learning disabled." Specific LDs in reading comprehension are rarely targeted by intervention studies.

There is strong evidence that instruction specifically targeting reading comprehension is associated with positive outcomes regardless of the source of difficulty, even in children with decoding problems. In Swanson's (1999) meta-analysis, strategy instruction was specifically effective with students with LDs who had comprehension difficulties. The NRP report (NRP, 2000) identified 47 studies involving vocabulary instruction and 203 studies that involved text comprehension. However, because many of the studies had limitations in their research designs, the final database was not adequate for empirical synthesis. It was difficult to separate and classify the many different variables and methodologies included in experimental research involving vocabulary instruction. The 203 studies on text comprehension instruction identified 16 different types of instruction, with 8 providing a firm scientific basis indicating that they improved comprehension. These included comprehension monitoring, cooperative learning, graphic and semantic organizers, instruction in story structure, question answering, question generating, summarization, and multiple strategy teaching.

For students with LDs, recent meta-analyses of cooperative learning (Jenkins & O'Connor, 2003) and the role of graphic organizers (Kim, Vaughn, Wanzek, & Wei, 2004) suggest moderate to large aggregated effect sizes for these kinds of interventions. In another review, Vaughn and Klingner (2004) found a variety of practices to show some evidence for facilitating reading comprehension of students with LDs. These included (1) assistance in activating background knowledge; (2) various aspects of comprehension monitoring during and after reading; (3) procedures using questioning; (4) various methods that focus on the main idea in summarization of text; (5) explicit teaching of vocabulary development that facilitates student understanding of concepts, as opposed to surface-level memorization; and (6) graphic organizers, including semantic maps, word maps, and semantic feature analysis. In addition, strategies that facilitate the understanding of unknown words, including the use of context cues, morphophonemic analysis, and external references, can be helpful. Explicit instruction in understanding the organization of text structure, particularly expository texts, has been effective. Finally, paralleling the findings of the NRP, the teaching of multiple strategies appears to be effective.

Methods used for students with LDs in reading, including reciprocal teaching, transactional strategies instruction, collaborative strategic reading, and PALS, have been found to be effective. Consistent with an older review by Mastropieri and Scruggs (1997), Vaughn and Klingner (2004) concluded that students with LDs can improve reading comprehension when teachers (1) provide instruction in strategies that have been documented as effective for reading comprehension; (2) design instruction that is explicit and not dependent on contextual or incidental learning; (3) model, support, and guide instruction; (4) provide opportunities to promote generalization across different kinds of text; and (5) systematically monitor student progress and make indicated adjustments in the instructional plan.

Collaborative Strategic Reading

A review of collaborative strategic reading is an interesting example of approaches that are used at the classroom level (Vaughn, Klingner, & Bryant, 2001). In collaborative strategic reading, the teacher presents strategies to the class as a whole, using modeling, role playing, and think-alouds. Students are explicitly taught to apply strategies involving why, when, and how events occur in the text they are reading. After they develop some proficiency with the strategies, they are divided into groups on the basis of their proficiency in applying the strategies. In the groups, students perform in defined roles as they collaboratively implement the strategies in expository text. In collaborative strategic reading, four strategies are taught to students, including (1) a *preview* component, in which students essentially attempt to activate background knowledge; (2) *comprehension monitoring* during reading by identifying difficult words and concepts in the passage and using strategies that address what to do when text does not make sense; (3) restudying the *most important idea* in the paragraph; and (4) *summarization/question asking*. The results of several studies showed that many students made significant gains in reading comprehension and academic content. However, some students showed little response, highlighting the importance of carefully monitoring the progress of students receiving a classroom-based intervention.

Peer-Assisted Learning Strategies

In a similar way, the line of work on PALS for reading at grades 2–6, in which the instructional focus is on comprehension strategies, has documented impressive effects for some students with LDs, as well as for their low-, average-, and high-performing classmates, in settings where English is the dominant language (Fuchs, Fuchs, Mathes, & Simmons, 1997; Saenz, Fuchs, & Fuchs, 2005). Of course, as with Vaughn et al. (2001), an unacceptable proportion of students with LDs demonstrate insufficient response to PALS.

Theme-Identification Program

Illustrating the research involving remediation of comprehension difficulties in primary-grade students with LDs, Williams and colleagues (see Williams, 2003) have completed studies that focused on middle school students with LDs (e.g., Wilder & Williams, 2001) as well as second- and third-grade students (Williams et al., 2005). This program used text structure to teach the strategies and processes that support proficient reading comprehension. This research is based on the Theme-Identification Program, which consists of 14 lessons (Williams, 2002, 2003). The goal of the program is to help students derive themes, the overall meaning of stories abstracted from the specific plot components. In the Theme-Identification Program, two introductory sessions focus on plot components; the remaining 12 lessons address the identification of a story's theme. Each lesson is organized around a single story and includes prereading discussion of the theme concept; reading the story aloud; discussing the important story information, using organizing questions as a guide (i.e., the "theme scheme"); transfer and application of the theme to other story examples and real-life situations; review; and activity. The heart of the program is the theme scheme, which provides a set of questions that organize the important story components to help students follow the plot and derive the theme. The teacher models how to answer the eight questions leading to a theme, and students gradually assume increasing responsibility for asking the questions and identifying the theme. In addition, the students rehearse and commit to memory these questions so they can apply the theme scheme guide to untaught stories. Toward that end of instruction, transfer instruction is provided in an explicit manner, with two additional questions employed to help students generalize the theme to other relevant situations.

Williams et al. (2002) applied this program in five second-grade and five third-grade inclusion classes in Harlem, New York City, representing high-, average-, and low-performing students relative to their classmates. Twelve of these 120 students had been identified with LDs. The 10 classrooms were assigned randomly to the Theme-Identification Program or to a more traditional comprehension program that emphasized vocabulary and plot. Results showed that, as a function of the Theme-Identification Program, students acquired the concept of a theme (effect size = 2.17) and learned the theme scheme questions (effect size = 2.11). More important, on novel passages, students in the experimental condition were more skilled at identifying themes (effect size = 0.68). Significant effects were apparent in high-, average-, and low-achieving classmates, as well as in students with LDs, in second and third grade.

Williams et al. (2005) tested the effectiveness of this program by contrasting theme identification, as a way of learning about animal classifications, with a more traditional content program on animal classification and with a no-treatment control group. Teachers of 10 second-grade classes in three New York City public schools volunteered to participate and were randomly assigned to treatments (text structure n = 4; content n = 4; no instruction n = 2). Figure 7.1 provides a comparison of the two programs, showing the overlap at the level of content. However, instruction in the experimental condition explicitly represented different aspects of text structure and was taught explicitly using principles from both direct instruction and strategy instruction. The content program used many of the same materials, but focused on facts and more general information on animals. Participants were 128 students, among whom approximately 6% had been identified as having LDs.

The researchers first looked at students' ability to summarize a compare/contrast paragraph that had been explicitly taught in the program. The text structure group outperformed the other two groups on the number of summary statements that were accurate and that included an appropriate clue word. The researchers also examined students' ability to transfer, with three novel compare/contrast texts that were structured analogously to those used for instruction but that incorporated novel content (the content of three texts was increasingly novel from the materials included in class). Across the near- and far-transfer measures, students in the text structure group scored significantly higher than both contrast groups. At the same time, the researchers also found that instruction on compare/contrast did not transfer to a new text structure, suggesting the need for explicit instruction on a variety of text structures.

Learning Strategies Curriculum

A long-term program of research from the Center for Research on Learning at Kansas University (Schumaker, Deshler, & McKnight, 2002)

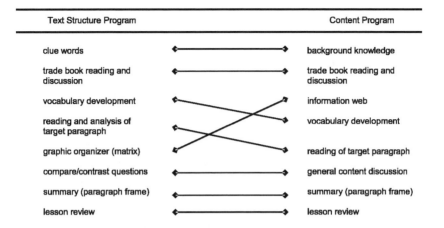

Text Structure Program		Content Program
clue words	◆————————————◆	background knowledge
trade book reading and discussion	◆————————————◆	trade book reading and discussion
vocabulary development		information web
reading and analysis of target paragraph		vocabulary development
graphic organizer (matrix)		reading of target paragraph
compare/contrast questions	◆————————————◆	general content discussion
summary (paragraph frame)	◆————————————◆	summary (paragraph frame)
lesson review	◆————————————◆	lesson review

FIGURE 7.1. An overview of the Theme-Identification and content programs. Solid lines with diamond end points indicate comparable sections in each of the two instructional programs. From Williams et al. (2005, p. 541). Copyright 2005 by the American Psychological Association. Reprinted by permission.

has identified a series of strategies, or teaching routines, that impact not only the learning of students with LDs, but all students in the classroom. These teaching routines involve a variety of domains, including reading comprehension and writing, as well as a variety of organizational skills in school and out of school (e.g., homework). Largely implemented in secondary school environments and at a classroom level, these routines have been organized into the Learning Strategies Curriculum, which focuses on three major demands presented by standard curriculum: acquisition, storage, and expression of information. For acquisition, the teaching routines involve strategies that facilitate word recognition and reading comprehension (paraphrasing, visual imagery, recall of narrative text, self-questioning, and related strategic activities). A series of research studies, many of them involving probe assessments in single case designs, have shown that adolescents with LDs can be taught complex learning strategies and that implementation of these strategies results in improved academic performance (Shumaker et al., 2002). Effect sizes are consistently in the large range for various strategies. Studies that involve classroom-level instruction of organizational skills not only show that such instruction improves organizational skills and overall performance in students with LDs, but also reveal that students without LDs who are showed these strategies also improve with explicit instruction in this domain (Hughes et al., 2002).

CONCLUSIONS

There is a strong evidence base that identifies how reading comprehension develops and the different sources of difficulty in reading comprehension. Although much research needs to be completed, the basis for this research program has been established (Snow, 2002). It is clear that there are children whose primary problems in reading reflect difficulties in comprehension, rather than decoding and fluency, and that oral language disorders do not account for all comprehension difficulties. Many issues remain concerning the measurement of reading comprehension and the core cognitive correlates of academic skill deficits associated with different approaches to measurement. Neurobiological studies of poor comprehenders are scant, and much of the understanding of this aspect of poor reading comprehension builds on studies of children with lower-level difficulties. Few intervention studies identify poor comprehenders as a specific subgroup. However, studies involving intervention in reading comprehension instruction show that comprehension can be improved, even in students with WLRD. In these studies, much of the impact on gains in reading comprehension stems from strategy instruction, often included as part of a comprehensive approach to reading instruction in children with word recognition and fluency difficulties.

In Chapter 9, the importance of strategic instruction for students with LDs is expanded to the written language domain. Although there is a role for "skills instruction," particularly in handwriting and spelling, it will be apparent that the overall impact of instruction involving written language for students with LDs largely focuses on the development of strategies. It is well known that students with LDs in a variety of domains do not spontaneously identify strategies. If they are taught strategies, they do not implement them in the absence of specific instruction that promotes generalization. Strategic instruction promotes self-regulation and raises the student's level of independence. Such instruction addresses the "executive function" deficiencies commonly observed in students with LDs in a variety of academic domains.

CHAPTER 8

Mathematics Disabilities

Unlike those in reading fluency and comprehension, definitions of LDs in mathematics have developed more like the exclusionary definitions historically characteristic of WLRD. As noted in Chapter 2, the federal statutory definition of LDs refers to disabilities in mathematical calculations and concepts, whereas the National Joint Committee on Learning Disabilities (NJCLD, 1988) definition of LDs refers to significant difficulties in "mathematics abilities." The DSM-IV (American Psychiatric Association, 1994) uses the term "mathematics disorder." The International Classification of Diseases-10 (ICD-10; World Health Organization, 1992) provides research criteria for the identification of a "specific disorder of arithmetical skills." All of these definitions of an LD in mathematics are based on assumptions of average- or above-average-ability IQ, normal sensory function, adequate educational opportunity, and absence of other developmental disorders and emotional disturbance. These definitions beg the question of the specific academic skill deficits that would identify a person with an LD in mathematics.

Because of this persistent vagueness and the parochial nature of the quality of extant definitions, no consistent standards have been established by which to judge the presence or absence of LDs in math. Adding to this dilemma is the fact that "LDs in mathematics," "developmental arithmetic disorder," "mathematics disabilities," and "specific mathematics disabilities" are broad terms used for a variety of impairments in mathematics skills ranging from computations to problem solving to word problems. As Fleishner (1994) suggested, in some cases the term "mathematics learning disability" has been used synonymously with the term "dyscalculia" to denote *specific* (as opposed to generalized) deficits in calculation or mathematical thinking. "Specific" usually implies that oral language, reading, and writing are intact (e.g., see Strang &

Rourke, 1985; World Health Organization, 1992). However, math deficits are frequently associated with other LDs (Fleishner, 1994; Fuchs,
Fuchs, & Prentice, 2004; Rourke & Finlayson, 1978). A major problem
in defining math LDs is the need to focus on identification of a set of key
academic skill deficits that represent markers for one or more LDs in
math. Ultimately, this identification would proceed from a model identifying critical components of math proficiency, much like reading can be
broken into component skills involving word recognition, fluency, and
comprehension.

ACADEMIC SKILL DEFICITS

Disorders of math occur in isolation and, by definition, involve difficulties with computations and often with problem solving. The importance
of focusing on problem solving is apparent, given the success of interventions targeted to these specific skills (Fuchs et al., 2004). Less clear is
whether there is a separate academic skill deficit involving math reasoning or concepts that cannot be explained by difficulties with reading and
language (see Chapter 3). In developmental models of math, conceptual
and procedural aspects of mathematical knowledge (e.g., understanding
the concept of cardinality versus the procedure of counting to 10) are assumed to be required for the performance of many mathematical tasks,
and the development of mathematical skills emerges from the reciprocal
nature of the relationship between conceptual and procedural knowledge (Rittle-Johnson, Siegler, & Alibali, 2001). This raises fundamental
questions about attempts to separate knowledge of mathematical concepts from mathematical computations in definitions of mathematical
disabilities.

In Chapter 5, we drew a distinction between academic skill deficits
in reading, in which word recognition is a specific marker of WLRD,
and core cognitive processes, such as phonological processing. It has
been important in the reading area to make this distinction and to show
that different cognitive processes predict different component skills in
reading: word recognition, fluency, and comprehension.

In the math area, this distinction among component academic skills
is also important (Geary, 2005), but the understanding of the numerical
competencies that characterize math and that may or may not be impaired in LDs involving math is not as well developed as in reading or
writing (Chapter 9). These components could be represented as separate
number-processing and calculation systems (McCloskey & Caramazza,
1985), a model that has arisen from studies of acquired acalculia. This
type of model tends to view numerical competency per se as an essen-

tially modular skill with specific neural correlates. Another perspective, which stems more from studies of children who are developing math skills, examines different math competencies and searches for cognitive mechanisms that explain why these competencies develop to different degrees in individual children. Thus, Geary (2004) distinguished competencies that involve conceptual knowledge, such as base-10 arithmetic, from procedural knowledge, such as rules and strategies for borrowing and carrying. He then argued that these forms of mathematical knowledge are supported by different cognitive systems.

These ideas about mathematical competencies reflect two different theoretical positions that have direct implications for how research will progress in math LDs. The view that mathematical competencies are themselves core, modular attributes has been expressed in the developmental literature by Butterworth (2005). The argument is that math derives from the ontogenetically ancient need to understand magnitude and quantities and to compare counts and numbers. These abilities are cross-species capabilities that can be observed in humans and nonhumans, representing what Dehaene and Cohen (1997) characterized as a "number sense." In studies of humans, infants at very early ages are able to discern differences in the numerosity of small sets (Starkey, Spelke, & Gelman, 1991), and infants appear to infer the numerical value of manipulations on numbers such as adding to small sets (Wynn, 1992). Preschoolers can accurately discriminate magnitude differences in small sets and numbers, and they can perform transformations on numbers such as adding to and taking away from small sets in nonverbal problem-solving situations (reviewed in Ginsburg, Klein, & Starkey, 1998). Butterworth (2005) interpreted this evidence as indicating that these early numerical abilities are not influenced by language (but see Hodent, Bryant, & Houde, 2005) and other aspects of the environment and that difficulty in these early math abilities eventuate in LDs involving math.

From this view, the key issue in defining and understanding LDs in math is identifying the competencies that make up this basic capacity of the human and nonhuman brain that are products of evolution and relate to specific brain circuits (Dehaene, Molko, Cohen, & Wilson, 2004). An adequate explanation of all mathematical competencies, especially those involving problem solving, would require an expansion into the language system, regardless of whether language is considered to simply *facilitate* the development of mathematical skills (Gelman & Butterworth, 2005) or whether it is thought to be *causally* implicated in the development of core mathematical skills and concepts (Carey, 2004). Whether the performance of infants and preschoolers in these quantitative tasks relies on innate or early numerical representations, or whether performance is, instead, a product of nonnumeric perceptual cues, language, and general attention mechanisms continues to be vigorously debated (e.g., Cohen & Marks, 2002, vs. Wynn, 2002; Hodent et al., 2005; Mix, Huttenlocher, & Levine, 2002). In any event, the predictiveness of these early abilities on quantitative tasks for individual differences in mathematical ability by school age is currently unknown.

A more traditional view is expressed by Geary (2004) and apparent in earlier work on LDs in math (Rourke, 1993). In this view, mathematical skills represent different domains of knowledge that are built on other general cognitive or neuropsychological systems such as the language system, the visual–spatial system, and the central executive that sustains attention and inhibits irrelevant information (Geary, 2004). Difficulties in math could arise from any of these cognitive systems or their interactions and could lead to different patterns of deficits in different math competencies or in the performance of various mathematical tasks.

There is some evidence for the framework (Geary, 2004, 2005), but the research base is not adequate to determine the value of this approach or that of the more modular approach discussed above. It is apparent that children with LDs in math vary in component math skills and in the cognitive processes related to these skills (Fuchs et al., 2005, 2006b; Hanich, Jordan, Kaplan, & Dick, 2001). However, regardless of the model of math disability, understanding the core processes underlying LDs in math begs the question of the academic skill deficits in math that identify LDs. Much of the research base has focused on children identified as having computational difficulties in math. This focus is not surprising, as the early neurological literature often described adults and children with "dyscalculia," based on their inability to perform simple arithmetic calculations either orally or in paper-and-pencil tasks. Yet, math is a domain that encompasses more than arithmetic computations.

One problem with the focus on dyscalculia or computations is that the ability to perform math computations requires multiple numerical competencies, just as proficient reading involves accurate word recognition, fluent word and text reading, and comprehension—with each of these components possibly determined by multiple core cognitive processes (Fuchs et al., 2006b). Mathematics involves computation, itself the product of knowledge and retrieval of facts, and application of procedural knowledge. Problem solving, particularly solving word problems, involves computation, language, reasoning, and reading skills, and perhaps visual–spatial skills as well (Geary, 1993). Any successful execution of math competencies requires that the person is attentive, organized, able to switch sets, and work quickly enough to avoid overloading working memory stores that retain information needed for on-line access of different kinds of information. Unlike reading achievement tests, in which the distinctions of different components of reading skills are clear and not necessarily confounded, the tests used to measure achievement in math tend to confound multiple components of math and to focus primarily on computation or problem solving. The value of the focus on basic numerical competencies is that it becomes possible to break down the components of math skills into more discrete components. If the investigator carefully specifies the component of math to be assessed and then looks at the cognitive correlates of that component in students who vary in such competencies, the links between breakdowns in math competencies and cognition may become more apparent. Thus, the two perspectives should be kept tightly linked (Geary, 2005). Researchers must carefully specify the component of numerical ability that is being evaluated because the cognitive correlates likely vary.

CORE COGNITIVE PROCESSES

Given the difficulty in defining a set of academic skill deficits that identify individuals with LDs in math, it is not surprising that research has not advanced to a level that allows the identification of a set of core cognitive processes that underlie LDs in math. At the very least, much will depend on the type of theoretical orientation and mathematical competencies that are used to identify the math LD. One established distinction is the importance of determining whether the person has a WLRD. Although it is less clear that numerical competencies actually vary between groups with mathematics disability (MD) only and those with MD and WLRD, it is clear that the cognitive correlates vary, if only because the child with math and reading LDs has impairments in language that are related to the reading problem. Moreover, the link of word reading and phonological processing is apparent regardless of whether math is impaired; the person with both word reading and math problems tends to have more severe language (and reading) difficulties. Figure 8.1 provides a comparison of groups with no LD, only LD in reading, only LD in math, and both reading and math LD. The more severe and pervasive impairment of the group with both reading and math difficulties is readily apparent, as is the striking similarity of the profiles for this group and the group with only reading problems on measures of phonological awareness and rapid naming. Similarly, the co-occurrence of reading and math LDs is associated with more severe reading and math difficulties.

Despite these difficulties with definition and differences in theoretical orientation, there is research on cognitive processes involving working memory/executive processes and language, which is reviewed in this section, along with a brief summary of other cognitive correlates.

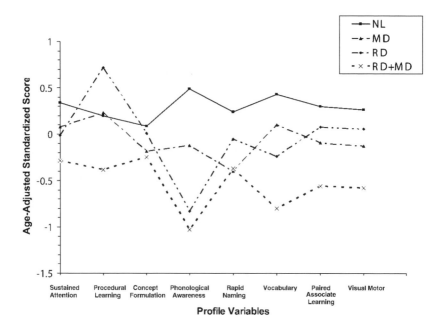

FIGURE 8.1. Cognitive profiles of typical achievers (NL), only LD in reading (RD), only LD in math (MD), and LD in both reading and math (RD + MD). Children with RD + MD show comorbid disabilities that are more severe than RD or MD in isolation. From Fletcher (2005, p. 310). Copyright 2005 by PRO-ED. Reprinted by permission.

Working Memory/Executive Processes

Regardless of numerical competency, deficits in working memory tasks (Bull & Johnston, 1997; Geary, Hoard, Byrd-Craven, & DeSoto, 2004) and executive function tasks (Sikora, Haley, Edwards, & Butler, 2002) are commonly observed in children with math LDs. In a series of studies by Swanson and associates (Keeler & Swanson, 2001; Swanson & Sachse-Lee, 2001; Swanson & Siegel, 2001), the contributions of both verbal and visual–spatial working memory, executive processes that involve strategy knowledge, and the ability to use working memory efficiently have been studied in children with specific math disabilities and with both reading and math disabilities.

Some studies have suggested that problems with visual–spatial working memory are more likely to characterize children with a specific math disability (Siegel & Ryan, 1989), whereas children with both reading and math disabilities have more pervasive language and verbal working memory difficulties. However, Keeler and Swanson (2001) found that math computational skills in individuals with a specific math disability were better predicted by verbal than by visual–spatial working memory. There was evidence for domain-specific working memory difficulties, as well as problems with executive control, that would lead to more pervasive problems with math. In contrast, Swanson and Sachse-Lee (2001) found that the domain-general system made a significant contribution to poor working memory in children with reading disabilities that was not directly related to their reading problems. Wilson and Swanson (2001) found that various measures of working memory that were both domain-general and domain-specific contributed to the ability to acquire strategies for math computations. As Geary and colleagues (Geary, Hamson, & Hoard, 2000; Geary et al., 2004) pointed out, the relation of working memory and math disabilities is complicated, and additional research is necessary to determine how this relationship relates to math disabilities in children with and without reading disabilities. Certainly, children who have both reading and math disabilities tend to have more severe problems in working memory than those who have problems in only reading or math (Fletcher et al., 2003). Similarly, relations between working memory and math disabilities are likely to be complex because different aspects of working memory may be related to different mathematical skills. In typically developing children, for example, numerical computation is related to short-term verbal memory or verbal working memory, depending on whether regrouping is required, but visual–spatial working memory is related to numerical estimation (Khemani & Barnes, 2005).

Language

Carey (2004) proposed that language is important in enabling formal math learning, as well as for development in areas of math like geometry that are often considered to be the least verbal (Spelke & Tsivkin, 2001). Language provides a set of symbols, such as the counting words that have no inherent meaning but which set the stage for the mappings between previously distinct representational systems, such as quantitative and language systems. The resulting integrated representations are more powerful and result in new mental structures.

Some evidence for the importance of language in the development of early math skills comes from studies of toddlers and preschoolers in which even the development of computation using small numbers varies according to linguistic quantifiers that differ across languages (Hodent et al., 2005). Although the role of language in mathematical competence has been explicated for typical development, aberrant development of the language system could be expected to result in deficits in certain aspects of mathematical function even from a very young age.

From a different perspective, other studies suggest that children who are impaired in both reading and math computations typically show more severe and pervasive disturbances of oral language than children who are impaired only in word recognition. Their difficulties reflect problems in learning, retaining, and retrieving math facts, which are essential to precise calculation. These lead to pervasive difficulties with math. Thus, Jordan and Hanich (2000) found that children with both reading and math difficulties showed problems in multiple domains of mathematical thinking. Language impairments clearly lead to difficulties in the acquisition of math skills.

Other Cognitive Correlates

Not surprisingly, a variety of other cognitive skills have been implicated in studies of LDs involving math. Fuchs et al. (2006b) determined how different child attributes are related to different math competencies. In terms of basic arithmetic skills, they reported evidence that processing speed, phonological processing, and attention were related to arithmetic ability. Working memory also emerged as a significant predictor, but only when reading and reading-related skills were omitted from the model. Some of the evidence relating working memory to arithmetic was reviewed above. Processing speed may be involved in arithmetic in terms of the speed with which numbers are counted; faster processing frees up cognitive resources and makes more efficient use of working memory. Bull and Johnston (1997) found that processing speed was a strong predictor of arithmetic skills in 7-year-olds, and Hecht, Torgesen, Wagner, and Rashotte (2001) found that processing speed was correlated with arithmetic skills even when controlling for language ability. Geary (1993) argued that phonological processing was important for arithmetic because successful computation requires the ability to create and maintain phonological representations. The evidence here is mixed, with Fuchs et al. (2005) finding that phonological processing was a unique predictor of arithmetic skills in a study of first-graders, whereas Swanson and Beebe-Frankenberger (2004) found that phonological processing did not determine arithmetic ability. Recent studies highlight the role of attention as a robust predictor of math skills. For example, Fuchs et al. (2005) found that teacher ratings of attention predicted arithmetic skills even when controlling for several other cognitive abilities. The question, of course, is exactly what teachers evaluate when they complete such scales; it may be that teachers are simply rating children according to academic competencies.

Fuchs et al. (2006b) also examined four attributes in children that may predict the ability to complete computations, which they termed "algorithmic computation" to represent the applications of procedural knowledge in which computations are completed by following a set of steps. Fuchs et al. (2005) found that teacher ratings of attention (i.e., distractibility) were a unique predictor of computation; paralleling findings were reported in other studies of children with ADHD (Ackerman, Anhalt, & Dykman,1986, Lindsay, Tomazic, Levine, & Accardo, 1999). Other research also implicates working memory and phonological processing for algorithmic problem solving (e.g., Hecht et al., 2001).

Finally, completing word problems that require arithmetic for a solution likely requires arithmetic skills as well as cognitive abilities connected to deciphering text. The major distinction between calculation and word problems is the addition of linguistic information, which requires children to construct a problem model. So whereas a calculation problem is already set up for solution, a word problem requires students to use the text to discern what information is missing, construct the number sentence, and derive the calculation problem for finding the missing information. Studies that address word problem solving also focus on working memory, language and reading ability, and different executive functions involving problem solving and concept formation. Thus, Desoete and Roeyers (2005) found evidence that a language factor involving semantic processing and a nonlanguage factor involving executive functions differentiated students with good and poor math problem-solving skills.

In an attempt to establish more formally the relation of numerical competencies involving arithmetic, algorithmic computation, and arithmetic word problems, Fuchs et al. (2006b) evaluated these three math competencies along with measures of language, nonverbal problem solving, concept formation, processing speed, long-term memory, working memory, phonological decoding, and sight word efficiency in a large sample of children in grade 3. They also obtained teacher ratings of inattention. A series of path analyses was used to test a model relating the three math competencies with different cognitive processes. Figure 8.2 depicts a final model, with unbolded lines indicating nonsignificant paths and bolded lines denoting significant predictors. The only attribute that independently predicted all three aspects of math performance was teacher ratings of inattention. In addition to inattention, phonological decoding and processing speed uniquely predicted arithmetic competency; nonverbal problem solving, concept formation, word reading efficiency, and language skills predicted competency in arithmetic word problems.

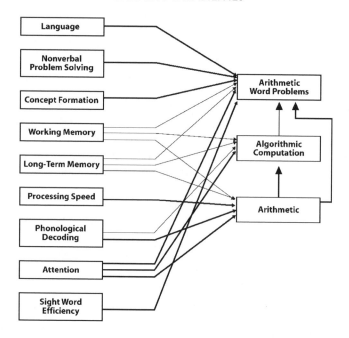

FIGURE 8.2. Path analysis of the relation of math competencies and cognitive correlates. Unbolded lines indicate nonsignificant paths. Significant predictors are in bold—for arithmetic: attentive behavior, phonological decoding, and processing speed; for algorithmic computation: arithmetic and attentive behavior; and for arithmetic word problems: arithmetic, attentive behavior, nonverbal problem solving, concept formation, sight word efficiency, and language. Although working memory was not a significant path in the overall model, it was a significant predictor of arithmetic and arithmetic word problems when the paths for reading and phonological processing were set to zero, suggesting that reading or reading-related processes may influence the relations between working memory and at least two aspects of math skill. From Fuchs et al. (2006b, p. 37). Copyright 2006 by the American Psychological Association. Reprinted by permission.

Subtypes of Math Disability

A final issue involves whether there are subtypes of math LD. To reiterate, there is clear evidence for a subset of children with LDs who have average word recognition skills and a general absence of phonological processing difficulties, but are markedly impaired in math computations. Such subgroups were empirically documented in a series of studies by Rourke and colleagues (Rourke & Finlayson, 1978; Rourke, 1993) and led to the current concept of nonverbal LDs (Rourke, 1989). The concept of nonverbal LDs is important because it suggests that some children with LDs have impairments in academic skills (i.e., math computations) due to impairments in core processes that are not based strictly in the language system and that lead to a variety of difficulties with math, social skills, and reading comprehension—a pattern quite different from WLRD. This is not to say that language is not involved in certain types of math capabilities or that children who read poorly invariably do well in math—neither view would be correct—but it highlights the older observation that some forms of LDs have less to do with the language system (Johnson & Myklebust, 1967).

Studies by Rourke (1993) and others compared groups based on patterns of word-reading, spelling, and math skills, representing LDs: (1) only in math but not reading; (2) in both math and reading; and (3) in reading but not math (see Figure 8.1). In Rourke's studies, those children with only low math performance demonstrated higher scores on auditory-verbal measures, those with poor reading and math showed problems in both domains, and those impaired only in reading had problems only in the verbal domain. In subsequent studies, there was support for distinctions of math and reading LDs based on these patterns (e.g., Ackerman & Dykman, 1995; Keller & Sutton, 1991; Morrison & Siegel, 1991).

Although these studies reveal the importance of considering the specificity and comorbidity of LDs, they do not permit an analysis of the mechanisms by which the cognitive marker skills influence mathematics learning. There are also hypothesized subtypes based on linkages of math competencies and cognitive processes. Geary (1993, 2004, 2005) identified three classes of problems based on different cognitive processes. The first, a semantic memory subtype, involves difficulties in learning, representing, and retrieving mathematics facts. These difficulties are often manifested in terms of slow, inaccurate, or inconsistent computational problem-solving abilities. In some instances, such children tend to use counting strategies because they do not appear to be able to retrieve a mathematics fact. The second, a procedural subtype, involves difficulties with concepts underlying different math procedures (such as understanding the base 10 system) and such children often use procedural strategies characteristic of younger children. Because these children use developmentally immature strategies and algorithms that are incorrectly applied to solve computational problems, Geary (2004) suggested that this group has a developmental delay in math skills. In contrast, the semantic memory subgroup is hypothesized to struggle because of a persistent deficit in math competencies. A third possible subtype involves spatial representation and manipulation of numerical information, representing a visual–spatial subtype. As the link of visual–spatial skills and math has not held up in research (Barnes et al., 2006; Cirino, Morris, & Morris, 2006; Geary et al., 2000; Rovet, Szekely, & Hockenberry, 1994), it is not further discussed here. Many children with specific MDs appear to have difficulties with visual–spatial processing, but efforts to link these difficulties specifically to mathematics competencies have yielded largely null results.

Geary (1993) hypothesized that difficulties with fact representation and retrieval were much more characteristic of individuals who have difficulties in both math and word recognition, which was supported by Robinson, Menchetti, and Torgesen (2002). Geary et al. (2000, 2004) found that in first grade, children with both mathematics and reading disabilities had problems with counting and number comprehension tasks. Problems with number comprehension did not characterize children with a specific mathematics disability, but these children had difficulties with counting knowledge in first and second grade. Furthermore, both types of children had more problems with counting procedures and retrieval of arithmetic facts in first grade. On tasks that were specifically designed to elicit retrieval errors, there was a clear tendency for children with comorbid reading and mathematics disabilities to have more difficulties than children with only an MD. Both these groups performed below the levels of children who had only a reading disability or no disability. What seemed to improve in math fact retrieval for children with procedural deficits was the type of strategies they used, leading Geary to hypothesize that procedural problems are delays, not deficits.

The idea that the two types of math difficulties represent distinct LDs with different kinds of math problems has not been supported by recent research in neurologically normal or brain-injured children (Barnes et al., 2006; Jordan, Hanich, & Kaplan, 2003b). Difficulties in representing and quickly retrieving mathematics facts, and problems in learning and implementing mathematics procedures do not appear to be orthogonal processes. In development, young children who experience mathematics difficulties commonly experience problems with both mathematics facts and procedural knowledge early in their schooling (Geary, Hoard, & Hamson, 1999; Geary et al., 2004). But these difficulties seem more a matter of severity and persistence than distinct math disorders. Although it is possible that the math problems in math LDs with and without word recognition problems are different, a more likely possibility is that LDs involving reading and math are comorbid—the cognitive correlates include those related to an MD and those related to a reading disability (RD). Furthermore, although basic reading abilities do predict achievement in mathematics, they do not add to the prediction of math outcomes at the end of grade 1 over and above measures of number sense at the beginning of kindergarten (Jordan, Kaplan, Olah, & Locuniak, 2006). As with other comorbid disorders, both the reading and the math problems are more severe when the disorders are comorbid. Deficits in math fact mastery in those who have both reading and math problems are not qualitatively different from those apparent when only math is a problem; that is, phonological deficits do *not* account for math fact problems in the comorbid group, and some other cognitive variable accounts for math fact problems in those with only math difficulties. Although children with reading and math difficulties may have particular problems with word problem solving because of their poor language and reading skills, comorbid and isolated math LDs on different math competencies are more similar than they are different and represent a continuum of severity as opposed to qualitatively different math LDs.

EPIDEMIOLOGY

Prevalence

MDs have been found to be about as prevalent as disabilities involving reading. In a review, Fleishner (1994) found that studies of the prevalence of math LDs have produced similar estimates. Earlier studies by Badian and Ghublikian (1983) and Norman and Zigmond (1980) reported that approximately 6% of school-age children have some form of LD in math. More recent studies give estimates of 5–6% (Shalev et al., 2000) and 3.6% (Lewis et al., 1994). The latter study broke prevalence into those who had only arithmetic disability (1.3%) and those with both arithmetic and reading disabilities (2.3%). These estimates contrasted with 3.9% for specific reading disabilities.

Most recent studies are European in origin, in which cutoff points tend to be more stringent (< 5th percentile) than in North American studies. A recent North American study (Barbaresi, Katusic, Colligan, Weaver, & Jacobsen, 2005) utilized three definitions of LDs in math (regression-based IQ–achievement discrepancy, unadjusted discrepancy of IQ and math achievement, and low achievement in math). The prevalence of math disability in this unselected birth cohort ranged from 5.9 to 13.8%, depending on the definition. Specific LDs in math that did not involve reading occurred in about one-third to one-half of the sample, depending on the definition. Fuchs et al. (2005), in a study of 564 first-graders, compared prevalence estimates based on 17 identification methods grouped into four categories: IQ–achievement discrepancy, low achievement with average IQ, and two categories tied to intervention response and growth over time that utilized benchmarks based on low achievement or change over time. Not surprisingly, prevalence estimates varied considerably within and across categories. Thus, definitions based on IQ–achievement discrepancy yielded a prevalence rate of 1.77%. A low achievement definition with a cut-point at the 10th percentile yielded a prevalence rate of 9.75%. The response to instruction method yielded prevalence of less than 1% if final low achievement was the benchmark and a standardized test was used, and 6–9% if the low achievement benchmark was derived from a curriculum-based assessment. Estimates based on both slope and low achievement yielded a prevalence rate of about 4%. The researchers emphasized the sources of variation, which reflected decisions about cut-points, the role of intervention, and the type of math skill that was assessed, as explaining the variability in prevalence estimates.

Gender Ratio

Most studies have not found gender differences in the prevalence of LDs in math (Shalev et al., 2000), although Barbaresi et al. (2005) did find male preponderance ratios of 1.6 to 2.2:1, depending on the definition. Because the latter study depended on access to records documenting a disability, there is always the possibility of bias in terms of who was referred for an evaluation. Spelke (2005) reviewed literature on gender differences in mathematical ability, failing to find differences between males and females in cognitive and neurobiological mechanisms at a variety of age levels.

DEVELOPMENTAL COURSE

A 3-year longitudinal study (grades 4–8) by Shalev, Manor, Auerbach, and Gross-Tsur (1998) reported that 47% of those with math disabilities in grade 5 met criteria for such disabilities (arithmetic scores 5th percentile) in grade 8. In a 6-year follow-up of this sample, Shalev, Manor, & Gross-Tsur (2005) found that 95% of those identified with math problems in grade 5 continued to perform in the bottom 25% of students in grade 11; 40% continued to meet the original definition of math disability (< 6th percentile). Thus, as in reading (S. E. Shaywitz et al., 1999), difficulties with math are persistent. Note that only 47% of students in grade 8 and 40% in grade 11 met the original definition, implying that students are moving in and out of disability categories. This phenomenon has also been observed in longitudinal studies of elementary school children (Gersten, Jordan, & Flojo, 2005; Mazzocco & Myers, 2003). The phenomenon is similar to that observed in studies of students with reading disabilities (Francis et al., 2005a; S. E. Shaywitz et al., 1992, 1999) and may simply represent the problems with the measurement error and the setting of a cut-point on a normal distribution observed in Chapter 3. As in reading, prevalence estimates of disabilities in math hinge on the definition and level of low achievement incorporated into the definition.

NEUROBIOLOGICAL FACTORS

Studies of adults with brain lesions show that fairly specific math skills can be lost or preserved, depending on the pattern of brain injury (Dehaene & Cohen, 1997). However, studies of either brain structure or brain function have not, to our knowledge, been carried out for children with LDs in math. Whether the development of math skills across different competencies can be fractionated in ways similar to those used in studies of adults with brain injury is not clear. Also emerging are studies of the familial segregation and heritability of math disability, which are reviewed in this section.

Brain Structure and Function

Acalculia

Research on the brain, math, and disorders of math has been driven by a model that focuses on the cross-species development of number sense that characterizes one of the theoretical orientations reviewed above. Developed initially by Dehaene, Spelke, Pinel, Staneseu, and Tsiukin (1999), it has continued to evolve (Dehaene et al., 2004). Feigenson, Dehaene, and Spelke (2004) characterized two core systems for representing numbers. One core system involves the ability to make approximations of numerical magnitude. This capability is observed early in development and across species (Dehaene et al., 2004). This system is eventually integrated with symbolic numerical systems supporting computation. The second system involves the ability to precisely represent distinct entities. This system involves small quantities, but is also apparent early in development and across species. At a neural level, Dehaene et al. (2004) summarized evidence suggesting that the intraparietal sulcus in both hemispheres is critically involved in approximate representations of number sense. Although Dehaene et al. (1999) hypothesized that exact representations would have more involvement with the left inferior frontal region and angular gyrus, identification of specific neural systems supporting exact calculation has proven elusive (Dehaene et al., 2004).

Studies of adults with acalculia seemed to support this distinction. To illustrate, Dehaene and Cohen (1997) described two patients with acalculia who experienced difficulties with calculations, but could read and write numbers. The first patient, who had a left subcortical lesion, had a selective problem in retrieving verbal knowledge that extended to arithmetic tables. In contrast, the second patient, who had a parietal lesion, had difficulties with multiple tasks involving numerical knowledge. Although knowledge of rote arithmetical facts was reserved, the patient had difficulty subtracting and completing number bisection tasks. The authors concluded that dissociable neural networks are involved in numerical knowledge. One network involves the left hemisphere, which contributes to the storage and retrieval of arithmetic facts. The second is a parietal network devoted to the ability to manipulate numerical quantities. These findings have been replicated in other studies (e.g., Lemer, Dehaene, Spelke, & Cohen, 2003).

Functional Neuroimaging

Functional imaging studies using PET and fMRI have also shown that the neural correlates of precise calculation and estimation/approximation may be different. Dehaene et al. (1999) found different imaging correlates for tasks that required exact answers and estimations. The former involved the inferior prefrontal cortex in the left hemisphere, as well as the left angular gyrus. These areas overlap substantially with those that mediate language functions. In contrast, estimation tasks showed bilateral activation in the inferior parietal lobes, which represent areas that overlap with spatial cognition and visual attention. Many children with LDs involving math have been found to have spatial cognition difficulties. This overlap in the neural representation of estimation and spatial cognition may help explain why the spatial processing difficulties do not seem to bear a strong relationship with math abilities in these children, but are often as profound as the math difficulties themselves. Any cognitive task that is sensitive to how these areas of the brain function will be deficient in children with a specific math disability, but this does not mean that the cognitive deficits themselves are tightly linked. What is not clear is whether the imaging correlates of children with both a math and reading disability differ when various math tasks are employed. These theories provide a strong basis for this research, and imaging work like that completed in WLRD is sorely needed.

Pediatric Brain Injury

Studies of populations with pediatric brain injury have been particularly useful in understanding math LDs. This is because many acquired brain disorders that affect children seem to produce subgroups in which reading is not affected, but math is severely impaired. For example, Turner syndrome is commonly characterized by intact word reading and poor math skills (Mazzocco, 2001). In a study of different arithmetic competencies, Bruandet, Molko, Cohen, and Dehaene (2004) found that the most significant differences between women with Turner syndrome and controls involved impairments in cognitive estimation, subitizing, and calculation. Difficulties were not apparent on tasks involving comprehension and production of numbers, oral counting, reading, and writing. Mazzocco (2001) also reported intact number processing and impaired arithmetic, and earlier studies found that multidigit calculation strategies were impaired in women with Turner syndrome (e.g., Rovet et al., 1994). Bruandet et al. (2004) interpreted this as a problem that affected regions of the brain in the parietal areas (i.e., intraparietal sulcus) known to be associated with numerical processing. In a subsequent study, Molko et al. (2004) completed structural MRIs on 14 patients with Turner syndrome and 14 controls. They found anomalies in a variety of brain areas, particularly in the intraparietal sulcus.

In studies of fragile X syndrome, boys tend to show generally deficient academic skills (Roberts et al., 2005), which is consistent with the higher rate of mental retardation in boys as compared with girls who have fragile X syndrome. Girls, however, are more likely to show specific math difficulties in the presence of intact intellectual and word reading skills (Keysor & Mazzocco, 2002). A functional imaging study of simple and complex arithmetic operations in females with fragile X found reduced activation in prefrontal and parietal brain regions that, unlike controls, did not differ for the two tasks (Rivera, Menon, White, Glaser, & Riess, 2002).

Simon, Bearden, Mc-Ginn, and Zackai (2005a) have studied math processing in children with velocardiofacial syndrome. They found difficulties in numerical magnitude judgment as well as on tasks involving visual attention orienting and enumeration. The difficulties could not be explained by global deficits in psychomotor speed. They related this pattern to deficiencies involving the posterior parietal lobe. Structural imaging studies of this disorder show reduced gray matter volumes in parietal and temporal regions, along with other white matter abnormalities across the brain (Zinkstok & van Amelsvoort, 2005). Simon et al. (2005b) used voxel-based morphometry to compare brain volumes in children with velocardiofacial syndrome and controls, finding especially marked reductions in gray matter volumes across a large segment of posterior brain regions, with increased gray matter in distinct regions of the frontal lobes. Diffusion tensor imaging showed lack of connectivity between the posterior aspect of the corpus callosum and posterior parietal regions.

In studies of children with spina bifida or hydrocephalus who have good word recognition skills and poor math ability, Barnes et al. (2002) found that those with spina bifida made more procedural errors than age-matched controls, but similar rates of math fact retrieval and visual–spatial errors. Furthermore, their procedural errors were similar to those of younger children who were matched in math ability with these older brain-injured children. Thus, children with hydrocephalus made errors in written computations that were developmentally immature for their age, but not different in kind from younger children with no math disability. These data are consistent with the hypothesis that children who are good at reading but poor at math can have a procedural deficit that involves the application of developmentally immature algorithms for solving written computations. In a more recent study of a large cohort of children with spina bifida myelomeningocele and hydrocephalus, children were classified into groups with reading decoding and math disability, only math disability, and no reading or math disability, and were compared with typically developing controls (Barnes et al., 2006). The researchers reported that visual–spatial errors in multidigit arithmetic were not more common in spina bifida; that deficits in accuracy, speed, and use of strategies in single-digit addition characterized both groups with math disability, regardless of reading ability; that phonological and visual–spatial abilities accounted for only a small amount of variance in math fact retrieval; and that accuracy and speed on single-digit addition were strong predictors of performance on tasks involving multidigit subtraction.

Different studies of adult and pediatric populations have converged in identifying the intraparietal sulcus as a region critical for the development of number sense (see Figure 8.3). In children, Issacs, Edmonds, Lucas, and Gadian (2001) found that the arithmetic computation difficulties that characterize many infants of very low birth weight were related to less development of gray matter in this region. The studies of children with velocardiofacial syndrome and Turner syndrome, and girls with fragile X syndrome, have also implicated this region of the brain, although the impairments are not restricted to this region. Altogether, these studies of children with early brain injury parallel studies of children with LDs in math, showing differences in subgroups who vary in reading skills. Although there do not appear to be any neuroimaging studies specifically addressing non-brain-injured children with math LDs, the studies of brain injury provide a risk base for study development.

Genetic Factors

As in reading disabilities, an emerging research base demonstrates heritable factors in math disabilities. However, in contrast to the findings for

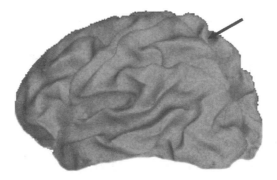

FIGURE 8.3. The left hemisphere of the human brain. The arrow represents the region around the intraparietal sulcus, a region bilaterally implicated in a variety of tasks involving numbers (Dehaene et al., 2004).

WLRD, specific genes have not yet been implicated. Math disabilities are more common in certain families. Gross-Tsur, Manor, and Shalev (1996) found that 10% of children with a specific math disability had at least one other family member who complained of difficulties with math. Another 45% had another type of LD. Those with a family history of math disabilities were more likely to have persistent difficulties in math. Shalev et al. (2001) found that prevalence of math disabilities was quite high in mothers (66%), fathers (40%), and siblings (53%) of probands with math disabilities. Shalev et al. concluded that the prevalence of math disabilities was about 10 times higher in those with family members who had math disabilities than in the general population.

Genetically sensitive studies of math are few in number and have focused on the comorbidity of reading and math disabilities, as well as specific math disabilities. In a twin study, Alarcon, DeFries, Light, and Pennington (1997) reported that 58% of monozygotic (MZ) twins shared a math disability, as compared with 39% of dizygotic twins. Knopik and DeFries (1999) found that genetic factors accounted for 83% of the shared variance between reading and math disabilities in a group of twins, as compared with 58% of the shared variance in a controlled group. The contribution of shared environmental influences was quite small. A recent study of 7-year-old twins in the TEDS study (Kovas, Harlaar, Petrill, & Plomin, 2005) reported that MZ twin correlations for math suggested substantial genetic influence and moderate environmental influence. The genetic correlations between math and reading were high, so that genes that predict individual differences in reading may also predict individual differences in math. This observation harks back to the discussion of general genes in WLRD in Chapter

5 (Plomin & Kovas, 2005). These findings suggest that genetic factors influence both reading and math disabilities. That there is substantial shared variance in heritability of reading and math disabilities is not surprising, given that many individuals tend to have problems in both areas. Plomin and Kovacs also observe evidence that math has independent genetic effects.

The comorbidity of ADHD and specific math disabilities has also been studied for a genetic perspective. Monuteaux, Faraone, Herzig, Navsaria, and Biederman (2005) reported that rates of ADHD were elevated in the relatives of children with ADHD regardless of the presence of math LDs. Similarly, rates of specific math LDs were elevated in relatives regardless of the presence of ADHD. The researchers concluded that math LDs and ADHD are independently transmitted and distant disorders. These findings are consistent with studies of the hereditability of LDs involving reading and ADHD (see Chapter 5).

SUMMARY: FROM ACADEMIC SKILL DEFICITS TO NEUROBIOLOGICAL FACTORS

As the Fuchs et al. study (2006b) demonstrates, the ability to link cognitive processes to LDs in math will require a multivariate approach with careful specification of the mathematic competencies and academic skill deficits that are involved in relation to multiple cognitive measures. In the reading area, such studies highlighted the unique relation of phonological processing and WLRD (Wagner et al., 1994). The distinction of math difficulties with and without reading problems needs to be maintained, if only because the math problems may be either qualitatively or quantitatively different in the two subgroups of math LD. Certainly, the interventions would be different, inasmuch as one group requires reading instruction and the other does not; the early predictors of later reading and math problems also appear to differ (Jordan et al., 2006). Thus, an important emphasis in research on math LDs is on the nature of the academic skill deficits because the cognitive correlates likely vary with different math competencies (Fuchs et al., 2006b). Particular emphasis should be placed on the role of inattention, as this is not an intuitive finding. The studies that have demonstrated strong relations to attention have relied on teacher ratings, but have not been completed with a strong cognitive model of attention. The application of such models may be illuminating, particularly because the neural basis for this type of inattention may represent a system in the posterior regions of the brain that overlaps with spatial processing, as well as with areas of the brain associated with numerical competencies (Dehaene et al., 2004; Simon et al., 2005a).

The neurobiological correlates of LDs in math are not well studied, but emerging, and there is a body of theory that will support these studies. Different parts of the brain appear to mediate different math skills, with the intraparietal sulcus commonly implicated as a region of interest in studies involving number sense and estimation. MDs have a significant heritable component, but specific genes have not been identified. The neural and genetic correlates are different from those that have been identified for reading, but there is overlap.

MATHEMATICS DISABILITIES INTERVENTIONS

Empirical Syntheses

Baker, Gersten, and Lee (2002) provided an empirical synthesis of the effects of interventions to improve the mathematics achievement of children considered learning disabled, low achieving in math, or at risk for math difficulties. They were able to find only 15 studies that met the methodological criteria for adequate rigor, including clear specification of low achievement in math. The results indicated that different interventions were associated with improvement in math achievement levels, especially (1) providing data on student performance to teachers and students (aggregated effect size; ES = 0.57); (2) peer tutoring (aggregated ES = 0.66); (3) providing feedback to parents on student achievement (aggregated ES = 0.42); and (4) explicit teaching of math concepts and procedures (aggregated ES = 0.58). Baker et al. noted that this was a small number of studies and that few explicitly included children with LDs. They called for more research on math intervention strategies, which does appear to be emerging.

Classroom Instruction

As with instruction in other content areas, the differentiated teaching of math skills should have the following characteristics: (1) the instruction takes place in groups; (2) it is teacher directed; (3) it is academically focused; and (4) it specifically takes into account individual student needs (Stevens & Rosenshine, 1981). Some basal or developmental programs used for students with LDs have many of these characteristics. For example, Connecting Mathematics Concepts (Engelmann, Carnine, Engelmann, & Kelly, 1991) is a basal program based on a behavioral/task-analytic model that is frequently used for primary- and elementary-age students with LDs. It contains highly structured lessons involving frequent teacher questions and student answers. A number of studies have demonstrated the efficacy of Direct Instruction approaches for math with students identified with LDs (Carnine, 1991). In a similar way, controlled studies on mathematics PALS documents the importance of explicit instruction targeting procedural skills as well as conceptual knowledge, with carefully guided peer-mediated practice. Such an approach can be used in general classrooms to improve outcomes for students with LDs, as well as their low-, average-, and high-performing classmates at kindergarten through grade 6 (e.g., Fuchs et al., 1997; Fuchs, Fuchs, & Karns, 2001b; Fuchs, Fuchs, Yazdian, & Powell, 2002b).

In addition to basal programs and specialized instructional programs, a number of classroom teaching techniques have been shown to be useful in helping students with LDs develop arithmetic and math concepts. For example, Rivera and Smith (1987), summarizing research on the value of modeling in teaching computational skills, found teacher demonstrations of calculation algorithms and higher-level procedural steps to be effective in increasing both computational and problem-solving behaviors in students. Lloyd (1980) tested the value of strategy training with students who are deficient in math skills. In this type of intervention, a task analysis of the relevant cognitive operation is demonstrated and explained to the students. When students have mastered the component skills, strategies are provided that help the students integrate the steps and apply them in different problem-solving contexts. Finally, cognitive-behavioral models of intervention have given rise to the development of self-instructional strategy techniques to help guide students with LDs through a variety of problem-solving contexts (Hallahan et al., 1996). A key component in this type of technique is to teach a student first to verbalize the steps that should be used in solving a particular math problem. Once the student has mastered the application of the problem-solving algorithm, the student is taught to self-instruct, but using subvocal directions. This type of technique has been shown to be useful with both elementary-age students (Lovitt & Curtiss, 1968) and adolescents (Seabaugh & Schumaker, 1993).

Tutorial Interventions

Fact Retrieval and Procedural Mathematics

Most previous intervention work for students with LDs in math focuses on lower-order skills, including fact retrieval and procedural mathematics (i.e., multidigit computation). This research provides guidance on how to structure effective remediation, which includes explicit explanations, pictorial or concrete representations, verbal rehearsal with fading, intensive timed practice on mixed problem sets, cumulative review of previously mastered skills, and self-regulation strategies.

With respect to explicit explanations, pictorial representations, verbal rehearsal with fading, intensive timed practice on mixed problem sets, and cumulative review, research substantiates benefits to student outcomes. For example, Fuchs and colleagues cumulatively designed and tested a set of instructional components for enhancing students' math competence involving fact retrieval (Fuchs et al., 1997; Fuchs, Fuchs, Phillips, Hamlett, & Karns, 1995) and procedural math (i.e., multidigit computation and estimation) (Fuchs et al., 2001b; Fuchs, Fuchs, Yazdian, & Powell, 2002b). Effects were assessed separately for students with LDs and students not identified with LDs who had low, average, and high initial achievement status. For students throughout the primary and intermediate grades, a combination of (1) explicit, procedurally clear, conceptually based explanations, (2) pictorial representations of the math, (3) verbal rehearsal with gradual fading, and (4) timed practice on mixed problem sets, which systematically provided cumulative review of previously mastered problem types, resulted in statistically significant effects across all four types of learners (learning disabled, low achieving, average achieving, and high achieving). Effect sizes ranged from 0.35 to 1.27.

This set of instructional principles was incorporated into an expert system, which was tested experimentally among 33 teachers who provided math instruction to students with LDs in grades 2–8 (Fuchs et al., 1991b). The focus of the study was procedural math, which represented a deficient area for all participating students with LDs. Teachers were assigned to three 20-week conditions: (1) ongoing, systematic assessment of student growth with descriptive profiles of students' strengths/weaknesses; (2) ongoing, systematic assessment of student growth with descriptive profiles of students' strengths/weaknesses plus use of an expert system incorporating task analyses for supplying clear explanations, pictorial representations, verbal rehearsal with fading, recommendations for instruction, and intensive timed practice that featured cumulative review with mixed problem sets; and (3) best practices controls. The results indicated that only the expert system condition effected superior learning, providing additional evidence for the effectiveness of this combination of instructional principles.

With respect to self-regulation strategies, studies demonstrate the contribution of ongoing monitoring of performance with student goal setting and feedback on fact retrieval and procedural math. For example, Fuchs, Bahr, and Rieth (1989a) randomly assigned 20 students with LDs who had a math fact retrieval deficit to self-selected versus assigned goals and to contingent versus noncontingent game play—all within the context of computer-mediated fact retrieval drill and practice. Performance was assessed prior to and following a 3-week treatment. Results indicated stronger learning for students who selected their own goals than for those who were assigned goals, with an effect size of 0.68. No differences were found between the contingency conditions.

Using similar methods, Fuchs, Fuchs, Hamlett, and Whinnery (1991c) examined the effects of student feedback. Twice weekly for 20 weeks, students completed math procedures tests on a computer and immediately received feedback. Each special educator ($n = 20$) identified two students with LDs who experienced chronic procedural math difficulties: One student was assigned to see a graph of performance over time, with a goal line superimposed over the graph, and the other student saw the graph without the goal line. Goal line feedback was associated with greater performance stability, with an effect size of 0.70. As these studies illustrate, engaging students in the monitoring of their own performance as they work via computer on math fact retrieval and procedural math provides substantial benefit.

Problem Solving

Most treatment research for students with LDs has focused on math fact retrieval and algorithmic computation (e.g., Cawley, Parmar, Yan, & Miller, 1998; Harris, Miller, & Mercer, 1995). At the same time that students acquire competence with foundational math skills, an additional challenge will be to improve their application of those skills to problem-solving situations (Catrambone & Holyoak, 1989). Toward that end, some attention has been allocated to arithmetic word problems, which exclude irrelevant information, keep syntactic structure straightforward, and require one-step solutions.

To promote competence with arithmetic word problems, Case, Harris, and Graham (1992) assessed the effects of self-regulated strategy development among four students with LDs. They found that overall performance improved, with less probability of applying the wrong operation, but that only two of the four students maintained effects. Hutchinson (1993) corroborated short-term effects of this sort of cognitive strategy instruction (see also Montague, Applegate, & Marquard, 1993).

Another line of work substantiates the value of concrete materials and diagrams in helping elementary-age students with LDs master arithmetic word problems (e.g., Jitendra & Hoff, 1996; Mercer & Miller, 1992). Jitendra et al. (1998) also tested and showed the value of combining diagrams with methods designed to induce schemas. Little attention, however, has been focused on math problem solving as it appears in school curricula, where problems are more varied and complex than arithmetic word problems. This more complex form of mathematical problem solving incorporates irrelevant information and more varied syntactic structures, with many problems requiring two or more computational steps and other related math skills, like computing halves or reading graphs, for solution.

This lack of attention to math problem solving, which is especially the case at the primary grades, is unfortunate on three counts. First, for students with LDs, the critical outcome of schooling in math is problem solving, as it occurs in the real world. Second, research with typical students reveals the challenges associated with effecting math problem solving. Researchers cannot assume that interventions designed to promote success with arithmetic word problems will translate into improved math problem solving (Catrambone & Holyoak, 1989). Finally, despite severe challenges with foundational mathematical skills (Jordan & Hanich, 2000), waiting for mastery of those foundational skills before beginning to develop math problem-solving competence may create math problem-solving deficits that are impossible to address later in school.

To address this gap in the literature, Fuchs and colleagues have focused on math problem solving at grade 3. This work falls into two categories. One strand of research has been conducted classwide in general education settings, exploring the effects of innovative math problem-solving treatments on students who enter grade 3 with varying achievement histories: LDs as well as low, average, and high initial math achievement. The second category of research examines the effects of tutoring treatments to enhance math problem solving among students with LDs. In both lines of work, the instruction has been explicit and systematic. That is, the teacher begins with worked examples illustrating the problem solution rules targeted for a particular problem type. The teacher explains the solutions in the worked examples and displays a poster listing the steps of a solution strategy. Moving to partially worked examples, with one step of the solution missing, the teacher asks students to complete the solution and then debriefs the activity, with students explaining their work and the teacher providing corrective feedback. Gradually, the teacher provides increasing opportunities for students to contribute more and more of the solutions to sample problems. Next, the teacher pairs higher- and lower-achieving students so they can help each other to complete entire problems and, as problems are completed, the teacher reviews solutions with correct feedback. Before the completion of each lesson, students complete problems independently, with teacher-led debriefing, and receive homework assignments. Instruction is clear and concise, with many opportunities for students to participate through choral and individual responding in the whole-class portions of the lessons and through peer interventions. Moreover, as mastery of the problem types is accomplished, cumulative review is routinely provided.

This form of explicit, systematic, scaffolded instruction is applied not only to instruction on problem solution rules but also when instruction is designed to enhance transfer. Theoretically, the instructional approach is based on schema theory. With schema theory, math problem solving is deemed a form of transfer because students are solving problems they have never seen before. To achieve this transfer, three kinds of development are required (Cooper & Sweller, 1987). First, for any given problem type, students must master the problem solution rules. Second, students must develop schemas—or generalized descriptions of two or more problems—which individuals use to sort problems into groups requiring similar solutions (Gick & Holyoak, 1980). The broader the schema, the greater the probability that individuals will recognize connections between familiar and novel problems (Cooper & Sweller, 1987). Third, students must be vigilant for the connections between teaching and transfer (Gick & Holyoak, 1980).

Salomon and Perkins (1989) provided a framework for broadening schemas and evoking independent searches for connections between novel and familiar tasks. With this framework, schemas provide the bridge from one context to the other, and metacognition is the conscious recognition and effortful application of that schema. Salomon and Perkins (1989) asserted that this framework represents an untapped instructional opportunity for explicitly teaching students to transfer.

CLASSROOM STUDIES

In addressing math problem solving at the third grade, Fuchs et al. (2003a, 2003b) operationalized Cooper and Sweller (1987) and Salomon and Perkins's (1989) frameworks: teaching problem solution rules, familiarizing students with the notion of transfer, teaching them to build schemas by showing how superficial problem features change without altering problem solution rules, and cautioning students to search novel-looking problems to recognize superficial problem features and thereby identify familiar problem types for which solutions are known. In a series of studies conducted classwide, Fuchs et al. (2003a) used this framework to explicitly teach students to transfer for math problem solving. Classrooms were assigned randomly to four study conditions: (1) teacher-designed instruction; (2) word-problem solution instruction (20 sessions); (3) word-problem solution instruction + explicit transfer instruction (20 sessions: half as much problem rule instruction to control for time); and (4) word-problem solution instruction + explicit transfer instruction (30 sessions with full doses of both components). Instruction was delivered in a whole-class arrangement over 16 weeks with strong fidelity. Effects were assessed on immediate, near, and far transfer on complex math problem-solving measures, with condition as a between-classroom variable, and student type (high, average, low) as a within-classroom variable. Effects were also explored for students with LDs ($n = 30$). Results showed that problem rule instruction was sufficient to improve performance on problems very similar to those used in intervention; that transfer instruction was necessary to enhance performance on less similar problems; and that for students with LDs and other low-performing students, the full dose of both components was most effective. For students without disability, effect sizes for the best condition (4) were 1.82 for immediate transfer, 2.25 for near transfer, and 1.16 for far transfer. For students with LDs, effect sizes for the best condition (also 4) were 1.78 for immediate transfer, 1.18 for near transfer, and 0.45 for far transfer.

To strengthen this prevention treatment, the contribution of self-regulation strategies was assessed in a subsequent study (Fuchs et al., 2003b). Classrooms were assigned randomly to three 16-week conditions: (1) teacher-designed instruction; (2) explicit transfer instruction (which included teaching rules for problem solutions); and (3) explicit transfer instruction (including teaching rules for problem solutions) + self-regulated learning strategies (graphing and monitoring performance and goal setting). Treatment fidelity was strong. Effects were assessed on immediate, near, and far transfer on complex word problem measures, with condition as a between-classroom variable, and student type (high, average, low) as a within-classroom variable. Effects were also explored for students with LDs ($n = 40$). Results supported the effectiveness of the combined treatment (3). Across all student types, effect sizes for the combined treatment were 2.81 on immediate transfer, 2.43 on near transfer, and 1.81 on far transfer. For students with LDs, effects on the three measures were 1.43, 0.95, and 0.58, respectively.

TUTORING

A second line of math problem-solving intervention research involving complex problems uses tutoring. Fuchs and colleagues have examined the effects of the schema-based explicit transfer approach to classroom-level math problem-solving intervention when the treatment is delivered in small-group tutoring. The goal is to remediate existing deficits among fourth-grade students with LDs in math, while exploring the potential for computer-assisted instruction to enhance effects (Fuchs, Fuchs, Hamlett, & Appleton, 2002a).

Stratifying by resource teacher/class, students were assigned randomly to (1) checking/labeling work (control); (2) checking/labeling work + computer-assisted practice on "far-transfer task"; (3) checking/

labeling work + small-group explicit tutoring on problem solutions rules and transfer; or (4) checking/labeling work + computer-assisted practice on "far-transfer task" + small-group explicit tutoring on problem solution rules and transfer. Instruction was delivered for 16 weeks with strong fidelity. Effects were assessed on immediate-, near-, and far-transfer word problem measures. Results documented the effectiveness of small-group tutoring on immediate and near transfer. On far transfer, moderate effects were revealed, but without statistical significance. Interestingly, findings revealed that computer work added little when small-group tutoring was in place. Effect sizes for tutoring versus control ranged from 0.64 to 2.10; for computer versus control, 0.51 to 0.64; for tutoring versus computer, −1.60 to 0.05 on far transfer; and for tutoring versus tutoring + computer, −0.03–0.14.

To extend this work, Fuchs et al. (2004) described responsiveness to the classroom-level schema-based treatment as a function of LDs subgroup: math disability, reading disability, or math and reading disability. Classrooms were assigned randomly to validated prevention or control (i.e., teacher-designed instruction) conditions. Instruction was delivered in a whole-class arrangement over 16 weeks with strong fidelity. Effects were assessed on immediate- and near-transfer math problem-solving measures, using performance dimension (problem solving, computation, communication) as a within-subjects variable and treatment condition as a between-subjects variable. All LD subgroups improved less than nondisabled students on computation and communication. However, only students with both reading and math disability improved less than nondisabled students on problem-solving accuracy.

To gain some insight into the relative role that reading versus math deficits play in the differentially poor problem-solving capacity of the students with reading and math disabilities, Fuchs et al. (2004) also conducted exploratory regression analyses. Results suggested that the multidigit computational deficits of these students explain a greater proportion of variance in responsiveness to problem-solving treatment than do reading comprehension deficits.

CONCLUSIONS

Children with LDs involving math are often represented in two distinct groups, depending on the presence of WLRD. However, the math problem—like the reading problem when both reading and math are involved—may be comorbid. The differences may be a matter of degree, inasmuch as the difficulties of children with both reading and math problems tend to be more severe in all academic areas (Jordan, Hanich, & Kaplan,

2003a; Rourke & Finlayson, 1978). It is critical to study different math competencies in children with both types of disabilities. Although mathematical computations may represent the primary academic skill deficit for identification of LDs in math, this is not a uniform continuum of proficiency. Resolution of definition issues depends on more systematic assessments of math competencies across subgroups of math-impaired children, especially in relation to different cognitive and neurobiological correlates.

A variety of cognitive processes are impaired in children with LDs in math, including working memory, language, inattention, and other child attributes. How these cognitive processes relate to different math competencies should be a focus for research. Neurobiological studies implicate different neural systems in association with different math competencies, especially in children and adults who sustain some form of injury to the brain. Such studies represent fertile sources of hypotheses for studies of math LDs in children without brain injury, but these studies are only emerging. However, in such populations, there is strong evidence for the heritability of math difficulties and for similarities and dissociations in the genetic loci of reading and math disabilities.

Our review of interventions for students with LDs in math shows that effective interventions are emerging for deficits in both foundational skills and higher-order skills involving problem solving. As in interventions for deficits in reading and writing, interventions for MDs often include not only "skills" instruction, but also explicit instruction in strategies that include a focus on self-regulation. In addition, many of the research studies specifically address the importance of transfer to the classroom environment, as well as broader environments that involve the application of academic skills. Given the evidence reviewed throughout this chapter for the efficacy of research-based intervention, the next set of questions concerns the translation of these kinds of interventions into practice.

CHAPTER 9

Written Expression Disabilities

Disorders involving the writing process have been discussed since Ogle (1867) used the term "agraphia" to distinguish an acquired writing disorder from aphasia, an acquired language disorder, indicating that the two disorders were dissociable. In the first half of the 20th century, Goldstein (1948), Head (1926), and others applied clinical observation and case study methodology to explore the association and dissociation between written and oral expression, but generally concluded that writing depended on speech and must therefore have similar neural correlates. As we discuss below, this hypothesis has not held up over time.

In aphasiology, reading and writing are distinguished by alexia, an acquired reading disorder, and agraphia, which may occur with or without alexia depending on the lesional pattern (Roeltgen, 2003). Both the alexias and agraphias have multiple subdivisions reflecting breakdowns in both overlapping and nonoverlapping components of written language and do not always occur with aphasia (Ralph & Patterson, 2005). However, the range of impairments is generally much greater in acquired than developmental disorders; the overlap of acquired and developmental disorders is not strong (Romani, Olson, & Betta, 2005). Patterns of impairment are not as distinct in developmental as in acquired disorders, with developmental disorders reflecting disruptions of development that have effects on subsequently developing skills. In contrast, acquired disorders are usually identified in adults who sustain relatively discrete lesions; even children with acquired disorders show much less distinct dissociations, again because the injury impacts a developing process (Dennis, 1988).

In developmental disorders of reading and writing that do not have a lesional basis, problems with spelling often accompany WLRD, but problems with handwriting and composition can occur in the absence of WLRD. Spelling and word reading are linked by problems involving phonological processing (Berninger, 2004). In a similar vein, Wong (1991) argued that deficits in written expression are frequently associated with reading disorders because of shared impairments that extend beyond phonological processing. Reading comprehension and composition, in particular, may be influenced by similar metacognitive processes, including planning, self-monitoring, self-evaluation, and self-modification. However, a variety of childhood disorders are associated with disorders of written expression in the absence of WLRD, including nonverbal learning disabilities (Rourke, 1989), oral language disorders (Bishop & Clarkson, 2003), and ADHD (Barkley, 1997).

Berninger (2004) argued that studies of acquired and developmental disorders of written expression support the dissociation of the two processes. Similarly, Abbott and Berninger (1993) found that written expression could not be explained just by oral expression; receptive written language ability always contributed uniquely to compositional ability. Berninger et al. (2006) compared the interrelations of listening comprehension, oral expression, reading comprehension, and written expression in a large sample of elementary school children in grades 1, 3, and 5. They found only moderate correlations among the four domains and that different neuropsychological tasks differentially predicted each domain, again suggesting that they are dissociable.

However, studies of written expression have not followed the lead of studies on math disabilities, and often do not separate children according to specific writing disabilities versus comorbidity with other LDs. This issue has hampered definitional efforts, so that the classification of disorders of written expression has lagged behind that of reading and math disabilities. There are still no clear operational definitions that address all components of the written language domain (see Berninger, 2004). Although the view that deficits in written expressions invariably co-occur with WLRD has not held up, emergent research on written language indicates that most children with LDs have problems with at least one academic skill in writing, whether it is handwriting, spelling, or written discourse (Hooper et al., 1994). Given the complexity of the writing process and the fact that it is the last language domain to develop in children (Johnson & Myklebust, 1967; Hooper et al., 1994), it should not be surprising that deficits in written expression can co-occur with deficits in oral language, reading, and mathematics. But it is not clear whether written language disorders are simple expressions of common underlying processes, as in the relation of word reading and spelling in children with WLRD, or represent additional, independent disorders.

A critical definitional issue relates to what is specific about disorders of written expression. In particular, is there a prototype for an isolated written expression disorder, or for academic skill deficits involving handwriting (likely), spelling (infrequently), and composition (not known)? In adults, writing difficulties often reflect an inability to spell that, even when remediated, is closely associated with difficulties in word recognition (Rourke, 1993). Some children with specific MDs have difficulty with handwriting, often because they have impairments in their motor development. Their spelling errors, interestingly, are typically phonetically constrained, in contrast to those of children who have word recognition difficulties (Rourke, 1993). Once these two difficulties (spelling and motor skills) are taken into account, is there a subgroup of children whose difficulties are restricted to composing? The classification research that is necessary to evaluate this hypothesis has not been completed, but there is some evidence for this possibility. In particular, some children have specific problems with handwriting and respond to preventative interventions (Graham, Harris, & Fink, 2000). Future research should target this possible subgroup in an effort to identify a prototype.

ACADEMIC SKILL DEFICITS

Despite difficulties with definition and the question of prototypes with isolated difficulties, progress has been made in understanding the academic skill deficits associated with written expression. Writing difficulties can involve problems with handwriting, spelling, and/or composition—the expression of ideas at the level of text. Berninger (2004) differentiated the "transcription" component of writing from its "generational" component. The transcription component involves the production of letters and spelling, which are necessary to translate ideas into a written product. The generational component translates ideas into language representations that must be organized, stored, and then retrieved from memory.

Over the past decade, progress has been made in research in both areas, although there has been more focus on the transcription than the generational component. This progress reflects in part the fact that transcription is specific to the writing process, whereas the generational component is applicable to many aspects of language and thought. Nonetheless, the transcription and generational components are closely linked. Just as word recognition problems constrain reading comprehension, problems with handwriting and spelling constrain composing. Graham, Berninger, Abbott, Abbott, and Whitaker (1997) conducted a structural modeling study of different measures of handwriting fluency, spelling, and composition in a sample of 600 children in grades 1–6. Handwriting fluency predicted compositional fluency and quality in primary and intermediate grades; handwriting fluency and spelling predicted compositional fluency in the primary grades. Across the age range, these latent variables accounted for 41–66% of the variance in compositional fluency and 25–42% in compositional quality. The researchers concluded that the transcription component of writing constrains the amount and quality of the generation component.

There are methods for assessing handwriting, spelling, and composition, although specific tests are not as well developed as many experts would desire. For handwriting, qualitative assessments of legibility of the writing sample are often employed. Spelling tests that involve the dictation of single words are common, but how the items are organized in terms of different orthographic conventions as well as the number of items at different levels of ability are often viewed as weaknesses. It is also possible to score spelling errors in context. Composition is usually evaluated through coding systems that require judgments about specific components of the written narrative. The Test of Written Language (Hammil & Larsen, 2003), which uses a spontaneous writing sample in response to complex pictures, represents a formal, published test; many approaches that involve the scoring of narratives are used in research. Interestingly, handwriting fluency is an effective predictor of composition, note taking, and other written language tasks in adults (Peverly, 2006). In a series of studies of elementary and middle school children, Berninger and colleagues (Berninger, 2004; Graham et al., 1997) found that a test involving printing of the lowercase letters of the alphabet as fast as possible for 15 seconds predicts a variety of written expression outcomes. Thus, transcription and generation are closely related. However, the core cognitive correlates of LDs in written expression vary, depending on the academic skill deficits used to define the writing problem.

CORE COGNITIVE PROCESSES

Handwriting

Berninger and her associates (Berninger, 1994, 2004; Berninger & Hart, 1993) and Graham and colleagues (Graham et al., 2000; Graham, Weintraub, & Berninger, 2001) reported that automaticity in the retrieval and production of alphabet letters, rapid coding of orthographic information, and speed of sequential finger movements were the best predictors of handwriting skills. Automaticity of handwriting predicted compositional fluency and quality. A deficit in fine motor skills also constrained handwriting, especially in the beginning stages of writing,

which may be why sequential motor movement is related to letter production and legibility (Berninger, 2004). Handwriting is more than a
motor act, so that knowledge of orthography and planning ability also
contribute to handwriting (and spelling) proficiency.

Spelling

Spelling abilities are predicted by language skills involving phonological
and orthographic mappings and motor skills, especially visual–motor
integration (Berninger, 2004). Because writing involves a mechanical act,
it is not surprising that assessments of the motor system predict spelling
abilities. Some controversy has arisen over whether phonological and orthographic processes are independent and whether orthographic processing can be reliably measured as a separate process (Vellutino,
Scanlon, & Tanzman, 1994). Romani et al. (2005) argued that spelling
development reflects two processes, one involving phonological processing at a sublexical level and the other representing a problem with stor-
ing adequate orthographic relations as a lexical pattern that leads to significant difficulties in the accurate spelling of irregular words. Romani et
al. (2005) questioned whether the lexical problem was due to problems
with (1) visual processing or (2) difficulties in creating lexical representations that reflect problems at a phonological and/or orthographic level
growing out of the language system.

The need for phonological representations of words for spelling is
obvious. Even in English, the phonological system is more predictive of
word spellings than is commonly understood, especially if the historical
origins of words are considered (Moats, 2005). Beyond alphabetic languages, writing in logographic languages like Chinese highlights the importance of orthographic and syntactic processes in spelling. Tan et al.
(2005) showed that learning to read in Chinese was strongly related to
the ability to write in Chinese. The relation of phonological awareness
to reading and writing was weaker in Chinese than in an alphabetic language. Tan et al. (2005) found that writing Chinese characters depends
on two interacting mechanisms: one involving orthographic awareness
that links visual, phonological, and semantic systems, the other involving motor programs that allow for the storage and retention of the characters. Across languages, those with more transparent relations of phonology and orthography seem to produce less severe difficulties with
word reading accuracy, but the spelling and fluency problems are more
marked, which suggests that the phonological and orthographic components of spelling (and word reading) are dissociable (Caravolas, 2005).

Linguistic skills involving both phonological and orthographic processes seem important at even the earliest development of spelling abili-

ties. Apel, Wolter, and Masterson (2006) examined the impact of phono-logical and orthographic processes on learning to spell. They found that young children quickly mapped orthographic information on letter patterns with minimal exposure to novel words. Letter patterns in the novel words that occurred more frequently were learned more easily, just as phonological information that occurred more frequently was mapped more rapidly. In concluding that both phonological and orthographic processes were important for spelling, Apel et al. (2006) countered other explanations for the relation of these processes in spelling that suggested that orthographic representations were simply mapped onto phonologi-cal representations (Treiman & Kessler, 2005).

Composition

Johnson and Myklebust (1967) presented a developmental model of lan-guage learning that posited that the ability to write is dependent on ade-quate development in listening, speaking, and reading, thus highlighting the link between different language skills and composition. Another do-main that seems critical involves executive functions. Hooper, Swartz, Wakely, de Kruif, and Montgomery (2002) documented a role of execu-tive functions in disorders of written expression. Controlling for level of decoding ability, comparisons of good and poor writers (identified on the basis of evaluations of narrative text) showed that poor writers had particular difficulties on measures involving initiating responses and shifting response set. De La Paz, Swanson, and Graham (1998) found that the difficulties experienced in revising written text by older (eighth-grade) students with writing problems were due in part to executive con-trol issues. However, mechanical difficulties also contributed to these problems with revision. In a study of note taking and report writing in third- and fourth-grade children, Altmeier, Jones, Abbot, and Berninger (2006) found that a measure of inhibition was a strong predictor of note taking, along with other reading and writing measures; for report writ-ing, measures of planning and fluency were among the best predictors. In examining different handwriting modes in third- and fifth-grade chil-dren, Berninger et al. (2006) found that inhibition and set switching were effective predictors. Obviously, the transcription and generation components must interact for an individual to produce high-quality written text. However, the role of executive functions in terms of plan-ning and organizing written expression at the level of handwriting and composition is clearly apparent and has had significant influence on the development of interventions in the written expression area (see below).

Attempting to link the language and executive function domains, Hooper et al. (1994) conceptualized writing as a complex problem-solving process reflecting the writer's declarative knowledge, procedural knowledge, and conditional knowledge, all of which are subserved by a network of neuropsychological factors, personality factors, and other conditions (including teacher–student relationships, amount of writing instruction, and the teacher's knowledge of the writing process). Within this context, "declarative knowledge" refers to the specific writing and spelling subskills that the learner has acquired, whereas "procedural knowledge" refers to the learner's competence in using such knowledge while writing for meaning. Similarly, Berninger (2004) suggested that neuropsychological, linguistic, and higher cognitive constraints may be recursive throughout the development of the writing process, but that each of these constraints may exert relatively more influence at different points in the developmental process (Hooper et al., 1994).

Subtypes of Written Expression LDs

The multivariate nature of the developmental writing process suggests that disorders in written language can be referable to multiple etiologies spanning biological, genetic, psychosocial, and environmental causes. Indeed, consider that in order to express thoughts in writing, one must formulate the idea; sequence relevant points in appropriate order; ensure that the written output is syntactically and grammatically correct; spell individual words correctly; and express the words, sentences, and passages in a legible manner via the graphomotor system. Given this multidimensional nature of the writing process, multiple-cause models for deficits in writing are the rule. For example, Gregg (1991) reported that a variety of language-based deficits in phonology and word retrieval could impair several aspects of the writing task, as could deficits in visual–spatial skills and problems with executive functions (including organization, planning, and evaluating). Similarly, Roeltgen (2003) proposed that deficits in linguistic, visual–spatial, and motor systems can interfere with the developmental writing process in distinct ways. The idea is that subtypes will emerge based on the stage or component of the writing process at which a breakdown occurs.

More recent studies have specifically examined written expression subtypes using empirical approaches to classification (see Chapter 5). Sandler et al. (1992) used cluster analysis to identify subtypes based on teacher responses to a questionnaire rating children on different cognitive skills. In addition, teachers rated student performance on a variety of dimensions involving writing, including legibility, mechanics, rate, and spelling. The sample largely included students with writing disorders ($n = 105$), but also included controls without writing disorders ($n = 56$). The cluster analysis yielded four writing disorder subtypes: (1) writing difficulties with both fine motor and linguistic deficits; (2) writing difficulties with predominantly visual-spatial deficits; (3) writing difficulties with attention and memory difficulties; and (4) writing difficulties characterized by sequencing problems. Most of the children were characterized by the first two subtypes.

Wakely, Hooper, de Kruif, and Schwartz (2006) evaluated 262 grade 4–5 students. Most of these students were viewed as typical achievers, with about 15% identified with an unspecified learning disability. The measures used with the cluster analysis included narrative writing assessments scored for the quality of written expression. Although assessments of the transcription component of writing were not included, the narratives were scored for grammar, semantics, and spelling. A reading comprehension measure was included as a classification attribute. For external validation, three self-report instruments were used, including measures of metacognitive awareness about writing, self-efficacy for writing, and self-regulated writing. Using a variety of procedures to ensure reliability and validity of the subtypes, six subtypes emerged, including (1) average writers; (2) poor writers with low semantics; (3) poor writers with low grammar; (4) expert writers; (5) poor writers with low spelling and reading; and (6) writers with poor quality of text. External validation studies based on the three indices reliably discriminated the four large subtypes, with the sample size too low to include the low grammar and low spelling-reading subtypes in the analysis. There were essentially two subtypes that showed normal variation in the writing process. The largest writing disability subtype, which composed a quarter of the sample, was characterized by difficulties in the quality of their narratives, but this subtype had a relatively low number of errors involving syntax, semantics, and spelling. Thus, this subtype appears to be relatively specific to composition, with the other subtypes demonstrating problems that occur on a more mechanical level. The strength of this approach is the focus on narrative productions and the attention to issues involving internal/external validity. Future research should continue to examine subtype variation, but would benefit from more specific assessments of the transcription component.

EPIDEMIOLOGY

Prevalence

Few epidemiological studies of disorders in written expression have been carried out (Hooper et al., 1994), which would be difficult inasmuch as the specific academic skill deficits of this type of LD are not well-established. Thus, the DSM-IV (American Psychiatric Association, 1994) explained that the prevalence rates for such disorders are difficult to establish, because "many studies focus on the prevalence of Learning Disorders in general without careful separation into specific disorders of reading, mathematics, or written expression. Disorder of Written Expression is rare when not associated with other Learning Disorders" (p. 52).

Basso, Taborelli, and Vignolo (1978) reported that acquired disorders of written expression occurred infrequently, at a rate of approximately 1 in every 250 people. For developmental disorders, Berninger and Hart (1992) found incidence rates of 1.3–2.7% for handwriting, about 4% for spelling, and 1–3% for written expression in a sample of 300 elementary school children. Hooper et al. (1993) evaluated the prevalence of composition problems in an epidemiological sample of 1,274 middle schoolers, finding rates of 6–22% with scores one standard deviation below average (about the 15th percentile) on the narrative subtest of the Test of Written Language; the variability reflected different sociodemographic factors, with higher rates in boys and minorities. Given the high rate of developmental language disorders in the general population (8–15%) and the significantly high rate of disorders in basic reading skills (10–15% of the general population), one could predict that written language disorders affect at least 10% of the school-age population, depending, as always, on the criteria used to define the LDs.

Gender Ratio

Berninger and Fuller (1992) and Hooper et al. (1993) reported that more boys than girls (about 1.5:1) displayed written language deficits when level of achievement was used as the comparison variable. In contrast, Berninger and Hart (1992) found no differences in gender ratio when IQ–achievement discrepancy criteria were used. Clearly, both the amount and accuracy of epidemiological data are lacking, particularly in comparison to studies of oral language and reading.

DEVELOPMENTAL COURSE

There are few, if any, studies of long-term outcomes in children identified specifically with disorders of written expression; we were not able to identify systematic long-term studies of written expression outcomes in a group specifically identified with LDs involving written expression. Most studies focus on children identified with language and reading problems, often reporting that writing problems are persistent (Bruck, 1987). In a recent study, Connelly, Campbell, Maclean, and Barnes (2006) found that college students identified with dyslexia had writing difficulties because of problems with handwriting speed and spelling in context. Addressing written expression in an unselected sample, Berninger et al. (2006) found that individual differences in writing ability were stable through grades 1–5 in a cross-sequential study following children in grades 1 and 3. It has long been known that oral language disorders are associated with significant long-term problems with written expression even when the oral language problems seem to have resolved or significantly improved, likely reflecting the later acquisition of written language skills (Bishop & Snowling, 2004). Bishop and Clarkson (2003) followed a large sample of twins in which one or both twins had an oral language disorder. Most of the twins could not spell well enough to attempt narrative production. Even twins of affected probands who had no evidence of oral language impairment on standardized tests showed more difficulties on written language narratives than age-matched controls. It is likely that written language problems are persistent across different populations and certainly in children defined with LDs in reading and oral language.

NEUROBIOLOGICAL FACTORS

Brain Structure

Agraphia

As with LDs in mathematics, few neuroimaging studies focus specifically on children with LDs in written expression. Studies of acquired disorders (i.e., agraphia) identify a number of disorders of writing that vary in their lesional patterns and may provide sources of hypotheses for anatomical MRI studies. In an overview, Roeltgen (2003) noted that classic neurological studies identified five forms of agraphia (see Table 9.1). However, he noted that lesional patterns were variable and coverage was poor. Using a neurolinguistic model, Roeltgen (2003) proposed an alternative classification based on disruptions of different aspects of the writing process that differentiated linguistic and motor components (see Table 9.2 for a partial list and description). Among the linguistically based agraphias, lexical and phonological agraphias show differential disruptions of the phonological and orthographic components of spelling. Lexical agraphia is often associated with lesions involving the posterior part of the angular gyrus and the occipitotemporal region, along with other regions of the left hemisphere, excluding the perisylvian region. In contrast, phonological agraphia involves lesions to the posterior perisylvian region, including the supramarginal gyrus and insula. These differences in lesion patterns appear related to the distinctions of the

TABLE 9.1. Traditional Classification of Agraphia

1. Pure agraphia: writing problems in the absence of any other language problem

2. Aphasic agraphia: writing problems in association with language problems

3. Agraphia with alexia: writing and reading problems in the absence of aphasia

4. Apraxic agraphia: writing problems characterized by difficulties in forming graphemes

5. Spatial agraphia: writing problems usually in association with visual neglect

Note. Data from Roeltgen (2003).

roles of these regions for phonological and orthographic processing in word reading (see Chapter 5). However, as in most studies of people with acquired disorders, the lesional pattern is variable.

For the motor components, the dissociations are based on the preservation of oral spelling and disturbances of writing. Apraxic agraphia is related to lesions involving the parietal lobe, either ipsilateral or contralateral to the hand used for writing. Spatial agraphia is usually associated with a lesion to the nondominant parietal lobes that often produces hemispatial neglect, in which the patient ignores visual information contralteral to the lesion (with a right hemisphere lesion, visual information to the patient's left side). The motor component of acquired disorders does not have any immediately obvious relevance for developmental disorders, with much of the focus on the role of the frontal lobes in motor programming (Barkley, 1997).

Brain Function

Berninger (2004) summarized findings from functional neuroimaging studies by the University of Washington group that addressed components of the writing process. She reported that components involved in fine motor control and language generation can be related to areas of the frontal lobes and the cerebellum. These areas are well known to be involved in support of core processes that underlie writing, including motor control and planning, executive functions, and language. Barkley (1997) used these findings to help explain why many children with ADHD have problems with writing.

In a more recent study, Richards et al. (2005, 2006) evaluated brain activation in response to two different spelling interventions in children in grades 4–6 identified with dyslexia. The treatments involved an orthographically based intervention that taught specific strategies for letter patterns. The second intervention focused on morphological components of spelling, teaching children to synthesize word parts to make

TABLE 9.2. Neurolinguistic Classification of Agraphia
_____

A. Linguistic components
  1. Lexical agraphia—impaired ability to spell irregular words, but not pseudowords
  2. Phonological agraphia—inability to spell pseudowords, but not familiar words (regular and irregular)
  3. Deep agraphia—inability to spell pseudowords and more trouble spelling function words than nouns
  4. Semantic agraphia—inability to spell and write with meaning

B. Motor components
  1. Apraxic agraphia—inability to write, but preservation of oral spelling
  2. Spatial agraphia—inability to copy writing legibly, but preservation of oral spelling
_____

Note. Data from Roeltgen (2003).

words and to break down words into constituent elements that supported the meaning of the words. These interventions were conducted in 14-hour-long sessions over 3 weeks with before and after fMRI based on four word reading tasks that manipulated phonological mapping, orthographic mapping, and morphological mapping with and without phonological shifts. The investigators found unique patterns of activation for each of the four tasks at baseline in controls, with common activation across tasks of structures often associated with reading: the left inferior frontal gyrus, bilateral lingual gyrus, bilateral fusiform gyrus, and left inferior temporal gyrus. A variety of cortical and cerebellum structures were uniquely activated. The patterns were different in the children with dyslexia, always involving underactivation, and were most apparent on tasks requiring phonological mapping. After intervention involving orthographic mapping, the right inferior frontal gyrus and the right posterior parietal gyrus showed significantly greater activation in the group with dyslexia, and little change in the controls. Morphological treatment did not lead to significant changes in activation. These changes were considered normalizing.

These studies notwithstanding, there do not appear to be any structural or functional neuroimaging studies of children specifically identified with LDs involving written language. Much work remains in this area.

Genetic Factors

There are a few studies of heritability of handwriting disability, which mostly involve spelling. Raskind, Hsu, Berninger, Thomson, and Wijsman (2000) found that spelling disorders, but not handwriting disorders, aggregate in families. Other studies have also found that spelling difficulties aggregate in families (Schulte-Korne, Deimel, Muller, Gutenbrunner, & Remschmidt, 1996). These findings are consistent with twin studies, which have found strong heritability of spelling abilities in twins, which exceeded that found for reading abilities (Stevenson, Graham, Fredman, & McLoughlin, 1987).

More recently, Bates et al. (2004) evaluated genetic and environmental influences on reading and spelling of real words, pseudowords, and irregular words. They reported heritabilities of .61 for real words, .71 for pseudowords, and .73 for irregular words; spelling yielded estimates of .76 for real and irregular words, and .52 for pseudowords. Evaluations of the environmental contributions were significant, representing variance due to unique environmental influences and not differences in families. In their study of adult twins reared apart, Johnson, Bouchard, Segal, and Samuels (2005) found heritabilities around .75 for different measures of word reading, .51 for reading comprehension, and .76 for spelling.

In linkage studies, Schulte-Korne (2001) found evidence linking spelling to a region of chromosome 15. Similarly, Nothen et al. (1999) reported a locus for spelling (and reading) on chromosome 15, which has also been reported for dyslexia (Grigorenko, 2005). As reading and spelling abilities are highly correlated and represent a common factor that shares heritability (Marlow et al., 2001), it remains to be seen how these findings really differ from those reported above for word reading. Grigorenko (2005) noted specifically that the issue of whether phenotypic variability reflected genotypic variability was not established even in the reading area.

SUMMARY: FROM ACADEMIC SKILL DEFICITS TO NEUROBIOLOGICAL FACTORS

Different academic skill deficits in written expression have different cognitive correlates: handwriting is correlated with fine motor, motor planning, and working memory skills; spelling with phonological analysis, knowledge of orthographic conventions specific to a child's language of instruction, and visual–motor skills; and composition with executive functions and a variety of oral language skills (Berninger, 2004; Hooper, Wakely, & de Kruif, 2006). Motor and phonological/orthographic difficulties correlated with handwriting and spelling especially constrain the transcription component, whereas difficulties with executive functions and language constrain the generational component. The motor and executive function problems help explain why so many children with ADHD have disorders of written expression (Barkley, 1997). Subtypes may exist, but the key classification question is whether written language difficulties occur in the absence of other LDs, oral language problems, or ADHD. Neurobiological correlates other than spelling have rarely been studied. Spelling shares considerable heritability with phonological decoding.

WRITTEN LANGUAGE INTERVENTIONS

Lyon and Cutting (1998) reported that interventions for LDs that affect handwriting, spelling, and written composition have been developed, but studied less extensively compared to those for reading disabilities. At the time, the relative paucity of intervention research in the area of written language was partly due to the complexity of the multiple linguistic tasks that must be negotiated in the writing process. In written expression, one has to formulate the ideas to be expressed, organize and sequence them in a coherent fashion, produce the ideas in a syntactically correct format, spell the words correctly, and produce the content legibly via motor response. Furthermore, after competence in these foundation skills is established, the skills must be integrated within a broader cognitive system that superimposes organizational strategies on issues of genre structure, text coherence and cohesion, and sense of audience. Given the number of variables that could be studied in written language intervention, it is not surprising that many investigations have focused on only parts of the process. In the past 10 years, a substantial research base on interventions addressing different components of written language has emerged.

Handwriting

Handwriting is composed of a set of complex behaviors that are developed over a period of time. Difficulties in both printing and cursive writing stem from a number of factors that include motor deficits, visual–motor coordination problems, visual memory deficits, and orthographic processing. The term "dysgraphia" has been used historically to refer to a developmental difficulty in transducing visual information to the motor system (Johnson & Myklebust, 1967), which manifests itself in an inability to copy.

Johnson and Myklebust (1967) conducted a substantial amount of clinical research involving written language disorders, including handwriting deficits. From their research, they developed a comprehensive task-analytic model for the treatment of handwriting difficulties. An older method for the remediation of written language deficits is the Gillingham and Stillman (1965) approach. This is a method used by many teachers working with students with LDs and is characterized by the following: (1) The teacher models a large letter on the blackboard, writing and saying the name; (2) the student traces the letter while saying the name (this tracing stage continues until the student is secure with both the letter formation and the name); (3) the student copies the letter while saying the name; and (4) the student writes the letter from memory while saying the name. In addition to these types of multisensory intervention methods, some studies have assessed the utility of improving handwriting by teaching students to verbally guide themselves through the process (Hayes & Flower, 1980).

Mechanically, letter formation and word spelling are necessary to express thoughts in written fashion. Graham, Struck, Santoro, and Berninger (2006) asked children in grades 1–2 who were weak and strong in handwriting to complete tasks involving writing alphabet letters from memory, copying letters in a passage, and composing specific topics. An evaluation of legibility revealed that poor handwriters generated more letters with extra strokes, tended to produce letters that were smaller, and were more variable in the spacing and alignment of letters. The results were interpreted as indicating problems with the execution of motor programs, visual-spatial arrangement, and letter formation that constrain the quality of composition. Thus, handwriting and spelling difficulties can have serious deleterious consequences for written expression. They can (1) result in misinterpretations of the author's meaning (Graham, Harris, & Chorzempa, 2002; Graham et al., 2000), (2) create negative perceptions about the writer, which taint overall impressions about the quality of an essay (Hughes, Keeling, & Tuck, 1983), (3) interfere with the execution of composing processes because cognitive resources are unduly allocated to the mechanical aspects of the process (Berninger, 2004), or (4) lead students to avoid writing, which constrains writing development (Graham & Harris, 2003). For these reasons, an explicit focus on the development of handwriting and spelling skills is important, especially for students with LDs who are most likely to experience these deficits. We describe a series of studies that illustrate critical instructional features for enhancing handwriting and spelling outcomes for students with learning disabilities.

Berninger and Amtmann (2003) reviewed a series of studies involving early intervention for handwriting difficulties. For example, Berninger et al. (1997) randomly assigned first-graders with poor legibility and automaticity in handwriting to one of five interventions: conventional repeated copying of letters; conventional imitating the motor components of letter formations; provision of visual cues for letter formations; writing letters from memory with increasing delays; and combinations of the visual cues/memory component. After 24 lessons over a 4-month period, the combined treatment was more effective than control or other conditions in improving handwriting. These findings were replicated by Graham et al. (2000) and Jones and Christensen (1999).

Berninger et al. (2005) completed three studies that evaluated different levels of intervention for first- and second-grade students. They found that intervention that provided either practice in motor activities with no letter component or practice in letters with no motor component led to some improvement in letter formation and legibility. However, explicit instruction in handwriting that combined motor and orthographic components with verbal mediation and visual cuing led to improved automaticity of writing and generalized to improved word recognition skills. In the second study, motor training or orthographic training in isolation did not add to outcomes produced by explicit instruction in automatic letter writing and composition. Finally, the third study showed that the addition of explicit instruction in handwriting to instruction in reading improved handwriting, but did not add to reading outcomes. Thus, explicitly teaching students handwriting is more beneficial than simply teaching different components, highlighting the importance of more integrative approaches that include considerable emphasis on actually producing letters and words.

Graham et al. (2000) conducted an experimental intervention study with first-grade students who were experiencing handwriting and writing difficulties. Thirty-eight students were assigned randomly to two groups: handwriting or phonological awareness instruction. Handwriting instruction comprised 27 15-minute lessons divided into nine units. In each unit, three lowercase letters, which shared common formational characteristics, were introduced and practiced. Each lesson incorporated four activities. The first activity, Alphabet Warm-Up, focused on learning to name each letter, matching the name with its letter, and knowing the sequence of the letters in the alphabet. The second activity, Alphabet Practice, provided tracing and writing individual letters. The third activity was Alphabet Rockets, designed to increase students' handwriting fluency, and the fourth activity, Alphabet Fun, allowed students to play with the letters in a creative manner. Across these four components, the instruction was explicit, relying on a task analysis of the letters to focus the child's attention on the critical features and demands of the task and to provide adequate support for the child to enjoy success until independent mastery was demonstrated. Results showed that students in the handwriting condition made greater handwriting gains by posttest (effect size = 1.39), which maintained 6 months later (effect size = 0.87). Effects were also demonstrated on posttest compositional fluency (effect size = 1.46), which dropped to a nonsignificant effect size of 0.45 at the 6-month maintenance assessment. This pattern held for these low-performing students with and without identified LDs. In addition, at posttest, students in the handwriting condition did not produce qualitatively better stories than their peers in the phonological awareness condition. This suggests that additional work in strengthening handwriting, perhaps in conjunction with composition tasks, may be needed.

Spelling

In Chapter 5, we indicated that the English spelling system, or orthography, is an alphabetic system in which phonemic units (speech sounds) are represented by graphemes (letters or letter combinations). For both students and primary-grade teachers, this fundamental relation between spoken and written language is the most important aspect underlying literacy development. Spelling is often not mastered by individuals with WLRD, who after appropriate intervention can usually improve their decoding skills, but typically continue to be poor spellers (Bruck, 1987). This finding, as well as the number of people who read well but spell poorly (Frith, 1980), suggests that reading and spelling are to some extent dissociated and that theoretical models of one skill will not necessarily explain the other (Moats, 2005).

In a more contemporary approach that involved rigorous evaluation, Graham et al. (2002) addressed spelling interventions for poor spellers in grade 2, who were randomly assigned to receive spelling or math supplementary instruction. Forty-eight sessions, each 20 minutes in duration, were conducted. The lessons were divided into eight units, each focusing on two or more related spelling patterns. The first lesson was a word-sorting activity, in which students categorized words by the spelling pattern featured in that unit. The teacher engaged the students in thinking about similarities and differences between the words—modeling the thinking process by which words might be sorted into their appropriate categories. Gradually, students assumed responsibility for sorting while articulating the features by which they categorized. Once all the words were sorted, the teacher provided the rule for the patterns emphasized in the word sort. After that, students generated words of their own. Then the pack of words was shuffled and students completed the sorting while trying to beat their previous times. During Lesson 2, the teacher gave each student eight study words that (1) occurred in the student's writing frequently and (2) the child had missed on the pretest. In Lessons 2–5, students employed two study procedures to learn these eight words: self-study using a set of steps and dyadic practice using games. Also as part of Lessons 2–5, teachers provided students explicit instruction and practice in identifying the sound patterns associated with the unit's content, and the students worked in pairs to build words that corresponded to the spelling pattern emphasized in that unit. In Lesson 6, students took a test to determine their mastery of the eight words. The students scored the test and plotted the score on a graph. They then set a goal for how many words they would spell correctly on the next unit test, which would be added to the graph. Students also completed a test assessing their spelling of nine words that contained the rimes emphasized during word sorting. Cumulative review was conducted systematically, beginning with the second unit. Results demonstrated the value of this systematic and explicit approach to spelling instruction. As compared with peers in the math control condition, students who received the spelling intervention made greater improvements on norm-referenced spelling tests (effect sizes = 0.64–1.05), a writing fluency test (effect size = 0.78), and a reading word attack measure (effect size = 0.82). Six months later, students in the spelling treatment maintained their advantage in spelling (effect sizes = 0.70–1.07) but not on the writing fluency (effect size = 0.57) or reading word attack (effect size = 0.47) measures. Spelling instruction did, however, have a positive effect at maintenance on the reading word recognition skills of students whose pretest scores on this measure were lowest.

Building on spelling intervention studies by Berninger et al. (1998, 2000), Berninger et al. (2002b) assigned third-graders to interventions that involved training only in spelling, training in essay composition, and a combined spelling/essay composition training, along with a control condition involving keyboard training. The spelling component emphasized orthographic patterns in words, particularly at the morphological level. Both interventions that included spelling instruction produced more gains in spelling than the essay condition that did not involve explicit intervention in spelling. Together, these latter studies highlight that many students with LDs do improve in spelling when it is taught and that gains are maximized with explicit focus on letter patterns (orthography) and opportunities to practice in writing.

Compensatory Devices

Berninger and Amtmann (2003) reviewed evidence for the efficacy of a variety of compensatory tools supporting handwriting and spelling, including keyboarding, dictation using a voice recognition system, and word prediction programs. Keyboarding did not seem to improve the mechanical components of writing if typing was slow. Students who had difficulty with automatic production of letters in a paper-and-pencil format also had difficulty with keyboard components. Ultimately, keyboarding may well be an effective bypass tool for students who write poorly, but a research base in terms of effective implementations has not emerged. In terms of dictating based on voice recognition methodologies, all students, including those with LDs, produced more material if they could dictate instead of write. Presently there is little evidence that indicates that such programs enhance written language performance, which may reflect the need to more fully develop voice recognition technologies. Finally, word prediction software for students that have written language difficulties has yet to show a significant impact on students with LDs. This may reflect comorbid difficulties with working memory or attention.

Altogether, there is a need to evaluate all forms of compensatory tools for individuals who have mechanical difficulties with the transcriptional component of written language. The weak results of compensatory tools likely reflect what has been learned in the reading area, which is the importance of integrating any type of compensatory tool into the actual process of writing (and reading).

Written Expression

The ability to produce one's thoughts in writing involves a complex form of communication requiring a number of cognitive abilities. In producing a written composition, the student must simultaneously attend to the subject, the text, and the reader. Deficits in oral language and reading are often precursors to difficulties in the writing process, and attention and memory play critical roles as well (Gregg, 1991). As simple as it sounds, some researchers (Higgins & Raskind, 2000) have found that increased writing practice can be a significant force in improving written composition that also impacts reading ability. In more detailed interventions, methods that require students to take two related sentences and write them as one (sentence combining) have produced significant gains in written composition (O'Hare, 1973).

Earlier studies focused on the characteristics of those who are good and poor at written expression. In these studies, several investigators (Bereiter, 1980; Berninger, 2004; Hayes & Flower, 1980; Hooper et al., 1994) reported that individuals who write well are goal directed; they understand the purpose of the writing assignment; they have a good knowledge of the topic prior to writing; they generate more ideas and use significant numbers of transitional ties; they produce a more cohesive text and flow of ideas; and they continuously monitor their written products for correctness of spelling and grammar. More recently, Hooper et al. (1994) and others (De La Paz et al., 1998; Graham, 2005) reported that writers with LDs demonstrate deficits in deploying strategies during production of written text and also have problems in generating text. As compared with "good" writers, those with LDs produce shorter and less interesting essays, with poorly organized text at the sentence and paragraph levels, and are less likely to review spelling, punctuation, grammar, or the body of their text to increase clarity (Hooper et al., 1994). These observations led directly to interventions addressing difficulties with composing.

The previously cited study by Berninger et al. (2002b) found that all active interventions, including groups that received spelling, composition, and both composition and spelling treatments, increased compositional fluency. Interventions that included spelling improved word-specific skills, and the interventions that included composing had the most effect on the quality of persuasive essays. Only the combined composing and spelling condition increased word-specific and essay skills.

Hooper et al. (2006) provided a metacognitive intervention for children in grades 4–5; about 35% met state criteria for LDs. Intervention was provided for 20 days for 20–45 minutes and included 15 minutes of explicit instruction and additional time in composing a story. The focus of the instruction was on increasing the students' awareness of writing as a problem-solving process that required planning, translating, and thinking about written products. Overall improvements were modest and varied, depending on membership in groups with four empirically derived subtypes. Few specific gains were noted for students who had problem-solving weaknesses, with or without co-occurring weaknesses in language. However, those with the latter subtype did show greater gains in spelling than those with the normal variant subtypes. Interestingly, those in the problem-solving subtypes were expected to show the greatest improvement because this domain was the target of the intervention, but such interactions were not apparent.

A number of cognitive-behavioral intervention techniques have been employed to increase composition skills. Graham and Harris (1996) developed Self-Regulated Strategy Development (SRSD) to assist students in mastering the higher-level cognitive processes involved in written composition and to develop the self-regulated use of these processes. Using SRSD, Graham and Harris stimulated significant gains in the length and quality of story writing in students with LDs (Graham & Harris, 1993) and found that such gains were maintained over time and generalized across settings and persons (Graham, Harris, MacArthur, & Schwartz, 1991). Although this body of work was initially conducted primarily at the intermediate and middle school levels (see Graham & Harris, 2003), Graham, Harris, and colleagues have moved their work on SRSD to second and third grades, targeting low-performing students with and without LDs for intervention. Effects with these younger struggling students are encouraging (Graham, 2005).

First targeting third-graders, Graham, Harris, and Mason (2005) taught struggling writers two genre-specific strategies. These genre-specific strategies were embedded in a more general strategy for planning and writing a paper, which reminded students to pick a topic, organize ideas into a writing plan, and use/upgrade this plan while writing. Within the second step of this general strategy (i.e., organize ideas into a writing plan), students were taught the two genre-specific strategies for generating ideas: the first for writing a story and the second for writing a persuasive essay. Further, students learned about the basic parts of a story and a persuasive essay, the importance of using words that make a paper more interesting, and self-talk to facilitate performance. Finally, a self-regulation component was overlaid on the instruction whereby students set goals to write complete papers, monitored and graphed their success in achieving this goal, compared their preinstructional performance with their performance during instruction, and credited their success to the use of the target strategies. At the same time, the study examined the effect of peer mediation in enhancing the effects of the strategy instruction, especially for the purpose of maintenance and generalization. In the peer-mediated condition, peers worked together to promote strategy use, identifying other places or instances in which they could apply the strategies and brainstorming about how they might need to modify the strategies for the new application. They were then encouraged to remind each other to apply what they were learning to those transfer situations, and in the next session, they identified when, where, and how they had applied the strategies. Thus, this study incorporated three conditions: Writers' Workshop (control condition), explicit and systematic SRSD, and SRSD with peer mediation. The control condition represents a popular approach to expressive writing in many public schools. Seventy-two students, screened into the study because of difficulty with writing, were assigned to pairs to ensure compatibility. Then, pairs (which were the unit of analysis for the study) were assigned randomly to the three conditions. Instructors worked with students three times weekly, for 20 minutes each time, with approximately 11 hours of total instruction across the two genres.

Results showed the advantage of both SRSD conditions over Writer's Workshop for planning and composing stories and persuasive essays. Students in the SRSD conditions wrote longer, more complete, and qualitatively better papers for both genres, with effect sizes ranging between 0.82 and 3.23. These effects were maintained over time for story writing and generalized to a third uninstructed genre, informative writing. The peer mediation component augmented SRSD by increasing students' knowledge of planning and enhancing generalization to informative and narrative writing.

With encouraging effects at grade 3, Harris, Graham, and Mason (in press) moved down to grade 2 with a parallel study that incorporated the same three conditions. Results were again strong. Among the struggling writers, SRSD produced greater knowledge about writing and stronger performance in the two instructed genres (story and persuasive writing) as well as two uninstructed genres (personal narrative and informative writing). Effect sizes were similarly strong. Peer support augmented SRSD by enhancing specific aspects of students' performance in the instructed and uninstructed genres. Across the two studies, findings revealed (1) the capacity to enhance relatively young students' writing performance, even within the high-poverty communities where this series of studies was conducted; (2) the added value of a peer support component to effect generalization of the targeted genres to untaught genres; and (3) the superiority of a structured, explicit, systematic approach to writing instruction over the more popular Writer's Workshop. The latter finding illustrates the hold of relatively unstructured instructional approaches to writing instruction despite persuasive evidence for more explicit, strategy-based approaches.

Saddler, Moran, Graham, and Harris (2004) provided supplemental strategy instruction to grade 2 students who were struggling with written expression. Learning to use a strategy for planning and writing a story that was explicitly taught to the students had a significant effect on compositional quality and fluency. The stories were more complete and rated much higher in assessments of narrative quality. At the individual level, improvement was apparent in all but one student, with generalization to other domains of writing. The effects persisted on follow-up, with evidence of continued growth in writing ability.

Research on SRSD in writing is a comprehensive, long-term program of research. Graham and Harris (2003) conducted a meta-analysis of 26 studies addressing strategy-based instruction in writing (see also Graham, 2005). Many of the studies included students identified with LDs, but actually involved a range of achievement levels as well as different comorbidities. Overall, strategic approaches to writing instruction yielded effect sizes in the large range for a variety of different components of writing (quality, elements, length, story grammar) across different groups, including students with LDs. For students with LDs, effect sizes ranged from 1.14 for quality to more than 2.0 for elements in story grammar. Similar effect sizes were found for average writers. There was evidence for maintenance and generalization of the effects, as well as large effect sizes with younger and older students and across instructional environments.

Evaluating the components of strategic instruction in writing showed that those that involve self-regulation are most significant in improving writing performance for students with LDs. These findings were noteworthy because SRSD is typically provided at a classroom level. As the provision of written language instruction is difficult for many teachers, it is not surprising that explicit teaching of writing strategies—like explicit teaching of comprehension strategies—is beneficial for all students in the classroom.

CONCLUSIONS

In contrast to our current understanding of oral language and reading disorders among children with LDs, less is known about the etiology, developmental course, prognosis, and treatment for disorders of written expression. The distinction of the transcription and generational components is very important and leads to the identification of academic skill deficits involving handwriting, spelling, and composition. Core cognitive processes have been identified, but these tend to be shared with other disorders. Neurobiological research is only in its infancy.

A key for the future is to attempt to identify subgroups of children with disorders of written expression that have some independence from other language-based disorders, with handwriting being the obvious example. But even here the comorbidity issue has not been adequately addressed, and the independence of ADHD and handwriting disorders is not established (Barkley, 1997). It is apparent that transcription and generation are separable, but also mutually interdependent—in particular, transcription constrains the quality of generation; many children with LDs involving reading or with oral language disorders cannot produce narrative text because they cannot spell (Bishop & Clarkson, 2003).

The intervention studies in handwriting and spelling demonstrate how systematic, explicit instruction can effect better outcomes for students with LDs on skills that are foundational to written expression. Results also suggest how work targeting these foundational skills may simultaneously enhance related skills, such as word attack and word recognition, as well as higher-order processes related to composition. There was clear evidence of transfer to reading and composing in many studies focusing on the transcription component.

There are many emerging intervention methods for the remediation of difficulties in composition. Reflecting the core cognitive impairment in executive functions that characterize many students who struggle with composing, teaching children explicit strategies for composing that focus on problem-solving, planning, and self-regulation in the context of writing leads to improvements in written expression.

As in other content areas, clinicians and teachers must be aware that written language is a complex domain, requiring the integration of oral language, written language, cognitive, and motor skills. Within this context, a combination of the different intervention methods discussed in this section is likely to net the greatest improvements in the writing skills of students with LDs. The key is to identify the basis for the impairment in this domain (handwriting, spelling, and written expression) and provide explicit instruction using one of the evidence-based approaches outlined in this section.

CHAPTER 10

Conclusions and
Future Directions

In this book, we have provided a selective review of research related to LDs. We have specifically attempted to integrate research across domains of inquiry based on the model presented in Chapter 1 (Figure 1.1). The value of this approach is most clearly illustrated in Chapter 5, which involves WLRD, the area in which research on LDs is most advanced. Here academic skill deficits and core cognitive correlates have been identified through converging scientific research, which has led to inclusionary definitions that have facilitated studies of the epidemiology, developmental course, and neurobiological correlates of dyslexia. As a consequence, research on treatment is flourishing in this area, with results from numerous intervention studies now informing practice and educational policies.

At the same time, there continue to be gaps in our knowledge of reading disabilities involving fluency and comprehension, math disabilities, and disorders of written language. These gaps are narrowing as research funding has increased. As with the research in WLRD, scientific inquiry in these areas may be facilitated by a clear distinction of specific academic skill deficits and core cognitive processes at the smallest grain size possible. This approach, when anchored in a framework that explicitly addresses the reliability and validity of the underlying classifications, will lead to the development of inclusionary definitions and the identification of prototypes. Neurobiological studies will be advanced by studying children identified with LDs specific to these domains, especially in reading fluency, comprehension, and written expression. Interventions that specifically address LDs in reading fluency and comprehension and that examine the range of academic impairments in LDs involving written expression and mathematics are sorely needed.

Although research on LDs continues to advance, practice and policy often do not integrate these research findings; moreover, the literature continues to incorporate studies that are methodologically deficient for reasons that we outline below. Accordingly, in this final chapter we consider why research to date has not yet effected more substantial benefits for students with LDs. Then we consider principles for designing high-quality intervention studies that might continue to provide the basis for guiding education practice. Finally, we synthesize across the narrative reviews in this book to offer 10 general principles for instructing people with LDs.

THE GAP BETWEEN RESEARCH AND PRACTICE: SCALING THE RESULTS OF EDUCATION RESEARCH

Considerable progress has been made in designing assessment and instruction that boost learning to an impressive degree for students with LDs. In light of the advances in what we know about best practices, it is disconcerting that so many students with LDs continue to suffer dramatic deficits in reading, writing, and math. We offer seven possible reasons to explain why moving this research into practice has proven difficult: (1) inadequate implementation, (2) insufficient reliance on screening and progress monitoring, (3) inadequate attention to prevention, (4) need for integration across instructional components, (5) insufficient consideration of multifaceted problems, (6) lack of sufficient engagement and practice, and (7) reliance on clinical experience and knowledge of craft over scientific evidence.

Implementation

The first reason why best practices instructional components fail to meet the needs of many students with LDs in schools today is inadequate implementation. Many interventions demonstrate efficacy when they are studied in controlled environments. However, when the interventions are translated into everyday practice in complex school and classroom settings, fidelity suffers, and contextual variables such as teacher preparation and commitment to the intervention, composition of students, and adequacy of resources dilute the efficacy that is apparent in a more controlled research setting (Denton, Vaughn, & Fletcher, 2003). Naturally, interventions will be only as effective as the fidelity with which they are implemented. Policy makers, administrators, and teachers require tools to help them build classroom contexts that support sound instructional practices, even as researchers must disseminate their methods in a manner that facilitates implementation (Vaughn & Fuchs, 2003).

Implementation is of particular concern, given the move toward full inclusion of students with LDs in general education classrooms in many schools. Although the goals of inclusion are laudatory, there is little evidence that students with LDs show significant academic growth in many standard general education settings (Vaughn, Moody, & Schumm, 1998; Zigmond, 2003).

These pessimistic findings are in stark contrast to the results of the classroom-based interventions reviewed in this book, which have been designed for inclusionary environments. Moreover, no single approach works with every student, and even successful classroom interventions fail to work adequately with up to 30% or more of students. A range of intervention strategies is therefore needed (Zigmond, 2003). This need supports the potential value of a multitiered intervention system.

Future research on interventions should carefully evaluate the conditions in which interventions can be scaled and implemented in everyday educational environments. Strategies that facilitate schools' and teachers' acceptance of evidence-based interventions should be delineated. Barriers to implementations of efficacious interventions should be identified and minimized. Clearly, there is a need to enhance personnel preparation, within both general and special education, to increase the effectiveness of services. The scaling issues in implementing response to instruction (RTI) specifically, and in preparing teachers to implement research-validated instructional and assessment practices more generally, are daunting.

Screening and Progress Monitoring

Sadly, outcomes for other practices, such as resource classes, are also not very positive. Bentum and Aaron (2003; see also Foorman et al., 1997) studied several hundred students with LDs in reading who received resource room instruction for 3–6 years. There was no evidence of improvement in word recognition or reading comprehension skills, with a decline in spelling skills. Verbal IQ scores actually declined over time. These results are similar to large scale studies of the effects of special education placement for students with LDs, which show little improvement in reading and only slight improvements in math in grades 3–6 (Hanushek, Kain, & Rivkin, 1998).

To implement any form of early intervention, or models based on RTI, different kinds of assessments need to be routinely implemented in schools. The first type is mass screening for academic and behavior problems. As Donovan and Cross (2002) indicated, screening technology is available for forecasting reading and behavioral difficulties. Such screening permits a quick assessment of every student to identify those who show risk characteristics much earlier than is possible in referral-based models. A variety of tools are available. It is also important to note that the Reading First component of No Child Left Behind requires universal screening of all students in kindergarten, grade 1, grade 2, and grade 3.

In addition to screening, progress monitoring of students who show risk characteristics or who demonstrate disabilities is critical. The technology for progress monitoring is well developed in reading and math through the elementary grades and into middle school (Stecker et al., 2005). Frequent monitoring to identify progress or lack thereof puts assessment data in the hands of teachers and provides informative data on who might need intensive interventions, such as those in special education (Fuchs & Fuchs, 1998). Routine progress monitoring for students identified as being at risk for LDs or who have LDs promises to have more impact than any other single scaling component because it provides immediate and ongoing feedback on student progress in ways that allow for more differentiation of instruction. Both screening and progress monitoring reflect assessments in the service of intervention and promise a dramatic modification in the focus of testing within schools.

Prevention

Given the evidence, the widespread lack of implementation of early intervention programs in general education is frustrating. Students vary in their instructional needs. Those who do not receive instruction addressing their needs early, in kindergarten through second grade, develop academic difficulties that parallel what is typically observed in students with LDs. When these students' needs go unaddressed over the primary grades, the commonly employed "wait and fail" model (1) creates large deficits in students who might have developed well with earlier prevention efforts and (2) exacerbates the difficulties of students with true LDs. Special education should be an opportunity to provide highly specialized and intensive interventions similar to those reviewed in the sections of this book on remediation, for which implementation may require the power and flexibility of IDEA. Wide implementation of early intervention programs could potentially reduce the number of students who emerge as eligible for special education at later ages. With more intensive and inductively formulated individualized instructional programming within special education, using systematic progress monitoring, the effectiveness of the most intensive instructional tier, special education, can be enhanced. All of this may be accomplished via universal screening for academic and behavior problems, progress monitoring of those who show risk characteristics, strong prevention for students who demonstrate inadequate response to general education instruction, and specialized intervention for those deemed in need of special education (Donovan & Cross, 2002; Vaughn & Fuchs, 2003).

The key is to embrace prevention when possible and to be prepared to respond with intensive specialized remediation when preventative efforts prove inadequate. Special education remediation can be effective, particularly if built upon a preventative effort. In this book, we have presented effect sizes for many remedial interventions that were similar in magnitude as those in prevention studies. But interventions of the type that are implemented in research are generally more intensive than those used in schools, where remedial instruction is frequently carried out in larger groups that make it difficult to ensure the level of intensity needed to accelerate growth in academic skills. The context within which special education is provided in the schools therefore requires reform, especially given the evidence for poor outcomes (Bentum & Aaron, 2003; Hanushek et al., 1998).

IDEA 2004 may provide the basis for this reform. The statute indicates that students should not be identified with LDs in the absence of appropriate instructional opportunities. In keeping with an RTI model, students might pass through a sequence of instructional opportunities in a multitiered process that begins at the general education classroom level, but could be part of the identification process for providing special education services to students with LDs or simply an effort to provide more intensive interventions in general education. With RTI, students may first be identified as being at risk for LDs and then provided with increasingly intensive interventions, which are monitored using curriculum-based assessments of progress. Students who do not show adequate response to quality instruction would be candidates for highly specialized interventions in special education. Moving this concept of RTI from research to practice, which requires the implementation of different assessments and validated interventions, will be a difficult, long-term process, but promises to highlight prevention and put remediation in a more manageable context.

Instructional Components

Even with adequate levels of implementation and strong fidelity, as well as a strong focus on screening and progress monitoring, and prevention, validated instructional components will fail to meet the needs of some students with LDs. Consider that, as demonstrated in research in which high levels of treatment fidelity are achieved, an unacceptably high pro-portion of students with LDs fail to profit. For example, with strong implementation of PALS, Fuchs et al. (1997) demonstrated statistically significant effects for students with LDs on a variety of reading mea-sures. Nevertheless, 2 of every 10 students with LDs failed to make ade-quate progress in terms of performance levels in the average range at the end of intervention. In a study by Foorman et al. (1998), about 30% of students in the bottom 20% of readers who received the most effective reading curriculum continued to struggle, with word reading scores be-low the 25th percentile after classroom-based instruction.

It should not be surprising to find that generally effective programs do not meet the needs of all students with LDs. Students with LDs have multifaceted problems, reflecting processing deficiencies that make fluent, generalized performances difficult to achieve, deficits in domain-relevant background knowledge, and poor self-regulation, metacognition, task persistence, and motivation (Gersten, White, Falco, & Carnine, 1982). Although each promising instructional component is designed to address one or more of these difficulties, none is sufficiently comprehensive to address the particular constellation of deficits and their severity that some children manifest. Moreover, there are domains for which instruc-tional components are not yet adequate, particularly in areas involving reading comprehension, writing, and math.

Finally, although many different instructional components have been developed, their integration into comprehensive instructional pack-ages remains to be addressed. Following the development of comprehen-sive, integrated reading programs for people with LDs in word recogni-tion, some examples are emerging in other domains. More integration of instruction that involves skills and strategies is needed, which is happen-ing in math (Fuchs et al., 2003a, 2003b), reading comprehension (Wil-liams et al., 2005), and written expression (Berninger & Amtmann, 2003; Graham & Harris, 2003). This integration should also begin to impact interventions for preschool children so that preventative efforts can begin as early as possible for those at highest risk owing to social and economic factors

Multifaceted Problems

In a related way, students with LDs are heterogeneous, even if they are identified in specific academic domains. Most students with LDs have problems that involve more than one domain. Even within a domain, students with LDs present with a variety of cognitive difficulties and comorbidities. In many instances, explaining the academic problem does not provide a full explanation of an LD, particularly if comorbidities are not addressed. Although variation at the level of major disorders (e.g., intellectual, academic, behavioral) accounts for much of the heterogeneity in people with LDs, variability remains substantial, largely because many with LDs have more than one problem.

Research on interventions has done an inadequate job of identifying and addressing the contributions of different sources of heterogeneity to outcomes. For example, one reason that strategy instruction emphasizing self-regulation may be effective is that many students with LDs have difficulties in areas involving "executive functions." However, executive function deficits are more dramatic in problems with math and reading than in problems with word recognition. Similarly, cognitive morbidity in students with ADHD without impairment of academic domains is much less significant than the cognitive morbidity associated when ADHD is combined with academic impairment (Fletcher et al., 1999b).

Understanding intervention outcomes in terms of major sources of heterogeneity may emerge as the next step in intervention design for a variety of childhood conditions. It seems wise, for example, to systematically evaluate students with ADHD for academic difficulties because treatment recommendations differ when attention and academic problems are present. Similarly, intervening for students with LDs without considering comorbid ADHD may dilute the effectiveness of academic interventions.

Engagement and Practice

We can make our prevention and remedial efforts more effective by applying some of the instructional methods and interventions reviewed in this book. However, for many students, much more time on task may be required to achieve adequate progress. Thus, the first step in accelerating academic development in a prevention or remedial mode is to increase the time devoted to instruction in the area in which the student struggles. To further accelerate development, it may be necessary to ensure that the student spends time engaging in academic tasks outside of school. Of course, this means that the student must become motivated to do so. More academic instruction and practice time in school can also be added. However, if that additional time reduces engagement in other important educational activities, especially in middle school and secondary school, overall achievement may suffer. In elementary school, learning to read, write, and do math are clear priorities, and some students need lots of time to become competent in these domains. However, as the studies of reading practice in Chapter 6 on fluency demonstrate, time spent in reading outside of school promotes practice, which in turn promotes the opportunity to develop vocabulary and other capabilities that support comprehension. Extra engagement also affords an opportunity to practice what is taught and to consolidate skills, promoting transfer from the remedial environment. Intervention programs must look more systematically at these practice and engagement issues.

Clinical Intuition

The field of LDs, like other areas of education, is in the process of transforming from a discipline based largely on clinical intuition and craft experience to a profession that relies on scientific research. Although intuition and experience influence teaching practices, especially with individual students, instruction also needs to be informed by research on effectiveness and the mechanisms that underlie efficacy. Education continues to be hampered by reliance on faddish interventions that persist despite the absence of evidence of efficacy or knowledge about mechanisms. Interventions based on learning styles, perceptual and motor training, instruction "tailored" for auditory or visual learners, the need for multisensory integration, and even less reasonable interventions involving special colored lenses, metronomes, neural patterning, and so on, continue to be promoted for LDs despite lack of evidence for efficacy and proposed mechanisms that are inconsistent with scientific understanding of cognitive processing and brain function. Some will testify that these interventions are effective. However, in the absence of scientific investigation, it is impossible to sort through competing claims about efficacy and the mechanisms underlying effectiveness, much less prescribe interventions specific to individual students. Consumers must have the information needed to make informed choices. Clinicians must be prepared to modify and update practice based on research, or at least to identify the shortcomings of research that contradicts traditional belief.

TREATMENT OF LDs

Nothing would facilitate effective scaling of research into practice more than continued demonstration that research-based intervention changes the course of development for persons at risk for or identified with LDs. The road to establishing the efficacy of treatment approaches and methods designed for students with LDs is a long one. Until the past decade, little progress had been made in developing an understanding of the core clinical and diagnostic features of each of the major LD types, and even now this understanding is unequally robust for the various types of LDs. Current knowledge about students' difficulties in learning academic concepts is most advanced for reading development, word-level skills in particular.

Our current knowledge of what works best for students with deficits in other reading domains and in written language and mathematics is less well developed. The reason is, in part, that we know less about the factors that presage such difficulties, the academic skill deficits that define the disorders, and the developmental courses associated with these types of LDs. A substantial increase in intervention research for different types of well-defined LDs in these domains will have to occur if students are to receive the best treatment we can offer.

Although the quality of intervention research has improved, the current treatment/intervention literature still includes studies that are difficult to interpret because of methodological problems. It is the responsibility of the developers of those intervention products to minimize the methodological shortcomings that make interpretation of intervention studies difficult and implementation of the results problematic. In this section of the chapter, we reiterate these research design considerations to help consumers make their own evaluations.

Appropriate Experimental Designs

As in much of education research, there continues to be a shortage of high-quality research designs, especially those that are most appropriate for inferring causality: randomized controlled experiments (RCEs) and regression discontinuity designs (Shadish, Cook, & Campbell, 2002). In RCEs, individuals are randomly assigned to one or more intervention and comparison groups so that the effects of the intervention can be objectively assessed. The value of RCEs is their ability to provide consumers of the research with a high degree of confidence that there are no systematic differences between groups in any observed or unobserved characteristics, except that the intervention groups receive the treatment and the control groups do not (Shadish et al., 2002). In contrast, pre–post intervention designs without control groups or appropriate statistical controls do not permit determination of whether improvements would have occurred over time without the intervention. In addition, these designs do not permit strong inferences concerning a causal role for the intervention. Although a variety of designs may support inferences about the causal effects of interventions, RCEs make the fewest assumptions about causality and are therefore strongest in supporting causal inferences (Shavelson & Towne, 2002).

Regression–discontinuity experiments (RDE) are emerging as a viable alternative for situations in which random assignment is not feasible (Shadish et al., 2002). An RDE is a quasi-experiment with a comparison group. What makes it unique is the method used to assign participants. In general, a cut-point is established on a continuously distributed measure. The cut-point may represent a critical level of the attribute of interest (e.g., 25th percentile on a reading measure), a benchmark believed to indicate a need for service (e.g., reading fewer than 35 words per minute at the end of the first grade), or something else entirely, such as a date of birth. The critical factor is that the attribute does not have natural discontinuities or breaks in its distribution. For assignment, those on one side of the cut-point receive the treatment; those on the other side of the cut-point do not. In the case of treatment for reading problems using a pretest measure of reading as the assignment variable, one would assign students below the cut-point to treatment and those above the cut-point as controls. Because the assignment attribute and the outcome of interest are continuously distributed, the experiment relies on the fact that, in the absence of any treatment effect, the bivariate distribution of the outcome and the assignment variable will be continuous. As such, it can be described with a single regression line that is the same for cases above and below the assignment score. In contrast, if the treatment is effective, then the regression line will be shifted up at the assignment score so that two regression lines will be needed to adequately explain the bivariate distribution of the assignment and outcome scores: one line for cases below the assignment score (i.e., the treated cases) and one line for cases above the assignment score (i.e., the untreated cases). The size of the difference in the intercept terms in the two regression lines is the measure of the treatment effect (assuming the two lines have the same slope).

The internal validity of an RDE may be as strong as that of an RCE because it contains a control group that is drawn from the same population as the group that is treated, but, most important, because assignment is controlled in such a way that chance enters into the difference between treated and untreated cases in a known way. The presence of a controlled assignment mechanism is why RDEs are less susceptible to inferential problems that could reflect selection or historical bias and statistical issues (e.g., regression to the mean) that make it difficult to infer causality from simple pre–post or quasi-experiments where assignment is less rigorously controlled. A main difference between RCEs and RDEs (other than in how they create the groups) is that RDEs have less power and require many more subjects than RCEs. However, given the emphasis throughout this book on the dimensional nature of LDs, RDEs may have particular advantages, especially when there are concerns about the appropriateness of randomization from either an ethical or logistical perspective.

We have described one type of RDE, but it is also possible to consider more complex examples, such as combining an RDE with an RCE, in which students above the cut-off are assigned to a no-treatment group and students below the cut-off are randomly assigned to two or more treatments. Such a design would allow one to determine the impact of treatment against no treatment through the RDE, but also to measure the differences between the active treatments. Even in situations in which a decision is made to implement a program without an RCE or RDE, some evaluation is better than none at all. At the very least, the effectiveness of school- or district-wide implementations should be evaluated locally. Of course, any causal inferences with simple pre–post or quasi-experiments are weak because of the number of assumptions that are required. Even the most powerful interventions may not result in reliable effects if traditional pretest–posttest designs are employed and only two measurement points are sampled, with no comparison groups. Multiple unknown factors may cloud inferences about "what works."

Heterogeneity of LDs

Many studies addressing the efficacy of different treatment intervention methods continue to enroll heterogeneous groups of students with LDs who are identified by vague and inconsistent criteria and who demonstrate unaccounted differences in demographics (e.g., socioeconomic status, race, ethnicity), in the severity of behavioral and academic disabilities, and in the comorbidity of these disabilities. As such, replication efforts have been impeded, and it has been difficult to determine specific treatment effects and outcomes due to the influence of uncontrolled variables, especially in the absence of an RCE or RDE. Moreover, this lack of clarity about students' demographic, academic, and behavioral characteristics has made it difficult to determine which intervention methods are most efficacious for which students and under what specific contextual conditions (Lyon & Moats, 1997).

Unpacking Effective Interventions

Intervention studies using methods that consist of several treatment components or procedures often do not address the question of which component or procedure, or which combination or sequence of procedures, is critical to promote learning gains (Zigmond, 1993). Likewise, intervention studies employing multimodal methods frequently fail to specify how and why different interventions are selected, or the roles different interventions play in achieving treatment gains. This information is critical, because some students with LDs may require a more intensive emphasis, a different sequence, or a longer duration of exposure to and teaching on particular components of the intervention program (Lyon & Moats, 1997).

Duration of Intervention

Many intervention studies conducted with students with LDs continue to be of relatively brief duration (Berninger, 2004; Lyon & Moats, 1997). Thus, when limited effects of an intervention are reported, it is not clear whether the limited efficacy is due to the intervention itself or to the fact that it was employed for a duration that was too short to promote long-term change, no matter how robust the intervention. Too few studies evaluate the conditions that promote the maintenance of a treatment effect.

Effects of Prior Intervention

Some studies assessing the efficacy of interventions are confounded by the effects of previous and concurrent interventions. It is unclear whether a history of a particular type of intervention significantly influences response to an ongoing intervention. Likewise, it is not well understood whether concurrent interventions or methods being used in either regular or special class settings influence response to ongoing experimental interventions. These issues must be addressed in order to separate specific treatment effects from additive practice or inhibitory effects produced by previous or concurrent interventions. Again, the use of RCEs and RDEs in assigning students to interventions would help in accounting for this type of bias.

Teacher and Contextual Variables

Many intervention studies involving students with LDs have not separated specific treatment effects from clinician or teacher effects. That is, limited attention has been paid to delineating those teacher and contextual variables (e.g., teacher experience and preparation, teacher–student relationship, etc.) that influence change within any treatment program (Lyon & Moats, 1997). This may include attention to the fidelity of implementation essential to employing the intervention in other contexts. Many intervention studies do not analyze the degree of fidelity needed to implement the intervention (Berninger, 2004). Even teachers who are prepared in similar ways have been found to deviate significantly in their application of a method outside the research setting (Vaughn & Fuchs, 2003).

Generalization and Maintenance

It is unclear in many intervention studies whether gains in academic skills developed under highly controlled intervention conditions generalize to less controlled naturalistic settings. In addition, with respect to maintenance of effects, some follow-up studies have typically shown a decrease in intervention gains, particularly when measurements are taken in settings that differ from those employed in the original intervention study (Lyon & Moats, 1997). Studies need to be designed so that they can be scaled in less controlled interventions (Denton et al., 2003).

TEN GENERAL PRINCIPLES
FOR INSTRUCTING STUDENTS WITH LDs

Across reading, written expression, and mathematics and within each domain, and across foundational skills and higher-order processes, the research we have reviewed in this book (along with other corroborating studies in the literature) provides the basis for drawing 10 conclusions about how to design instruction to enhance academic outcomes for students with LDs.

1. The first step in any intervention is to increase time on task. Interventions for students with LDs should supplement instructional opportunities, not supplant them.

2. Students with LDs require an instructional approach that is explicit, well organized, and routinely provides opportunity for cumulative review of previously mastered content. This conclusion applies whether teachers are addressing foundational skills and/or higher-order processes for which transfer and generalization are critical challenges.

3. Self-regulation strategies, whereby students monitor their academic progress and set goals for their academic performance, provide an added value over and beyond systematic, explicit instruction.

4. Peer mediation provides a potentially feasible and effective method for extending scaffolded instruction, creating structured opportunities for supported practice in ways that enhance acquisition of knowledge and extend transfer of learned content.

5. It is possible to produce impressive growth in higher-order processes even when students' foundational skills are weak. This argues that educators should integrate systematic instruction on both dimensions so that as foundational skills are strengthened, teachers are simultaneously working explicitly to improve students' text comprehension, written expression, and mathematical problem solving.

6. Gains are specific to what is taught. If interventions do not teach academic content, little transfer occurs. Similarly, if academic content in one domain is learned, it does not lead to improvement in another domain if that domain is not explicitly taught. As the research in this book demonstrates, academic therapies are most effective for LDs; other intervention approaches are not well grounded and do not show the systematic efficacy of academic therapies. Basing intervention on processing deficits, theories of brain function, vision, acoustic processing, perceptual skills, and so forth, with no attention to specific academic skills and content, leads to a morass of pseudoscientific interventions that do not result in improved outcomes for people with LDs and are often simply deceptive in their appeal to parents and teachers.

7. Instructional programs need to be integrated. It is not enough to simply provide "skills" instruction. The focus should be on the ultimate set of competencies that are desirable for students with LDs. In reading, for example, intervention programs ultimately need to account for word recognition, fluency, and comprehension. The goal of any instructional program in reading is the development of proficient reading comprehension, so only teaching word recognition and fluency is not adequate. Adequate proficiency requires that opportunities for engagement and practice be incorporated into the intervention.

8. Research must increasingly take into account the heterogeneity of students with LDs. The strongest formulation of this issue is to focus on heterogeneity at the level of major comorbidities, especially those that involve combinations of academic difficulties and those behaviors subsumed under ADHD. In addition, the multifaceted nature of LDs in many students needs to be taken into account.

9. Progress must be frequently monitored and used to inform instruction at all levels of intervention. All assessments should be oriented to intervention. The field of LDs has matured to a point where testing for the sake of diagnosis is outmoded and potentially iatrogenic. People with LDs or at risk for academic difficulties, including LDs, need to move into treatment as quickly and efficiently as possible. Funds should be systematically diverted from testing to treatment.

10. Interventions designed for students with LDs must be systematically integrated with general education practices. Practice must be grounded in and modified on the basis of scientific evidence that, in turn, must be tempered by experience and judgment.

The last conclusion recognizes the explosion of systematic, empirical research on interventions that work for students who have LDs in reading, written language, and mathematics, and the need to integrate instructional design across special and general education. In a related way, major changes in identification procedures for LDs can be expected that will require a closer working relationship between special education and general education. It is likely that the current practice of waiting for students to fail before identifying LDs and then placing them in educational environments that are not capable of closing the gap will begin to change, and that greater emphasis on preventing disabilities through multiple tiers of effective general education will emerge.

For this change to occur, general education and special education must share responsibility for preventing academic difficulties whenever possible (President's Commission on Excellence in Special Education, 2002). Students likely to struggle must be identified and instructed earlier in their development than is presently the case, which will require more systematic screening and assessment, as well as better teacher preparation programs in both general education and special education. Teachers need to become experts in implementing research-based assessments and interventions. The ultimate goal of identifying students with LDs should be to provide instructional experiences that will allow them to overcome the difficulties associated with LDs. Special education therefore needs to be reformed so that it is expected to address the needs of a smaller subset of students, for whom the power of the legislation underlying special education is used to individually design and deliver more intensive interventions that could not be provided in the classroom or through small-group instruction in general education.

The research reviewed in this book illustrates that many interventions already exist that would work with many students if effectively implemented; moreover, the evidence base for achieving these outcomes is apparent. To be sure, the past decade has brought about a major convergence of scientific evidence that has the capacity to revolutionize how we address LDs and design general and special education. But research is only as good as its implementation. Perhaps for the first time in education, scientific evidence is not only informing instruction, but is also playing a major role in federal education legislation. These strides provide the basis for optimism about the future for students with LDs, a future that requires the integration of science, practice, and policy.

References

Aaron, P. G. (1997). The impending demise of the discrepancy formula. *Review of Educational Research, 67,* 461–502.

Aaron, P. G., Joshi, M., & Williams, K. A. (1999). Not all reading disabilities are alike. *Journal of Learning Disabilities, 32,* 120–137.

Aaron, P. G., Kuchta, S., & Grapenthin, C. T. (1988). Is there a thing called dyslexia? *Annals of Dyslexia, 38,* 33–49.

Abbott, R. D., & Berninger, V. W. (1993). Structural equation modeling of relationships among developmental skills and writing skills in primary- and intermediate-grade writers. *Journal of Educational Psychology, 85,* 478–508.

Ackerman, P. T., Anhalt, J. M., & Dykman, R. A. (1986). Arithmetic automatization failure in children with attention and reading disorders: Associations and sequelae. *Journal of Learning Disabilities, 19,* 222–232.

Ackerman, P. T., & Dykman, R. A. (1995). Reading disabled adolescents with and without comorbid arithmetic disability. *Developmental Neuropsychology, 11,* 351–371.

Adams, G., & Carnine, D. (2003). Direct Instruction. In H. L. Swanson, K. R. Harris, & S. Graham (Eds.), *Handbook of learning disabilities* (pp. 403–416). New York: Guilford Press.

Adams, G. L., & Engelmann, S. (1996). *Research on Direct Instruction: 25 years beyond DISTAR.* Portland, OR: Educational Achievement Systems.

Alarcon, M., DeFries J. C., Light, J. C., & Pennington, B. F. (1997). A twin study of mathematics disability. *Journal of Learning Disabilities, 30,* 617–623.

Al Otaiba, S. D. (2000). Children who do not respond to early literacy intervention: A longitudinal study across kindergarten and first grade. *Dissertation Abstracts International, 61*(04), 1354A. (UMI No. 9970028)

Altemeier, L., Jones, J., Abbott, R. D., & Berninger, V. W. (2006). Executive functions in becoming writing readers and reading writers: Note taking and report writing in third and fifth graders. *Developmental Neuropsychology, 29,* 161–173.

American Psychiatric Association. (1980). *Diagnostic and statistical manual of mental disorders* (3rd ed.). New York: Author.

American Psychiatric Association. (1994). *Diagnostic and statistical manual of mental disorders* (4th ed.). Washington, DC: Author.

Amitay, S., Ben-Yehudah, G., Banai, K., & Ahissar, M. (2002). Disabled readers suffer

from visual and auditory impairments but not from a specific magnocellular deficit. *Brain, 125,* 2272–2285.

Apel, K., Wolter, J. A., & Masterson, J. J. (2006). Effects of phonotactic and orthotactic
probabilities during fast mapping on 5–year-olds' learning to spell. *Developmental Neuropsychology, 29,* 21–42.

Aro, M., & Wimmer, H. (2003). Learning to read: English in comparison to six more
regular orthographies. *Applied Psycholinguistics, 24,* 621–635.

Aylward, E. H., Richards, T. L., Berninger, V. W., Nagy, W. E., Field, K. M., Grimme, A.
C., et al. (2003). Instructional treatment associated with changes in brain activation in children with dyslexia. *Neurology, 22,* 212–219.

Badian, N. A. (1999). Reading disability defined as a discrepancy between listening and
reading comprehension: A longitudinal study of stability, gender differences, and
prevalence. *Journal of Learning Disabilities, 32,* 138–148.

Badian, N. A., & Ghublikian, M. (1983). The personal-social characteristics of children
with poor mathematical computation skills. *Journal of Learning Disabilities, 16,*
154–157.

Baker, S., Gersten, R., & Lee, D. (2002). A synthesis of empirical research on teaching
mathematics to low-achieving students. *Elementary School Journal, 103,* 51–73.

Barbaresi, W. J., Katusic, S. K., Colligan, R. C., Weaver, A. L., & Jacobsen, S. J. (2005).
Math learning disorder: Incidence in a population-based birth cohort, 1976–82,
Rochester, Minn. *Ambulatory Pediatrics, 5,* 281–289.

Barkley, R. A. (1997). *ADHD and the nature of self-control.* New York: Guilford Press.

Barkley, R. A. (2006). *Attention-deficit hyperactivity disorder: A handbook for diagnosis and treatment* (3rd ed.). New York: Guilford Press.

Barnes, M. A., & Dennis, M. (1996). Reading comprehension deficits arise from diverse
sources: Evidence from readers with and without developmental brain pathology.
In C. Cornoldi & J. Oakhill (Eds.), *Reading comprehension difficulties* (pp. 251–
278). Hillsdale, NJ: Erlbaum.

Barnes, M. A., & Dennis, M. (2001). Knowledge-based inferencing after childhood
head injury. *Brain and Language, 76,* 253–265.

Barnes, M. A., Dennis, M., & Haefele-Kalvaitis, J. (1996). The effects of knowledge
availability and knowledge accessibility on coherence and elaborative inferencing
from six to fifteen years of age. *Journal of Experimental Child Psychology, 61,*
216–241.

Barnes, M. A., Dennis, M., & Wilkinson, M. (1999). Reading after closed head injury in
childhood: Effects on accuracy, fluency, and comprehension. *Developmental
Neuropsychology, 15,* 1–24.

Barnes, M. A., Johnston, A., & Dennis, M. (in press). Text comprehension in a
neurodevelopmental disorder, spina bifida myelomeningocele. In K. Cain & J.
Oakhill (Eds.), *Cognitive bases of children's language comprehension difficulties.*
New York: Guilford Press.

Barnes, M. A., Pengelly, S., Dennis, M., Wilkinson, M., Rogers, T., & Faulkner, H.
(2002). Mathematics skills in good readers with hydrocephalus. *Journal of the International Neuropsychological Society, 8,* 72–82.

Barnes, M. A., Wilkinson, M., Khemani, E., Boudousquie, A., Dennis, M., & Fletcher,
J. M. (2006). Arithmetic processing in children with spina bifida: Calculation accuracy, strategy use, and fact retrieval fluency. *Journal of Learning Disabilities,
39,* 174–187.

Basso, A., Taborelli, A., & Vignolo, L. A. (1978). Dissociated disorders of speaking and writing in aphasia. *Journal of Neurology, Neurosurgery, and Psychiatry, 41,* 556–563.

Bastian, H. C. (1898). *Aphasia and other speech defects.* London: Lewis.

Bates, T. C., Castles, A., Coltheart, M., Gillespie, N., Wright, M., & Martin, N. G. (2004). Behaviour genetic analyses of reading and spelling: A component processes approach. *Australian Journal of Psychology, 56,* 115–126.

Bear D. R., & Barone, D. (1991). The relationship between rapid automatized naming and orthographic knowledge. *National Reading Conference Yearbook, 40,* 179–184.

Beaton, A. A. (2002). Dyslexia and the cerebellar deficit hypothesis. *Cortex, 38,* 479–490.

Beaulieu, C., Plewes, C., Pauson, L. A., Roy, D., Snook, L., Concha, L., et al. (2005). Imaging brain connectivity in children with diverse reading ability. *NeuroImage, 25,* 1266–1271.

Bennett, D. E., & Clarizio, H. F. (1988). A comparison of methods for calculating a severe discrepancy. *Journal of School Psychology, 26,* 359–369.

Benton, A. L., & Pearl, D. (Eds.). (1978). *Dyslexia.* New York: Oxford University Press.

Bentum, K. E., & Aaron, P. G. (2003). Does reading instruction in learning disability resource rooms really work?: A longitudinal study. *Reading Psychology, 24,* 361–382.

Bereiter, C. (1967). Some persisting dilemmas in the measurement of change. In C. W. Harris (Ed.), *Problems in the measurement of change.* Madison: University of Wisconsin Press.

Bereiter, C. (1980). Toward a developmental theory of writing. In L. W. Gregg & E. R. Steinberg (Eds.), *Cognitive processes in writing* (pp. 73–93). Hillsdale, NJ: Erlbaum.

Berninger, V. W. (1994). *Reading and writing acquisition: A developmental neuropsychological perspective.* Madison, WI: Brown & Benchmark.

Berninger, V. W. (2004). Understanding the graphia in developmental dysgraphia: A developmental neuropsychological perspective for disorders in producing written language. In D. Dewey & D. Tupper (Eds.), *Developmental motor disorders: A neuropsychological perspective* (pp. 189–233). New York: Guilford Press.

Berninger, V. W., Abbott, R. D., Brooksher, R., Lemos, Z., Ogier, S., Zook, D., et al. (2000). A connectionist approach to making the predictability of English orthography explicit to at-risk beginning readers: Evidence for alternative, effective strategies. *Developmental Neuropsychology, 17,* 241–271.

Berninger, V. W., Abbott, R. D., Jones, J., Wolf, B. J., Gould, L., Anderson-Youngstrom, M., et al. (2006). Early development of language by hand: Composing, reading, listening, and speaking connections; three letter-writing modes; and fast mapping in spelling. *Developmental Neuropsychology, 29,* 61–92.

Berninger, V. W., Abbott, R. D., Vermeulen, K., Ogier, S., Brooksher, R., Zook, D., et al. (2002a). Comparison of faster and slower responders to early intervention in reading: Differentiating features of their language profiles. *Learning Disability Quarterly, 25,* 59–76.

Berninger, V. W., Abbott, R. D., Zook, D., Ogier, S., Lemons-Britton, Z., & Brooksher, R. (1999). Early intervention for reading disabilities: Teaching the alphabet principle in a connectionist framework. *Journal of Learning Disabilities, 32,* 491–503.

Berninger, V. W., & Amtmann, D. (2003). Preventing written expression disabilities through early and continuing assessment and intervention for handwriting and/or spelling problems: Research into practice. In H. L. Swanson, K. R. Harris, & S.

Graham (Eds.), *Handbook of learning disabilities* (pp. 345–363). New York: Guilford Press.

Berninger, V. W., & Fuller, F. (1992). Gender differences in orthographic, verbal, and compositional fluency: Implications for assessing writing disabilities in primary grade children. *Journal of School Psychology, 30,* 363–382.

Berninger, V. W., & Hart, T. (1992). A developmental neuropsychological perspective for reading and writing acquisition. *Educational Psychologist, 27,* 415–434.

Berninger, V. W., & Hart, T. (1993). From research to clinical assessment of reading and writing disorders: The unit of analysis problem. In R. M. Joshi & C. K. Leong (Eds.), *Reading disabilities: Diagnosis and component processes* (pp. 33–61). Dordrecht, the Netherlands: Kluwer Academic.

Berninger, V. W., Judith, V., Rutberg, E., Abbott, R. D., Garcia, N., Anderson-Youngstrom, M., et al. (2005). Tier 1 and Tier 2 early intervention for handwriting and composing. *Journal of School Psychology, 44,* 3–30.

Berninger, V. W., Nagy, W. E., Carlisle, J., Thomson, J., Hoffer, D., Abbott, S., et al. (2003a). Effective treatment for children with dyslexia in grades 4–6: Behavioral and brain evidence. In B. R. Foorman (Ed.), *Preventing and remediating reading difficulties* (pp. 381–418). Baltimore: York Press.

Berninger, V. W., Vaughan, K., Abbott, R. D., Begay, K., Coleman, K. B., Curtin, G., et al. (2002b). Teaching spelling and composition alone and together: Implications for the simple view of writing. *Journal of Educational Psychology, 94,* 291–304.

Berninger, V. W., Vaughan, K., Abbott, R., Abbott, S., Brooks, A., Rogan, L., et al. (1997). Treatment of handwriting fluency problems in beginning writing: Transfer from handwriting to composition. *Journal of Educational Psychology, 89,* 652–666.

Berninger, V. W., Vaughan, K., Abbott, R. D., Brooks, A., Abbott, S. P., Rogan, L., et al. (1998). Early intervention for spelling problems: Teaching functional spelling units of varying size with a multiple-connections framework. *Journal of Educational Psychology, 90,* 587–605.

Berninger, V. W., Vermeulen, K., Abbott, R. D., McCutchen, D., Cotton, S., Cude, J., et al. (2003b). Comparison of three approaches to supplementary reading instruction for low-achieving second-grade readers. *Language, Speech, and Hearing Services in Schools, 34,* 101–116.

Biancarosa, G., & Snow, C. E. (2004). *Reading Next—A vision for action and research in middle and high school literacy: A report to Carnegie Corporation of New York.* Washington, DC: Alliance for Excellent Education.

Birsh, J. (Ed.). (1999). *Multi-sensory teaching of basic language skills.* Baltimore: Brookes.

Bishop, D. V. M., & Clarkson, B. (2003). Written language as a window into residual language deficits: A study of children with persistent and residual speech and language impairments. *Cortex, 39,* 215–237.

Bishop, D. V. M., & Snowling, M. J. (2004). Developmental dyslexia and specific language impairment: Same or different? *Psychological Bulletin, 130,* 858–886.

Blachman, B. A. (1997). Early intervention and phonological awareness: A cautionary tale. In B. Blachman (Ed.), *Foundations of reading acquisition and dyslexia* (pp. 408–430). Mahwah, NJ: Erlbaum.

Blachman, B. A., Ball, E. W., Black, R. S., & Tangel, D. M. (1994). Kindergarten teachers develop phoneme awareness in low-income, inner-city classrooms: Does it make a difference? *Reading and Writing: An Interdisciplinary Journal, 6,* 1–18.

Blachman, B. A., Schatschneider, C., Fletcher, J. M., Francis, D. J., Clonan, S., Shaywitz, B., et al. (2004). Effects of intensive reading remediation for second and third graders. *Journal of Educational Psychology, 96,* 444–461.

Blashfield, R. K. (1993). Models of classification as related to a taxonomy of learning disabilities. In G. R. Lyon, D. B. Gray, J. F. Kavanagh, & N. A. Krasnegor (Eds.), *Better understanding learning disabilities: New views from research and their implications for education and public policies* (pp. 17–26). Baltimore: Brookes.

Bos, C. S., & Anders, P. L. (1990). Interactive teaching and learning: Instructional practices for teaching content and strategic knowledge. In T. E. Scruggs & B. Y. L. Wong (Eds.), *Intervention research in learning disabilities* (pp. 161–185). New York: Springer-Verlag.

Bowers, P. G., & Wolf, M. (1993). Theoretical links among naming speed, precise timing mechanisms, and orthographic skill in dyslexia. *Reading and Writing, 5,* 69–86.

Bradley, R., Danielson, L., & Hallahan, D. P. (Eds.). (2002). *Identification of learning disabilities: Research to practice.* Mahwah, NJ: Erlbaum.

Brambati, S. M., Termine, C., Ruffino, M., Stella, G., Fazio, F., Cappa, S. F., et al. (2004). Regional reductions of gray matter volume in familial dyslexia. *Neurology, 63,* 742–745.

Breier, J. I., Fletcher, J. M., Denton, C., & Gray, L. C. (2004). Categorical perception of speech stimuli in children at risk for reading difficulty. *Journal of Experimental Child Psychology, 88,* 152–170.

Breier, J. I., Fletcher, J. M., Foorman, B. R., & Gray, L. C. (2002). Perception of speech and nonspeech stimuli by children with and without reading disability and attention deficit hyperactivity disorder. *Journal of Experimental Child Psychology, 82,* 226–250.

Breier, J. I., Simos, P. G., Fletcher, J. M., Castillo, E. M., Zhang, W., & Papanicolaou, A. C. (2003). Abnormal activation of temporoparietal language areas during phonetic analysis in children with dyslexia. *Neuropsychology, 17,* 610–621.

Broca, P. P. (1865). Sur la siège du faculté de langage articule. *Bulletin de la Société d'Anthropologie de Paris, 6,* 377–393.

Bruandet, M., Molko, N., Cohen, L., & Dehaene, S. (2004). A cognitive characterization of dyscalculia in Turner syndrome. *Neuropsychologia, 42,* 288–298.

Bruck, M. (1987). The adult outcomes of children with learning disabilities. *Annals of Dyslexia, 37,* 252–263.

Bryan, T., Burstein, K., & Ergul, C. (2004). The social-emotional side of learning disabilities: A science-based presentation of the state of the art. *Learning Disability Quarterly, 27,* 45–51.

Bull, R., & Johnston, R. S. (1997). Children's arithmetical difficulties: Contributions from processing speed, item identification, and short-term memory. *Journal of Experimental Child Psychology, 65,* 1–24.

Burns, M. K., Appleton, J. J., & Stehouwer, J. D. (2005). Meta-analytic review of responsiveness-to-intervention research: Examining field-based and research-implemented models. *Journal of Psychoeducational Assessment, 23,* 381–394.

Burt, C. (1937). *The backward child.* London: University of London Press.

Butterworth, B. (2005). Developmental dyscalculia. In J. I. D. Campbell (Ed.), *Handbook of mathematical cognition* (pp. 455–467). New York: Psychology Press.

Byrne, B., Delaland, C., Fielding-Barnsley, R., Quain, P., Samuelsson, S., Hoien, T., et al.

(2002). Longitudinal twin study of early reading development in three countries: Preliminary results. *Annals of Dyslexia, 52*, 49–74.

Byrne, B., Samuelsson, S., Wadsworth, S., Hulslander, J., Corley, R., DeFries, J. C., et al. (in press). Longitudinal twin study of early literacy development: Preschool through Grade 1. *Reading and Writing*.

Cain, K., & Oakhill, J. V. (1999). Inference making and its relation to comprehension failure in young children. *Reading and Writing: An Interdisciplinary Journal, 11*, 489–503.

Cain, K., Oakhill, J. V., Barnes, M. A., & Bryant, P. E. (2001). Comprehension skill, inference-making ability, and the relation to knowledge. *Memory and Cognition, 29*, 850–859.

Cain, K., Oakhill, J. V., & Bryant, P. (2000). Phonological skills and comprehension failures: A test of the phonological processing deficits hypothesis. *Reading and Writing, 13*, 31–56.

Cain, K., Oakhill, J. V., & Bryant, P. (2004a). Children's reading comprehension ability: Concurrent prediction by working memory, verbal ability, and component skills. *Journal of Educational Psychology, 96*, 31–42.

Cain, K., Oakhill, J. V., & Lemmon, K. (2004b). Individual differences in the inference of word meanings from context: The influence of reading comprehension, vocabulary knowledge, and memory capacity. *Journal of Educational Psychology, 96*, 671–681.

Canning, P. M., Orr, R. R., & Rourke, B. P. (1980). Sex differences in the perceptual, visual–motor, linguistic and concept-formation abilities of retarded readers? *Journal of Learning Disabilities, 13*, 563–567.

Caplan, D. (2004). Functional neuroimaging studies of written sentence comprehension. *Scientific Studies of Reading, 8*, 225–240.

Caravolas, M. (2005). The nature and causes of dyslexia in different languages. *The science of reading: A handbook* (pp. 336–356). Oxford, UK: Blackwell.

Caravolas, M., Volin, J., & Hulme, C. (2005). Phoneme awareness is a key component of alphabetic literacy skills in consistent and inconsistent orthographies: Evidence from Czech and English children. *Journal of Experimental Child Psychology, 92*, 107–139.

Carey, S. (2004). Bootstrapping and the origin of concepts. *Daedalus, 133*, 59–68.

Carlson, C. D., & Francis, D. J. (2002). Increasing the reading achievement of at-risk children through Direct Instruction: Evaluation of the Rodeo Institute for Teacher Excellence (RITE). *Journal of Education for Students Placed at Risk, 7*, 141–166.

Carnine, D. (1991). Reforming mathematics instruction: The role of curriculum materials. *Journal of Behavioral Education, 1*, 37–57.

Casby, M. W. (1992). The cognitive hypothesis and its influence on speech–language services in schools. *Language, Speech, and Hearing Services in Schools, 23*, 198–202.

Case, L. P., Harris, K. R., & Graham, S. (1992). Improving the mathematical problem solving skills of students with learning disabilities: Self-regulated strategy development. *Journal of Special Education, 26*, 1–19.

Castles, A., & Coltheart, M. (1993). Varieties of developmental dyslexia. *Cognition, 47*, 149–180.

Castles, A., & Coltheart, M. (2004). Is there a causal link from phonological awareness to success in learning to read? *Cognition, 91*, 77–111.

Cataldo, M. G., & Cornoldi, C. (1998). Self-monitoring in poor and good reading comprehenders and their use of strategy. *British Journal of Developmental Psychology, 16*, 155–165.

Catrambone, R., & Holyoak, K. J. (1989). Overcoming contextual limitations on problem-solving transfer. *Journal of Experimental Psychology: Learning, Memory, and Cognition, 15*, 1127–1156.

Catts, H., Hogan, T., & Adlof, S. M. (2005). Developmental changes in reading and reading disabilities. In H. Catts & A. Kamhi (Eds.), *Connections between language and reading disabilities* (pp. 25–40). Mahwah, NJ: Erlbaum.

Catts, H. W., Adlof, S. M., Hogan, T. P., & Weismer, S. E. (2005). Are specific language impairment and dyslexia distinct disorders? *Journal of Speech, Language, and Hearing Research, 48*, 1378–1396.

Catts, H. W., Fey, M. E., Tomblin, J. B., & Zhang, X. (2002a). A longitudinal investigation of reading outcomes in children with language impairments. *Journal of Speech, Language, and Hearing Research, 45*, 1142–1155.

Catts, H. W., Gillispie, M., Leonard, L. B., Kail, R. V., & Miller, C. A. (2002b). The role of speed processing, rapid naming, and phonological awareness in reading achievement. *Journal of Learning Disabilities, 35*, 510–525.

Catts, H. W., & Hogan, T. P. (2003). Language basis of reading disabilities and implications for early identification and remediation. *Reading Psychology, 24*, 223–246.

Catts, H. W., Hogan, T. P., & Fey, M. E. (2003). Subgrouping poor readers on the basis of individual differences in reading-related abilities. *Journal of Learning Disabilities, 36*, 151–164.

Catts, H., Taylor, P., & Zhang, X. (2006, February 4). *Individual differences in reading achievement: Application of growth mixture modeling and latent profile analyses.* Paper presented at the annual Pacific Coast Research Conference, San Diego, CA.

Cawley, J. F., Parmar, R. S., Yan, W., & Miller, J. H. (1998). Arithmetic computation performance of students with learning disabilities: Implications for curriculum. *Learning Disabilities Research and Practice, 13*, 68–74.

Chapman, J. W., Tunmer, W. E., & Prochnow, J. E. (2001). Does success in the Reading Recovery program depend on developing proficiency in phonological processing skills?: A longitudinal study in a whole language instruction context. *Scientific Studies of Reading, 5*, 141–176.

Chard, D. J., Vaughn, S., & Tyler, B. (2002). A synthesis of research on effective interventions for building reading fluency with elementary students with learning disabilities. *Journal of Learning Disabilities, 35*, 386–406.

Cirino, P. T., Israelian, M. K., Morris, M. K., & Morris, R. D. (2005). Evaluation of the double-deficit hypothesis in college students referred for learning difficulties. *Journal of Learning Disabilities, 38*, 29–44.

Cirino, P. T., Morris, M. K., & Morris, R. D. (2006). Neuropsycholological concomitants of calculation skills in college students referred for learning disabilities. *Developmental Neuropsychology, 21*, 201–218.

Cisek, G. J. (2001). Conjectures on the rise and call of standard setting: An introduction to context and practice. In G. J. Cisek (Ed.), *Setting performance standards: Concepts, methods, and perspectives* (pp. 3–18). Mahwah, NJ: Erlbaum.

Clairborne, J. H. (1906). Types of congenital symbol amblyopia. *Journal of the American Medical Association, 47*, 1813–1816.

Clark, D. B., Hulme, C., & Snowling, M. (2005). Individual differences in RAN and reading: A response timing analysis. *Journal of Research in Reading, 28*, 73–86.

Clark, D. B., & Uhry, J. K. (1995). *Dyslexia: Theory and practice of remedial instruction*. Baltimore, MD: York Press.

Clay, M. M. (1993). *Reading Recovery: A guidebook for teachers in training*. Portsmouth, NH: Heinemann.

Clay, M. M. (2002). *An observation survey of early literacy achievement* (2nd ed.). Portsmouth, NH: Heinemann.

Clements, S. D. (1966). *Minimal brain dysfunction in children* (NINDB Monograph No. 3). Washington, DC: U.S. Department of Health, Education and Welfare.

Cohen, J. (1983). The cost of dichotomization. *Applied Psychological Measurement, 7*, 249–253.

Cohen, L. D., & Marks, K. S. (2002). How infants process addition and subtraction events. *Developmental Science, 5*, 186–201.

Coltheart, M. (2005a). Modeling reading: The dual-route approach. In M. J. Snowling & C. Hulme (Eds.), *The science of reading: A handbook* (pp. 6–23). Oxford, UK: Blackwell.

Coltheart, M. (2005b). Analyzing developmental disorders of reading. *Advances in Speech Language Pathology, 7*, 49–57.

Compton, D. L., DeFries, J. C., & Olson, R. K. (2001). Are RAN and phonological awareness deficits additive in children with reading disabilities? *Dyslexia, 3*, 125–149.

Connelly, V., Campbell, S., MacLean, M., & Barnes, J. (2006). Contribution of lower order skills to the written composition of college students with and without dyslexia. *Developmental Neuropsychology, 29*, 175–196.

Cooley, E. J., & Ayers, R. R. (1988). Self-concept and success–failure attributions of nonhandicapped students and students with learning disabilities. *Journal of Learning Disabilities, 21*, 174–178.

Cooper, G., & Sweller, J. (1987). Effects of schema acquisition and rule automation on mathematical problem solving transfer. *Journal of Educational Psychology, 79*, 347–362.

Cornoldi, C., DeBeni, R., & Pazzaglia, F. (1996). Profiles of reading comprehension difficulties: An analysis of single cases. In C. Cornoldi & J. Oakhill (Eds.), *Reading comprehension difficulties: Processes and intervention* (pp. 113–136). Mahwah, NJ: Erlbaum.

Coyne, M. D., Kame'enui, E. J., Simmons, D. C., & Harn, B. A. (2004). Beginning reading intervention as inoculation or insulin: First-grade reading performance of strong responders to kindergarten intervention. *Journal of Learning Disabilities, 37*, 90–104.

Critchley, M. (1970). *The dyslexic child*. Springfield, IL: Charles C Thomas.

Cruickshank, W. M., Bice, H. V., & Wallen, N. E. (1957). *Perception and cerebral palsy*. Syracuse, NY: Syracuse University Press.

Cunningham, A. E., & Stanovich, K. E. (1999). What reading does for the mind. *American Educator, 4*, 8–15.

D'Agostino, J. V., & Murphy, J. A. (2004). A meta-analysis of Reading Recovery in United States schools. *Educational Evaluation and Policy Analysis, 26*, 23–38.

Davis, C. J., Gayan, J., Knopik, V. S., Smith, S. D., Cardon, L. R., Pennington, B. F., et al. (2001). Etiology of reading difficulties and rapid naming: The Colorado Twin Study of Reading Disability. *Behavior Genetics, 31*, 625–635.

DeFries, J. C., & Fulker, D. W. (1985). Multiple regression analysis of twin data. *Behavior Genetics, 15*, 467–478.

DeFries, J. C., & Gillis, J. J. (1991). Etiology of reading deficits in learning disabilities: Quantitative genetic analyses. In J. E. Obrzut & G. W. Hynd (Eds.), *Neuropsychological foundations of learning disabilities: A handbook of issues, methods, and practice* (pp. 29–48). San Diego, CA: Academic Press.

Dehaene, S., & Cohen, L. (1997). Cerebral pathways for calculation: Double disassociation between rote verbal and quantitative knowledge of arithmetic. *Cortex, 33,* 219–250.

Dehaene, S., Cohen, L., Sigman, M., & Vinckier, F. (2005). The neural code for written words: A proposal. *Trends in Cognitive Sciences, 9,* 335–341.

Dehaene, S., Molko, N., Cohen, L., & Wilson, A. L. (2004). Arithmetic and the brain. *Current Opinion in Neurobiology, 14,* 218–224.

Dehaene, S., Spelke, E., Pinel, P., Stanescu, R., & Tsiukin, S. (1999). Sources of mathematical thinking: Behavioral and brain-injury evidence. *Science, 284,* 970–974.

de Jong, P. F., & van der Leij, A. (2003). Developmental changes in the manifestation of a phonological deficit in dyslexic children learning to read a regular orthography. *Journal of Educational Psychology, 95,* 22–40.

de Jong, P. F., & Vrielink, L. O. (2004). Rapid automatic naming: Easy to measure, hard to improve (quickly). *Annals of Dyslexia, 54,* 65–88.

De La Paz, S., Swanson, P. M., & Graham, S. (1998). The contribution of executive control to the revising by students with writing and learning difficulties. *Journal of Educational Psychology, 90,* 448–460.

Denckla, M. B., & Cutting, L. E. (1999). Historical significance of rapid automatized naming. *Annals of Dyslexia, 49,* 29–42.

Dennis, M. (1988). Language and the young damaged brain. In T. Boll & B. K. Bryant (Eds.), *Clinical neuropsychology and brain function: Research, measurement and practice* (Vol. 7, pp. 85–123). Washington DC: American Psychological Association.

Deno, S. L., & Marston, D. (2001). *Test of Oral Reading Fluency.* Minneapolis, MN: Educators Testing Service.

Denton, C. A., Ciancio, D. J., & Fletcher, J. M. (2006). Validity, reliability, and utility of the Observation Survey of Early Literacy Achievement. *Reading Research Quarterly, 41,* 8–34.

Denton, C. A., Fletcher, J. M., Anthony, J. L., & Francis, D. J. (in press). An evaluation of intensive intervention for students with persistent reading difficulties. *Journal of Learning Disabilities.*

Denton, C. A., & Mathes, P. G. (2003). Intervention for struggling readers: Possibilities and challenges. In B. R. Foorman (Ed.), *Preventing and remediating reading difficulties* (pp. 229–252). Baltimore: York Press.

Denton, C. A., Vaughn, S., & Fletcher, J. M. (2003). Bringing research-based practice in reading intervention to scale. *Learning Disabilities Research and Practice, 18,* 201–211.

Desoete, A., & Roeyers, H. (2005). Cognitive skills in mathematical problem solving in grade 3. *British Journal of Educational Psychology, 75,* 119–138.

Deutsch, G. K., Doughtery, R. F., Bammer, R., Siok, W. T., Gabrieli, J. D. E., & Wandell, B. (2005). Children's reading performance is correlated with white matter structure measured by diffusion tensor imaging. *Cortex, 41,* 354–363.

Doehring, D. G. (1978). The tangled web of behavioral research on developmental dyslexia. In A. L. Benton & D. Pearl (Eds.), *Dyslexia* (pp. 123–137). New York: Oxford University Press.

Donovan, M. S., & Cross, C. T. (2002). *Minority students in special and gifted education*. Washington, DC: National Academy Press.

Doris, J. L. (1993). Defining learning disabilities: A history of the search for consensus. In G. R. Lyon, D. B Gray, J. F. Kavanagh, & N. A. Krasnegor (Eds.), *Better understanding learning disabilities: New views from research and their implications for education and public policies* (pp. 97–116). Baltimore: Brookes.

Duara, R., Kuslch, A., Gross-Glenn, K., Barker, W., Jallad, B., Pascal, S., et al. (1991). Neuroanatomic differences between dyslexic and normal readers on magnetic resonance imaging scans. *Archives of Neurology, 48,* 410–416.

Dykman, R. A., Ackerman, P., Clements, S. D., & Peters, J. E. (1971). Specific learning disabilities: An attentional deficit syndrome. In H. R. Myklebust (Ed.), *Progress in learning disabilities* (Vol. 2, pp. 56–93). New York: Grune & Stratton.

Eckert, M. A., Leonard, C. M., Richards, T. L., Aylward, E. H., Thomson, J., & Berninger, V. W. (2003). Anatomical correlates of dyslexia: Frontal and cerebellar findings. *Brain, 126,* 482–494.

Eden, G. F., Jones, K. M., Cappell, K., Gareau, L., Wood, F. B., Zeffiro, T. A., et al. (2004). Neural changes following remediation in adult developmental dyslexia. *Neuron, 44,* 411–422.

Eden, G. F., Stern, J. F., Wood, M. H., & Wood, F. B. (1995). Verbal and visual problems in dyslexia. *Journal of Learning Disabilities, 28,* 282–290.

Eden, G. F., & Zeffiro, T. A. (1998). Neural systems affected in developmental dyslexia revealed by functional neuroimaging. *Neuron, 21,* 279–282.

Elbaum, B., & Vaughn, S. (2003). For which students with learning disabilities are self-concept interventions effective? *Journal of Learning Disabilities, 36,* 101–108.

Elbaum, B., Vaughn, S., Hughes, M. T., & Moody, S. W. (2000). How effective are one-to-one tutoring programs in reading for elementary students at risk for reading failure?: A meta-analysis of the intervention research. *Journal of Educational Psychology 92,* 605–619.

Ellis, A. W. (1984). The cognitive neuropsychology of developmental (and acquired) dyslexia: A critical survey. *Cognitive Neuropsychology, 2,* 169–205.

Engelmann, S., Becker, W. C., Hanner, S., & Johnson, G. (1978). *Corrective Reading Program: Series guide.* Chicago: Science Research Associates.

Engelmann, S., Carnine, D. W., Engelmann, O., & Kelly, B. (1991). *Connecting math concepts.* Chicago: Science Research Associates.

Feigenson, L., Dehaene, S., & Spelke, E. (2004). Core systems of numbers. *Trends in Cognitive Sciences, 8,* 307–314.

Fernald, G. (1943). *Remedial techniques in basic school subjects.* New York: McGraw-Hill.

Filipek, P. (1996). Structural variations in measures in the developmental disorders. In R. Thatcher, G. Lyon, J. Rumsey, & N. Krasnegor (Eds.), *Developmental neuroimaging: Mapping the development of brain and behavior* (pp. 169–186). San Diego: Academic Press.

Finch, A. J., Nicolson, R. I., & Fawcett, A. J. (2002). Evidence for a neuroanatomical difference within the olivo-cerebellar pathway of adults with dyslexia. *Cortex, 38,* 529–539.

Fisher, S. E., & DeFries, J. C. (2002). Developmental dyslexia: Genetic dissection of a complex cognitive trait. *Neuroscience, 3,* 767–780.

Fleishner, J. E. (1994). Diagnosis and assessment of mathematics learning disabilities. In

G. R. Lyon (Ed.), *Frames of reference for the assessment of learning disabilities: New views on measurement issues* (pp. 441–458). Baltimore: Brookes.

Fletcher, J. M. (2005). Predicting math outcomes: Reading predictors and comorbidity. *Journal of Learning Disabilities, 38,* 308–312.

Fletcher, J. M., Denton, C., & Francis, D. J. (2005a). Validity of alternative approaches for the identification of LD: Operationalizing unexpected underachievement. *Journal of Learning Disabilities, 38,* 545–552.

Fletcher, J. M., Foorman, B. R., Boudousquie, A. B., Barnes, M. A., Schatschneider, C. & Francis, D. J. (2002). Assessment of reading and learning disabilities: A research-based, intervention-oriented approach. *Journal of School Psychology, 40,* 27–63.

Fletcher, J. M., Foorman, B. R., Shaywitz, S. E., & Shaywitz, B. A. (1999a). Conceptual and methodological issues in dyslexia research: A lesson for developmental disorders. In H. Tager-Flusberg (Ed.), *Neurodevelopmental disorders* (pp. 271–306). Cambridge, MA: MIT Press.

Fletcher, J. M., Francis, D. J., Morris, R. D., & Lyon, G. R. (2005b). Evidence-based assessment of learning disabilities in children and adolescents. *Journal of Clinical Child and Adolescent Psychology, 34,* 506–522.

Fletcher, J. M., Francis, D. J., Stuebing, K. K., Shaywitz, B. A., Shaywitz, S. E., Shankweiler, D. P., et al. (1996a). Conceptual and methodological issues in construct definition. In G. R. Lyon & N. A. Krasnegor (Eds.), *Attention, memory, and executive functions* (pp. 17–42). Baltimore: Brookes.

Fletcher, J. M., Lyon, G. R., Barnes, M., Stuebing, K. K., Francis, D. J., Olson, R., et al. (2002). Classification of learning disabilities: An evidence-based evaluation. In R. Bradley, L. Danielson, & D. P. Hallahan (Eds.), *Identification of learning disabilities: Research to practice* (pp. 185–250). Mahwah, NJ: Erlbaum.

Fletcher, J. M., Morris, R. D., & Lyon, G. R. (2003). Classification and definition of learning disabilities: An integrative perspective. In H. L. Swanson, K. R. Harris, & S. Graham (Eds.), *Handbook of learning disabilities* (pp. 30–56). New York: Guilford Press.

Fletcher, J. M., Shaywitz, S. E., Shankweiler, D., Katz, L., Liberman, I. Y., Steubing, K. K., et al. (1994). Cognitive profiles of reading disability: Comparisons of discrepancy and low achievement definitions. *Journal of Educational Psychology, 86,* 6–23.

Fletcher, J. M., Shaywitz, S. E., & Shaywitz, B. A. (1999b). Comorbidity of learning and attention disorders: Separate but equal. *Pediatric Clinics of North America, 46,* 885–897.

Fletcher, J. M., Simos, P. G., Papanicolaou, A. C., & Denton, C. (2004). Neuroimaging in reading research. In N. Duke & M. Mallette (Eds.), *Literacy research methods* (pp. 252–286). New York: Guilford Press.

Fletcher, J. M., Stuebing, K. K., Shaywitz, B. A., Brandt, M. E., Francis, D. J., & Shaywitz, S. E. (1996b). Measurement issues in the interpretation of behavior-brain relationships. In R. W. Thatcher, G. R. Lyon, J. Rumsey, & N. Krasnegor (Eds.), *Developmental neuroimaging: Mapping the development of brain and behavior* (pp. 255–262). San Diego: Academic Press.

Florida Center for Reading Research. (2005). Spell Read P.A.T. Retrieved May 29, 2006, from http://www.fcrr.org/FCRRReports/PDF/spell_read_pat.pdf.

Florida Center for Reading Research. Retrieved June 5, 2006, from http://www.fcrr.org/.

Flowers, L., Meyer, M., Lovato, J., Wood, F., & Felton, R. (2001). Does third grade discrepancy status predict the course of reading development? *Annals of Dyslexia*, *51*, 49–71.

Flynn, J. M., & Rahbar, M. H. (1993). The effects of age and gender on reading achievement: Implications for pediatric counseling. *Journal of Developmental and Behavioral Pediatrics, 14*, 304–307.

Flynn, J. M., & Rahbar, M. H. (1994). Prevalence of reading failure in boys compared with girls. *Psychology in the Schools, 31*, 66–70.

Foorman, B. R. (1994). The relevance of a connectionist model of reading for "the great debate." *Educational Psychology Review, 16*, 25–47.

Foorman, B. R., Fletcher, J. M., & Francis, D. J. (2004). Early reading assessment. In W. Evans & H. J. Walberg (Eds.), *Student learning, evaluating teaching effectiveness* (pp. 81–125). Stanford, CA: Hoover Press.

Foorman, B. R., Francis, D. J., Fletcher, J. M., Schatschneider, C., & Mehta, P. (1998). The role of instruction in learning to read: Preventing reading failure in at-risk children. *Journal of Educational Psychology, 90*, 37–55.

Foorman, B. R., Francis, D. J., Winikates, D., Mehta, P., Schatschneider, C., & Fletcher, J. M. (1997). Early interventions for children with reading disabilities. *Scientific Studies of Reading, 1*, 255–276.

Francis, D. J., Fletcher, J. M., Catts, H., & Tomblin, B. (2005b). Dimensions affecting the assessment of reading comprehension. In S. G. Paris & S. A. Stahl (Eds.), *Current issues in reading comprehension and assessment* (pp. 369–394). Mahwah, NJ: Erlbaum.

Francis, D. J., Fletcher, J. M., Stuebing, K. K., Lyon, G. R., Shaywitz, B. A., & Shaywitz, S. E. (2005a). Psychometric approaches to the identification of learning disabilities: IQ and achievement scores are not sufficient. *Journal of Learning Disabilities, 38*, 98–110.

Francis, D. J., Shaywitz, S. E., Stuebing, K. K., Shaywitz, B. A., & Fletcher, J. M. (1996). Developmental lag versus deficit models of reading disability: A longitudinal, individual growth curves analysis. *Journal of Educational Psychology, 88*, 3–17.

Frith, U. (Ed.). (1980). *Cognitive processes in spelling*. New York: Academic Press.

Fuchs, D., & Fuchs, L. S. (2005). Peer-Assisted Learning Strategies: Promoting word recognition, fluency, and reading comprehension in young children. *Journal of Special Education, 39*, 34–44.

Fuchs, D., & Fuchs, L. S. (2006). Introduction to response to intervention: What, why, and how valid is it? *Reading Research Quarterly, 41*, 93–99.

Fuchs, D., Fuchs, L. S., Mathes, P., & Simmons, D. (1997). Peer-Assisted Learning Strategies: Making classrooms more responsive to student diversity. *American Educational Research Journal, 34*, 174–206.

Fuchs, D., Fuchs, L. S., Thompson, A., Al Otaiba, S., Yen, L., Yang, N. Y., et al. (2001a). Is reading important in reading-readiness programs?: A randomized field trial with teachers as field implementers. *Journal of Educational Psychology, 93*, 251–267.

Fuchs, L. S., Bahr, C. M., & Rieth, H. J. (1989a). Effects of goal structures and performance contingencies on the math performance of adolescents with learning disabilities. *Journal of Learning Disabilities, 22*, 554–560.

Fuchs, L. S., Compton, D. L., Fuchs, D., Hamlett, C. L., & Bryant, J. (2006a). *Modeling the development of math competence in first grade*. Paper presented at the annual meeting of the Pacific Coast Research Conference.

Fuchs, L. S., Compton, D. L., Fuchs, D., Paulsen, K., Bryant, J. D., & Hamlett, C. L.

(2005). The prevention, identification, and cognitive determinants of math difficulty. *Journal of Educational Psychology, 97*, 493–513.

Fuchs, L. S., Deno, S. L., & Mirkin, P. K. (1984). The effects of frequent curriculum-based measurement and evaluation on student achievement, pedagogy, and student awareness of learning. *American Educational Research Journal, 21*, 449–460.

Fuchs, L. S., & Fuchs, D. (1998). Treatment validity: A simplifying concept for reconceptualizing the identification of learning disabilities. *Learning Disabilities Research and Practice, 4*, 204–219.

Fuchs, L. S., & Fuchs, D. (2000). Building student capacity to work productively during peer-assisted reading activities. In B. Taylor, M. Graves, & P. van den Broek (Eds.), *Reading for meaning: Fostering comprehension in the middle grades* (pp. 95–115). New York: Teachers College Press.

Fuchs, L. S., Fuchs, D., Compton, D. L., Powell, S. R., Seethaler, P. M., Capizzi, A. M., et al. (2006b). The cognitive correlates of third-grade skill in arithmetic, algorithmic computation, and arithmetic word problems. *Journal of Educational Psychology, 98*, 29–43.

Fuchs, L. S., Fuchs, D., & Hamlett, C. L. (1989b). Effects of alternative goal structures within curriculum-based measurement. *Exceptional Children, 55*, 429–438.

Fuchs, L. S., Fuchs, D., & Hamlett, C. L. (1989c). Effects of instrumental use of curriculum-based measurement to enhance instructional programs. *Remedial and Special Education, 102*, 43–52.

Fuchs, L. S., Fuchs, D., & Hamlett, C. L. (1989d). Monitoring reading growth using student recalls: Effects of two teacher feedback systems. *Journal of Educational Research, 83*, 103–111.

Fuchs, L. S., Fuchs, D., Hamlett, C. L., & Allinder, R. M. (1991a). Effects of expert system advice within curriculum-based measurement on teacher planning and student achievement in spelling. *School Psychology Review, 20*, 49–66.

Fuchs, L. S., Fuchs, D., Hamlett, C. L., & Appleton, A. C. (2002a). Explicitly teaching for transfer: Effects on the mathematical problem solving performance of students with disabilities. *Learning Disabilities Research and Practice, 17*, 90–106.

Fuchs, L. S., Fuchs, D., Hamlett, C. L., & Stecker, P. M. (1991b). Effects of curriculum-based measurement and consultation on teacher planning and student achievement in mathematics operations. *American Educational Research Journal, 28*, 617–641.

Fuchs, L. S., Fuchs, D., Hamlett, C. L., & Whinnery, K. (1991c). Effects of goal line feedback on level, slope, and stability of performance within curriculum-based measurement. *Learning Disabilities Research and Practice, 6*, 65–73.

Fuchs, L. S., Fuchs, D., & Karns, K. (2001b). Enhancing kindergartners' mathematical development: Effects of Peer-Assisted Learning Strategies. *Elementary School Journal, 101*, 495–510.

Fuchs, L. S., Fuchs, D., Phillips, N. B., Hamlett, C. L., & Karns, K. (1995). Acquisition and transfer effects of class wide Peer-Assisted Learning Strategies in mathematics for students with varying learning histories. *School Psychology Review, 24*, 604–620.

Fuchs, L. S., Fuchs, D., & Prentice, K. (2004). Responsiveness to mathematical-problem-solving treatment among students with risk for mathematics disability, with and without risk for reading disability. *Journal of Learning Disabilities, 27*, 273–306.

Fuchs, L. S., Fuchs, D., Prentice, K., Burch, M., Hamlett, C. L., Owen, R., et al. (2003a).

Explicitly teaching for transfer: Effects on third-grade students' mathematical problem solving. *Journal of Educational Psychology, 95,* 293–305.

Fuchs, L. S., Fuchs, D., Prentice, K., Burch, M., Hamlett, C. L., Owen, R., et al. (2003b). Enhancing third-grade students' mathematical problem solving with self-regulated learning strategies. *Journal of Educational Psychology, 95,* 306–326.

Fuchs, L. S., Fuchs, D., Yazdian, L., & Powell, S. R. (2002b). Enhancing first-grade children's mathematical development with peer-assisted learning strategies. *School Psychology Review, 31,* 569–584.

Galaburda, A. M. (1993). The planum temporale. *Archives of Neurology, 50,* 457.

Galaburda, A. M., Sherman, G. P., Rosen, G. D., Aboitiz, F., & Geschwind, N. (1985). Developmental dyslexia: Four consecutive patients with cortical anomalies. *Annals of Neurology, 18,* 222–233.

Gayan, J., & Olson, R. K. (2001). Genetic and environmental influences on orthographic and phonological skills in children with reading disabilities. *Developmental Neuropsychology, 20,* 483–507.

Geary, D. C. (1993). Mathematical disabilities: Cognitive, neuropsychological, and genetic components. *Psychological Bulletin, 114,* 345–362.

Geary, D. C. (2004). Mathematics and learning disabilities. *Journal of Learning Disabilities, 37,* 4–15.

Geary, D. C. (2005). Role of cognitive theory in the study of learning disability in mathematics. *Journal of Learning Disabilities, 38,* 305–307.

Geary, D. C., Hamson, C. O., & Hoard, M. K. (2000). Numerical and arithmetical cognition: A longitudinal study of process and concept deficits in children with learning disability. *Journal of Experimental Child Psychology, 77,* 236–263.

Geary, D. C., Hoard, M. K., Byrd-Craven, J., & DeSoto, M. C. (2004). Strategy choices in simple and complex addition: Contributions of working memory and counting knowledge for children with mathematical disability. *Journal of Experimental Child Psychology, 88,* 121–151.

Geary, D. C., Hoard, M. K., & Hamson, C. O. (1999). Numerical and arithmetical cognition: Patterns of functions and deficits in children at risk for a mathematical disability. *Journal of Experimental Child Psychology, 74,* 213–239.

Gelman, R., & Butterworth, B. (2005). Number and language: How are they related? *Trends in Cognitive Sciences, 9,* 6–10.

Gernsbacher, M. A., & Kaschak, M. P. (2003). Neuroimaging studies of language production and comprehension. *Annual Reviews of Psychology, 54,* 91–114.

Gersten, R., Jordan, N. C., & Flojo, J. R. (2005). Early identification and interventions for students with mathematics difficulties. *Journal of Learning Disabilities, 38,* 293–304.

Gersten, R. M., White, W. A., Falco, R., & Carnine, D. (1982). Teaching basic discriminations to handicapped and non-handicapped individuals through a dynamic presentation of instructional stimuli. *Analysis and Intervention in Developmental Disabilities, 2,* 305–317.

Geschwind, N., & Levitsky, W. (1968). Human brain: Left–right asymmetries in temporal speech region. *Science, 161,* 186–187.

Gick, M. L., & Holyoak, K. J. (1980). Analogical problem solving. *Cognitive Psychologist, 12,* 306–355.

Gillingham, A., & Stillman, B. (1965). *Remedial training for children with specific disability in reading, spelling and penmanship* (7th ed.). Cambridge, MA: Educators.

Ginsburg, H. P., Klein, A., & Starkey, P. (1998). The development of children's mathematical thinking: Connecting research with practice. In W. Damon (Series Ed.), & I. E. Siegal & K. A. Renninger (Vol. Eds.), *Handbook of child psychology: Vol. 4. Child psychology in practice* (5th ed., pp. 401–476). New York: Wiley.

Gleitman, L. R., & Rosen, P. (1973). Teaching reading by use of a syllabary. *Reading Research Quarterly, 8,* 447–483.

Goldstein, K. (1948). *Language and language disorders.* New York: Grune & Stratton.

Good, R. H., III, Simmons, D. C., & Kame'enui, E. J. (2001). The importance and decision-making utility of a continuum of fluency-based indicators of foundational reading skills for third-grade high-stakes outcomes. *Scientific Studies of Reading, 5,* 257–288.

Goswami, U. (2002). Phonology, reading development and dyslexia: A cross-linguistic perspective. *Annals of Dyslexia, 52,* 141–163.

Gough, P. B. (1984). Word recognition. In P. D. Pearson, R. Barr, M. L. Kamil, & P. Mosenthal (Eds.), *Handbook of reading research* (pp. 225–253). New York: Longman.

Gough, P. B., & Tunmer, W. E. (1986). Decoding, reading and reading disability. *Remedial and Special Education, 7,* 6–10.

Graham, S. (2005). Strategy instruction and the teaching of writing: A meta-analysis. In C. MacArthur, S. Graham, & J. Fitzgerald (Eds.), *Handbook of writing research.* New York: Guilford Press.

Graham, S., Berninger, V. W., Abbott, R. D., Abbott, S. P., & Whitaker, D. (1997). Role of mechanics in composing of elementary school students: A new methodological approach. *Journal of Educational Psychology, 89,* 170–182.

Graham, S., & Harris, K. R. (1993). Self-regulated strategy development: Helping students with learning problems develop as writers. *Elementary School Journal, 94,* 169–181.

Graham, S., & Harris, K. R. (1996). Addressing problems in attention, memory, and executive function. In G. R. Lyon & N. A. Krasnegor (Eds.), *Attention, memory, and executive function* (pp. 349–366). Baltimore: Brookes.

Graham, S., & Harris, K. R. (2003). Students with learning disabilities and the process of writing: A meta-analysis of SRSD studies. In H. L. Swanson, K. R. Harris, & S. Graham (Eds.), *Handbook of learning disabilities* (pp. 323–344). New York: Guilford Press.

Graham, S., Harris, K. R., & Chorzempa, B. F. (2002). Contribution of spelling instruction to the spelling, writing, and reading of poor spellers. *Journal of Educational Psychology, 94,* 669–686.

Graham, S., Harris, K. R., & Fink, B. (2000). Is handwriting causally related to learning to write?: Treatment of handwriting problems in beginning writers. *Journal of Educational Psychology, 92,* 620–633.

Graham, S., Harris, K. R., MacArthur, C., & Schwartz, S. (1991). Writing and writing instruction with students with learning disabilities: A review of a program of research. *Learning Disability Quarterly, 14,* 89–114.

Graham, S., Harris, K. R., & Mason, L. (2005). Improving the writing performance, knowledge, and motivation of struggling young writers: The effects of self-regulated strategy development. *Contemporary Educational Psychology, 30,* 207–241.

Graham, S., Struck, M., Santoro, J., & Berninger, V. W. (2006). Dimensions of good and poor handwriting legibility in first and second graders: Motor programs, visual–

spatial arrangement, and letter formation parameter setting. *Developmental Neuropsychology, 29,* 43–60.

Graham, S., Weintraub, N., & Berninger, V. (2001). Which manuscript letters do primary grade children write legibly? *Journal of Educational Psychology, 93,* 488–497.

Gregg, N. (1991). Disorders of written expression. In A. Bain, L. Bailet, & L. Moats (Eds.), *Written language disorders: Theory into practice* (pp. 65–97). Austin, TX: PRO-ED.

Gresham, F. M. (2002). Response to treatment. In R. Bradley, L. Danielson, & D. Hallahan (Eds.), *Identification of learning disabilities: Research to practice* (pp. 467–519). Mahwah, NJ: Erlbaum.

Griffiths, Y. M., Hill, N. I., Bailey, P. J., & Snowling, M. J. (2003). Auditory temporal order discrimination and backward recognition masking in adults with dyslexia. *Journal of Speech, Language, and Hearing Research, 46,* 1352–1366.

Griffiths, Y. M., & Snowling, M. J. (2002). Predictors of exception word and nonword reading in dyslexic children: The severity hypothesis. *Journal of Educational Psychology, 94,* 34–43.

Grigorenko, E. L. (2001). Developmental dyslexia: An update on genes, brains, and environments. *Journal of Child Psychology and Psychiatry, 42,* 91–125.

Grigorenko, E. L. (2005). A conservative meta-analysis of linkage and linkage-association studies of developmental dyslexia. *Scientific Studies of Reading, 9,* 285–316.

Gross-Tsur, V., Manor, O., & Shalev, R. S. (1996). Developmental dyscalculia: Prevalence and demographic features. *Developmental Medicine and Child Neurology, 38,* 25–33.

Hale, J. B., Naglieri, J. A., Kaufman, A. S., & Kavale, K. A. (2004). Specific learning disability classification in the new Individuals with Disabilities Education Act: The danger of good ideas. *School Psychologist, 58,* 6–13, 29.

Hallahan, D. P., Kauffman, J., & Lloyd, J. (1996). *Introduction to learning disabilities.* Needham Heights, MA: Allyn & Bacon.

Hammill, D. D. (1993). A brief look at the learning disabilities movement in the United States. *Journal of Learning Disabilities, 26,* 295–310.

Hammill, D. D., & Larsen, S. (2003). *Test of Written Language–III.* Austin, TX: PRO-ED.

Hanich, L. B., Jordan, N. C., Kaplan, D., & Dick, J. (2001). Performance across different areas of mathematical cognition in children with learning difficulties. *Journal of Educational Psychology, 93,* 615–626.

Hanley, J. R. (2005). Learning to read in Chinese. In M. J. Snowling & C. Hulme (Eds.), *The science of reading: A handbook* (pp. 316–335). Oxford, UK: Blackwell.

Hanushek, E. A., Kain, J. F., & Rivkin, S. G. (1998). *Does special education raise academic achievement for students with disabilities?* Cambridge, MA: National Bureau of Economic Research, Working Paper No. 6690.

Harcourt Assessment. (2002). *Stanford Achievement Test* (10th ed.). New York: Author.

Harris, C. A., Miller, S. P., & Mercer, C. D. (1995). Teaching initial multiplication skills to students with disabilities in general education classrooms. *Learning Disabilities Research and Practice, 10,* 190–195.

Harris, K. R., Graham, S., & Mason, L. (in press). Improving the writing performance, knowledge, and self-efficacy of struggling writers in second grade: The effects of self-regulated strategy development. *American Educational Research Journal.*

Hart, B., & Risley, T. R. (1995). *Meaningful differences in the everyday experience of young American children.* Baltimore: Brookes.

Hasbrouck, J. E., Ihnot, C., & Rogers, G. (1999). Read Naturally: A strategy to increase oral reading fluency. *Reading Research and Instruction, 39,* 27–37.

Hatcher, P., & Hulme, C. (1999). Phonemes, rhymes, and intelligence as predictors of children's responsiveness to remedial reading instruction. *Journal of Experimental Child Psychology, 72,* 130–153.

Hayes, J. R., & Flower, L. S. (1980). Identifying the organization of the writing process. In L. W. Gregg & E. R. Steinbery (Eds.), *Cognitive processes in writing* (pp. 3–30). Hillsdale, NJ: Erlbaum.

Head, H. (1926). *Aphasia and kindred disorders of speech.* London: Cambridge University Press.

Hecht, S. A., Torgesen, J. K., Wagner, R. K., & Rashotte, C. A. (2001). The relations between phonological processing abilities and emerging individual differences in mathematical computation skills: A longitudinal study from second to fifth grades. *Journal of Experimental Child Psychology, 79,* 192–227.

Hessler, G. L. (1987). Educational issues surrounding severe discrepancy. *Learning Disabilities Research, 3,* 43–49.

Hiebert, E. H. (1994). Reading Recovery in the United States: What difference does it make to an age cohort? *Educational Researcher, 23,* 15–25.

Hiebert, E. H., Colt, J. M., Catto, S. L., & Gury, E. C. (1992). Reading and writing of first grade students in a restructured Chapter I program. *American Educational Research Journal, 29,* 545–572.

Higgins, E., & Raskind, M. (2000). Speaking to read: A comparison of continuous vs. discrete speech recognition in the remediation of learning disabilities. *Journal of Special Education Technology, 15,* 19–30.

Hinshelwood, J. (1895). Word-blindness and visual memory. *Lancet, ii,* 1564–1570.

Hinshelwood, J. (1917). *Congenital word-blindness.* London: Lewis.

Hodent, C., Bryant, P., & Houde, O. (2005). Language-specific effects on number computation in toddlers. *Developmental Science, 8,* 420–423.

Holland, J., McIntosh, D., & Huffman, L. (2004). The role of phonological awareness, rapid automatized naming, and orthographic processing in word reading. *Journal of Psychoeducational Assessment, 22,* 233–260.

Hooper, S. R., Montgomery, J., Swartz, C., Reed, M., Sandler, A., Levine, M., et al. (1994). Measurement of written language expression. In G. R. Lyon (Ed.), *Frames of reference for the assessment of learning disabilities: New views on measurement issues* (pp. 375–418). Baltimore: Brookes.

Hooper, S. R., Swartz, C. W., Montgomery, J., Reed, M. S., Brown, T. T., Wasileski, T. J., et al. (1993). Prevalence of writing problems across three middle school samples. *School Psychology Review, 22,* 610–622.

Hooper, S. R., Swartz, C. W., Wakely, M. B., de Kruif, R. E. L., & Montgomery, J. W. (2002). Executive functions in elementary school children with and without problems in written expression. *Journal of Learning Disabilities, 35,* 57–68.

Hooper, S. R., Wakely, M. B., de Kruif, R. E. L., & Swartz, C. W. (2006). Aptitude–treatment interactions revisited: Effect of meta-cognitive intervention on subtypes of written expression in elementary school students. *Developmental Neuropsychology, 29,* 217–241.

Hooper, S. R., & Willis, W. G. (1989). *Learning disability subtyping: Neuropsychological foundations, conceptual models, and issues in clinical differentiation.* New York: Springer-Verlag.

Hoover, A. N., Hieronymous, A. N., Frisbie, D. A., & Dunbar, S. B. (2001). *Iowa Test of Basic Skill*. Itasca, IL: Riverside Press.

Horwitz, B., Rumsey, J. M., & Donohue, B. C. (1998). Functional connectivity of the angular gyrus in normal reading and dyslexia. *Proceedings of the National Academy of Sciences USA, 95*, 8939–8944.

Hoskyn, M., & Swanson, H. L (2000). Cognitive processing of low achievers and children with reading disabilities: A selective meta-analytic review of the published literature. *School Psychology Review, 29*, 102–119.

Hugdahl, K., Heiervang, E., Ersland, L., Lundervold, A., Steinmetz, H., & Smievoll, A. I. (2003). Significant relation between MR measures of planum temporal area and dichotic processing of syllables in dyslexic children. *Neuropsychologia, 41*, 666–675.

Hughes, C. A., Ruhl, K. L., Schumaker, J. B., & Deshler, D. D. (2002). Effects of instruction in an assignment completion strategy on the homework performance of students with learning disabilities in general education classes. *Learning Disabilities Research, 17*, 1–18.

Hughes, D. C., Keeling, B., & Tuck, B. F. (1983). Effects of achievement expectations and handwriting quality on scoring essays. *Journal of Educational Measurement, 20*, 65–70.

Hulme, C. (1988). The implausibility of low-level visual deficits as a cause of children's reading difficulties. *Cognitive Neuropsychology, 5*, 369–374.

Hulme, C., Snowling, M., Caravolas, M., & Carroll, J. (2005). Phonological skills are (probably) one cause of success in learning to read: A comment on Castles and Coltheart. *Scientific Studies of Reading, 9*, 351–365.

Humphreys, P., Kaufmann, W. E., & Galaburda, A. M. (1990). Developmental dyslexia in women: Neuropathological findings in three patients. *Annals of Neurology, 28*, 727–738.

Hunter, J. V., & Wang, Z. J. (2001). MR spectroscopy in pediatric neuroradiology. *MRI Clinics of North America, 9*, 165–189.

Hutchinson, N. L. (1993). Effects of cognitive strategy instruction on algebra problem solving of adolescents with learning disabilities. *Learning Disability Quarterly, 16*, 34–63.

Hynd, G. W., Hall, J., Novey, E. S., Etiopulos, D., Black, K., Gonzales, J. J., et al. (1995). Dyslexia and corpus callosum morphology. *Archives of Neurology, 52*, 32–38.

Hynd, G. W., & Semrud-Clikeman, M. (1989). Dyslexia and brain morphology. *Psychological Bulletin, 106*, 447–482.

Hynd, G. W., Semrud-Clikeman, M., Lorys, A. R., Novey, E. S., & Eliopulos, D. (1990). Brain morphology in developmental dyslexia and attention deficit disorder/hyperactivity. *Archives of Neurology, 47*, 919–926.

Hynd, G. W., & Willis, W. G. (1988). *Pediatric neuropsychology*. Orelando, FL: Grune & Stratton.

Ihnot, C. (2000). *Read Naturally*. St. Paul, MN: Read Naturally.

Iovino, I., Fletcher, J. M., Breitmeyer, B. G., & Foorman, B. R. (1999). Colored overlays for visual perceptual deficits in children with reading disability and attention deficit/hyperactivity disorder: Are they differentially effective? *Journal of Clinical and Experimental Neuropsychology, 20*, 791–806.

Isaacs, E. B., Edmonds, C. J., Lucas, A., & Gadian, D. G. (2001). Calculation difficulties in children of very low birth weight: A neural correlate. *Brain, 124*, 1701–1707.

Iverson, S., & Tunmer, W. (1993). Phonological processing skills and the Reading Recovery program. *Journal of Educational Psychology, 85,* 112–120.

Iverson, S., Tunmer, W. E., & Chapman, J. W. (2005). The effects of varying group size on the Reading Recovery approach to preventive early intervention. *Journal of Learning Disabilities, 38,* 456–472.

Jenkins, J. R., Fuchs, L. S., van den Broek, P., Espin, C., & Deno, S. L. (2003). Accuracy and fluency in list and context reading of skilled and RD groups: Absolute and relative performance levels. *Learning Disabilities Research and Practice, 18,* 237–245.

Jenkins, J. R., & O'Connor, R. E. (2003). Cooperative learning for students with learning disabilities: Evidence from experiments, observations, and interviews. In H. L. Swanson, K. R. Harris, & S. Graham (Eds.), *Handbook of learning disabilities* (pp. 417–430). New York: Guilford Press.

Jitendra, A. K., Griffin, C. C., McGoey, K., Gardill, M. C., Bhat, P., & Riley, T. (1998). Effects of mathematical word problem-solving by students at risk or with mild disabilities. *Journal of Educational Research, 91,* 345–355.

Jitendra, A. K., & Hoff, K. (1996). The effects of schema-based instruction on the mathematical problem solving performance of students with learning disabilities. *Journal of Learning Disabilities, 29,* 422–431.

Joanisse, M. F., Manis, F. R., Keating, P., & Seidenberg, M. S. (2000). Language deficits in dyslexic children: Speech perception, phonology, and morphology. *Journal of Experimental Child Psychology, 77,* 30–60.

Johnson, D. J., & Blalock, J. (Eds.). (1987). *Adults with learning disabilities.* Orlando, FL: Grune & Stratton.

Johnson, D. J., & Myklebust, H. (1967). *Learning disabilities.* New York: Grune & Stratton.

Johnson, W., Bouchard, T. J., Jr., Segal, N. L., & Samuels, J. (2005). General intelligence and reading performance in adults: Is the genetic factor structure the same as for children? *Personality and Individual Differences, 38,* 1413–1428.

Jones, D., & Christensen, C. (1999). The relationship between automaticity in handwriting and students' ability to generate written text. *Journal of Educational Psychology, 91,* 44–49.

Jordan, N. C., & Hanich, L. B. (2000). Mathematical thinking in second-grade children with different forms of LD. *Journal of Learning Disabilities, 33,* 567–578.

Jordan, N. C., Hanich, L. B., & Kaplan, D. (2003a). A longitudinal study of mathematical competencies in children with specific mathematics difficulties versus children with comorbid mathematics and reading difficulties. *Child Development, 74,* 834–850.

Jordan, N. C., Hanich, L. B., & Kaplan, D. (2003b). Arithmetic fact mastery in young children: A longitudinal investigation. *Journal of Experimental Child Psychology, 85,* 103–119.

Jordan, N. C., Kaplan, D., Olah, L. N., & Locuniak, M. N. (2006). Number sense growth in kindergarten: A longitudinal investigation of children at risk for mathematics difficulties. *Child Development, 77,* 153–175.

Jorm, A. F., Share, D. L., Matthews, M., & Matthews, R. (1986). Cognitive factors at school entry predictive of specific reading retardation and general reading backwardness: A research note. *Journal of Child Psychology, 27,* 45–54.

Joshi, R. M. (2003). Misconceptions about the assessment and diagnosis of reading disability. *Reading Psychology, 24,* 247–266.

Joshi, R. M., & Aaron, P. G. (2000). The component model of reading: Simple view of reading made a little more complex. *Reading Psychology, 21,* 85–97.

Kamin, L. J. (1974). *The science and politics of I.Q.* Potomac, MD: Erlbaum.

Kavale, K. A. (1988). Learning disability and cultural disadvantage: The case for a relationship. *Learning Disability Quarterly, 11,* 195–210.

Kavale, K., & Forness, S. (1985). *The science of learning disabilities.* San Diego: College-Hill Press.

Kavale, K. A., & Forness, S. R. (2000). What definitions of learning disability say and don't say: A critical analysis. *Journal of Learning Disabilities, 33,* 239–256.

Kavele, K. A., & Mostert, M. P. (2004). Social skills interventions for individuals with learning disabilities. *Learning Disability Quarterly, 27,* 31–43.

Kavale, K. A., & Reese, L. (1992). The character of learning disabilities: An Iowa profile. *Learning Disability Quarterly, 15,* 74–94.

Keeler, M. L., & Swanson, H. L. (2001). Does strategy knowledge influence working memory in children with mathematical disabilities? *Journal of Learning Disabilities, 34,* 418–434.

Keenan, J. M., Betjemann, R. S., Wadsworth, S. J., DeFries, J. C., & Olson, R. K. (2006). Genetic and environmental influences on reading and listening comprehension. *Journal of Research on Reading, 29,* 75–91.

Kellam, S. G., Rebok, G. W., Mayer, L. S., Ialongo, N., & Kalodner, C. R. (1994). Depressive symptoms over first grade and their response to a developmental epidemiologically based preventive trial aimed at improving achievement. *Development and Psychopathology, 6,* 463–481.

Keller, C. E., & Sutton, J. P. (1991). Specific mathematics disorders. In J. E. Obrzut & G. W. Hynd (Eds.), *Neuropsychological foundations of learning disabilities: A handbook of issues, methods, and practice* (pp. 549–572). New York: Academic Press.

Keysor, C. S., & Mazzocco, M. M. (2002). A developmental approach to understanding fragile X syndrome in females. *Microscopy Research and Technique, 57,* 179–186.

Khemani, E., & Barnes, M. A. (2005). Calculation and estimation in typically developing children from grades 3 to 8. *Canadian Psychology, 46,* 219.

Kibby, M. Y., Francher, J. B., Markanen, R., Lewandowski, A., & Hynd, G. W. (2003). A test of the cerebellar deficit hypothesis of dyslexia. *Journal of the International Neuropsychological Society, 9,* 219.

Kim, A., Vaughn, S. R., Wanzek, J., & Wei, S. (2004). Graphic organizers and their effects on the reading comprehension of students with LD: A synthesis of research. *Journal of Learning Disabilities, 37,* 105–118.

Kirk, S. A. (1963). Behavioral diagnosis and remediation of learning disabilities. *Conference on Exploring Problems of the Perceptually Handicapped Child, 1,* 1–23.

Klingberg, T., Hedehus, M., Temple, E., Salz, T., Gabrieli, J. D., Moseley, M. E., et al. (2000). Microstructure of temporo-parietal white matter as a basis for reading ability: Evidence from diffusion tensor magnetic resonance imaging. *Neuron, 25,* 493–500.

Knapp, M. S. (1995). *Teaching for meaning in high-poverty classrooms.* New York: Teachers College Press.

Knopik, V. S., & DeFries, J. C. (1999). Etiology of covariation between reading and mathematics performance: A twin study. *Twin Research, 2,* 226–234.

Kovas, Y., Harlaar, N., Petrill, S. A., & Plomin, R. (2005). "Generalist genes" and mathematics in 7-year-old twins. *Intelligence, 33,* 473–489.

Kriss, I., & Evans, B. J. W. (2005). The relationship between dyslexia and Meares-Irlen syndrome. *Journal of Research in Reading, 28,* 350–365.

Kroesbergen, E. H., Van Luit, J. E. H., & Naglieri, J. A. (2003). Mathematical learning difficulties and PASS cognitive processes. *Journal of Learning Disabilities, 36,* 574–562.

Kuhn, M. R., & Stahl, S. A. (2003). Fluency: A review of developmental and remedial practices. *Journal of Educational Psychology, 95,* 3–21.

Kussmaul, A. (1877). Disturbance of speech. *Cyclopedia of Practical Medicine, 14,* 581–875.

Lambe, E. K. (1999). Dyslexia, gender, and brain imaging. *Neuropsychologia, 37,* 521–536.

Larsen, J. P., Hoien, T., Lundberg, I., & Ödegaard, H. (1990). MRI evaluation of the size and symmetry of the planum temporale in adolescents with developmental dyslexia. *Brain and Language, 39,* 289–301.

Leach, J. M., Scarborough, H. S., & Rescorla, L. (2003). Late-emerging reading disabilities. *Journal of Educational Psychology, 95,* 211–224.

Lemer, C., Dehaene, S., Spelke, E., & Cohen, L. (2003). Approximate quantities and exact number words: Dissociable systems. *Neuropsychologia, 41,* 1942–1958.

Leonard, C. M., Eckert, M. A., Lombardino, L. J., Oakland, T., Franzier, J., Mohr, C. M., et al. (2001). Anatomical risk factors for phonological dyslexia. *Cerebral Cortex, 11,* 148–157.

Leonard, C. M., Lombardino, L. J., Mercado, L. R., Browd, S. R., Breier, J. I., & Agee, O. F. (1996). Cerebral asymmetry and cognitive development in children: A magnetic resonance imaging study. *Psychological Science, 7,* 89–95.

Lerner, J. (1989). Educational intervention in learning disabilities. *Journal of the American Academy of Child and Adolescent Psychiatry, 28,* 326–331.

Levy, B. A. (2001). Moving the bottom: Improving reading fluency. In M. Wolf (Ed.), *Dyslexia, fluency, and the brain* (pp. 357–382). Timonium, MD: York Press.

Lewis, C., Hitch, G. J., & Walker, P. (1994). The prevalence of specific arithmetic difficulties and specific reading difficulties in 9- to 10-year-old boys and girls. *Journal of Child Psychology and Psychiatry, 35,* 283–292.

Liberman, I. Y. (1971). Basic research in speech and lateralization of language. *Bulletin of the Orton Society, 21,* 72–87.

Liberman, I. Y., & Shankweiler, D. (1991). Phonology and beginning reading: A tutorial. In L. Rieben & C. A. Perfetti (Eds.), *Learning to read: Basic research and its implications* (pp. 3–17). Hillsdale, NJ: Erlbaum.

Lindamood, P., & Lindamood, P. (1998). *The Lindamood Phoneme Sequencing Program for Reading, Spelling, and Speech.* Austin, TX: PRO-ED.

Lindsay, R. L., Tomazic, T., Levine, M. D., & Accardo, P. J. (1999). Impact of attentional dysfunction in dyscalculia. *Developmental Medicine and Child Neurology, 41,* 639–642.

Livingstone, M. S., Rosen, G. D., Drislane, F. W., & Galaburda, A. M. (1991). Physiological and anatomical evidence for a magnocellular defect in developmental dyslexia. *Proceedings of the National Academy of Sciences USA, 88,* 7943–7947.

Lloyd, J. W. (1980). Academic instruction and cognitive- behavior modification. *Exceptional Education Quarterly, 1,* 53–63.

Logan, G. D. (1997). Automaticity and reading: Perspectives from the instance theory of automatization. *Reading and Writing Quarterly, 13,* 123–146.

Lonigan, C. J. (2003). Development and promotion of emergent literacy skills in children at-risk of reading difficulties. In B. R. Foorman (Ed.), *Preventing and remediating reading difficulties* (pp. 23–50). Baltimore: York Press.

Lovegrove, W., Martin, F., & Slaghuis, W. (1986). A theoretical and experimental case for a visual deficit in specific reading disability. *Cognitive Neuropsychology, 3,* 225–267.

Lovett, M. W. (1987). A developmental approach to reading disability: Accuracy and speed criteria of normal and deficient reading skill. *Child Development, 58,* 234–260.

Lovett, M. W., Barron, R. W., & Benson, N. J. (2003). Effective remediation of word identification and decoding difficulties in school-age children with reading disabilities. In H. L. Swanson, K. Harris, & S. Graham (Eds.), *Handbook of learning disabilities* (pp. 273–292). New York: Guilford Press.

Lovett, M. W., Lacerenza, L., Borden, S. L., Frijters, J. C., Steinbach, K. A., & DePalma, M. (2000a). Components of effective remediation for developmental reading disabilities: Combining phonological and strategy-based instruction to improve outcomes. *Journal of Educational Psychology, 92,* 263–283.

Lovett, M. W., Ransby, M. J., Hardwick, N., & Johns, M. S. (1989). Can dyslexia be treated?: Treatment-specific and generalized treatment effects in dyslexic children's response to remediation. *Brain and Language, 37,* 90–121.

Lovett, M. W., Steinbach, K. A., & Frijters, J. C. (2000b). Remediating the core deficits of reading disability: A double-deficit perspective. *Journal of Learning Disabilities, 33,* 334–358.

Lovett, M. W., Warren-Chaplin, P., Ransby, M., & Borden, S. (1990). Training the word recognition skills of reading disabled children: Treatment and transfer effects. *Journal of Educational Psychology, 82,* 769–780.

Lovitt, T. C., & Curtiss, K. A. (1968). Effects of manipulating an antecedent event on mathematics response rate. *Journal of Applied Behavior Analysis, 1,* 329–333.

Lukatela, G., & Turvey, M. T. (1998). Reading in two alphabets. *American Psychologist, 53,* 1057–1072.

Lyon, G. R. (1983). Learning-disabled readers: Identification of subgroups. In H. R. Myklebust (Ed.), *Progress in learning disabilities* (Vol. 5, pp. 103–134). New York: Grune & Stratton.

Lyon, G. R. (1987). Learning disabilities research: False starts and broken promises. In S. Vaughn & C. Bos (Eds.), *Research in learning disabilities: Issues and future directions* (pp. 69–85). Boston: College-Hill Press.

Lyon, G. R. (1995). Toward a definition of dyslexia. *Annals of Dyslexia, 45,* 3–27.

Lyon, G. R. (1996). Learning disabilities. In E. J. Mash & R. A. Barkley (Eds.), *Child psychopathology* (pp. 390–435). New York: Guilford Press.

Lyon, G. R., & Cutting, L. E. (1998). Treatment of learning disabilities. In E. J. Mash & R. A. Barkley (Eds.), *Treatment of childhood disorders* (pp. 468–500). New York: Guilford Press.

Lyon, G. R., Fletcher, J. M., & Barnes, M. C. (2003a). Learning disabilities. In E. J. Mash & R. A. Barkley (Eds.), *Child psychopathology* (2nd ed., pp. 520–588). New York: Guilford Press.

Lyon, G. R., Fletcher, J. M., Fuchs, L., & Chhabra, V. (2006). Treatment of learning disabilities. In E. J. Mash & R. A. Barkley (Eds.), *Treatment of childhood disorders* (3rd ed., pp. 512–591). New York: Guilford Press.

Lyon, G. R., Fletcher, J. M., Shaywitz, S. E., Shaywitz, B. A., Torgesen, J. K., Wood, F. B.,

References

297

Lyon, G. R., Fletcher, J. M., Shaywitz, S. E., Shaywitz, B. A., Torgesen, J. K., Wood, F. B.,
et al. (2001). Rethinking learning disabilities. In C. E. Finn, Jr., R. A. J. Rotherham,
& C. R. Hokanson, Jr. (Eds.), Rethinking special education for a new century (pp.
259–287). Washington, DC: Thomas B. Fordham Foundation and Progressive
Policy Institute.

Lyon, G. R., & Moats, L. C. (1997). Critical conceptual and methodological considerations in reading intervention research. Journal of Learning Disabilities, 30, 578–
588.

Lyon, G. R., Shaywitz, S. E., & Shaywitz, B. A. (2003b). A definition of dyslexia. Annals
of Dyslexia, 53, 1–14.

MacMillan, D. L., & Siperstein, G. N. (2002). Learning disabilities as operationally defined by schools. In R. Bradley, L. Danielson, & D. Hallahan (Eds.), Identification
of learning disabilities: Research to practice (pp. 287– 340). Mahwah, NJ:
Erlbaum.

Manis, F. R., Doi, L. M., & Bhadha, B. (2000). Naming speed, phonological awareness,
and orthographic knowledge in second graders. Journal of Learning Disabilities,
33, 325–333.

Manis, F. R., Seidenberg, M. S., Doi, L. M., McBride-Chang, C., & Peterson, A. (1996).
On the basis of two subtypes of developmental dyslexia. Cognition, 58, 157–195.

Maria, K. (1990). Reading comprehension instruction: Issues and strategies. Parkton,
MD: York Press.

Marlow, A. J., Fisher, S. E., Richardson, A. J., Talcott, J. B., Monaco, A. P., Stein, J. F., et
al. (2001). Investigation of quantitative measures related to reading disability in a
large sample of sib-pairs from the UK. Behavior Genetics, 31, 219–230.

Mastropieri, M. A., & Scruggs, T. E. (1997). Best practices in promoting reading comprehension in students with learning disabilities: 1976 to 1996. Remedial and Special Education, 18, 197–214.

Mathes, P. G., Denton, C. A., Fletcher, J. M., Anthony, J. L., Francis, D. J., &
Schatschneider, C. (2005). An evaluation of two reading interventions derived
from diverse models. Reading Research Quarterly, 40, 148–183.

Mathes, P. G., Howard, J. K, Allen, S., & Fuchs, D. (1998). Peer-assisted learning strategies for first-grade readers: Making early reading instruction responsive to the
needs of diverse learners. Reading Research Quarterly, 33, 62–94.

Mazzocco, M. M. (2001). Math learning disability and math LD subtypes: Evidence
from studies of Turner syndrome, fragile X syndrome, and neurofibromatosis
type 1. Journal of Learning Disabilities, 34, 520–533.

Mazzocco, M. M., & Myers, G. F. (2003). Complexities in identifying and defining
mathematics learning disability in the primary school-age years. Annals of Dyslexia, 53, 218–253.

McBride-Chang, C., & Manis, F. R. (1996). Structural invariance in the associations of
naming speed, phonological awareness, and verbal reasoning in good and poor
readers: A test of the double-deficit hypothesis. Reading and Writing, 8, 323–339.

McCloskey, M., & Caramazza, A. (1985). Cognitive mechanisms in number processing
and calculation: Evidence from dyscalculia. Brain and Cognition, 4, 171–196.

McCrory, E., Frith, U., Brunswick, N., & Price, C. (2000). Abnormal functional activation during a simple word repetition task: A PET study of adult dyslexics. Journal
of Cognitive Neuroscience, 12, 753–762.

McCrory, E., Mechelli, A., Frith, U., & Price, C. J. (2005). More than words: A common neural basis for reading and naming deficits in developmental dyslexia? *Brain, 128,* 261–267.

McGuiness, C., McGuiness, D., & McGuiness, G. (1996). Phono-Graphix: A new method for remediating reading difficulties. *Annals of Dyslexia, 46,* 73–96.

McMaster, K. L., Fuchs, D., Fuchs, L. S., & Compton, D. L. (2005). Responding to nonresponders: An experimental field trial of identification and intervention methods. *Exceptional Children, 71,* 445–463.

Mercer, C. D., & Miller, S. P. (1992). Teaching students with learning problems in math to acquire, understand, and apply basic math facts. *Remedial and Special Education, 13,* 19–35, 61.

Meyer, M. S. (2002). Repeated reading: An old standard is revisited and renovated. *Perspectives, 28,* 15–18.

Miles, T. R., & Haslum, M. N. (1986). Dyslexia: Anomaly or normal variation. *Annals of Dyslexia, 36,* 103–117.

Misra, M., Katzir, T., Wolf, M., & Poldrack, R. A. (2004). Neural systems for rapid automatized naming in skilled readers: Unraveling the RAN–reading relationship. *Scientific Studies of Reading, 8,* 241–256.

Mix, K. S., Huttenlocher, J., & Levine, S. C. (2002). Multiple cues for quantification in infancy: Is number one of them? *Psychological Bulletin, 128,* 278–294.

Moats, L. C. (2005). How spelling supports reading: And why it is more regular and predictable than you many think. *American Educator, 29,* 12–43.

Moats, L. C., & Farrell, M. L. (1999). Multi-sensory instruction. In J. Birsh (Ed.), *Multi-sensory teaching of basic language skills* (pp. 1–18). Baltimore: Brookes.

Mody, M., Studdert-Kennedy, M., & Brady, S. (1997). Speech perception deficits in poor readers: Auditory processing or phonological coding? *Journal of Experimental Child Psychology, 64,* 199–231.

Molko, N. Cachia, A., Riviere, D., Mangin, J. F., Bruandet, M., LeBihan, D., et al. (2004). Brain anatomy in Turner syndrome: Evidence for impaired social and spatial–numerical networks. *Cerebral Cortex, 14,* 840–850.

Montague, M., Applegate, B., & Marquard, K. (1993). Cognitive strategy instruction and mathematical problem-solving performance of students with learning disabilities. *Learning Disabilities Research and Practice, 8,* 223–232.

Monuteaux, M. C., Faraone, S. V., Herzig, K., Navsaria, N., & Biederman, J. (2005). ADHD and dyscalculia: Evidence for independent familial transmission. *Journal of Learning Disabilities, 38,* 86–93.

Morgan, W. P. (1896). A case of congenital word blindness. *British Medical Journal, ii,* 1378.

Morris, R. D., & Fletcher, J. M. (1988). Classification in neuropsychology: A theoretical framework and research paradigm. *Journal of Clinical and Experimental Neuropsychology, 10,* 640–658.

Morris, R. D., Fletcher, J. M., & Francis, D. J. (1993) Conceptual and psychometric issues in the neuropsychological assessment of children: Measurement of ability discrepancy and change. In I. Rapin & S. Segalovitz (Eds.), *Handbook of neuropsychology* (Vol. 7, pp. 341–352). Amsterdam: Elsevier.

Morris, R. D., Lovett, M. W., Wolf, M., Sevcik, R. A., Steinbach, K. A., Frijters, J. C., et al. (2006). *Multiple component remediation of developmental reading disabilities: A controlled factorial evaluation of the influence of IQ, socioeconomic statues, and race on outcomes.* Manuscript under review.

Morris, R. D., Stuebing, K. K., Fletcher, J. M., Shaywitz, S. E., Lyon, G. R., Shankweiler,

D. P., et al. (1998). Subtypes of reading disability: Variability around a phonological core. *Journal of Educational Psychology, 90,* 347–373.

Morrison, S. R., & Siegel, L. S. (1991). Learning disabilities: A critical review of definitional and assessment issues. In J. E. Obrzut & G. W. Hynd (Eds.), *Neuropsychological foundations of learning disabilities: A handbook of issues, methods, and practice* (pp. 79–98). New York: Academic Press.

Murphy, L., & Pollatsek, A. (1994). Developmental dyslexia: Heterogeneity without discrete subgroups. *Annals of Dyslexia, 44,* 120–146.

Myers, C. A. (1978). Reviewing the literature on Fernald's technique of remedial reading. *Reading Teacher, 31,* 614–619.

Naglieri, J. A., & Das, J. P. (1997). *Cognitive Assessment System interpretive handbook.* Itasca, IL: Riverside.

Naglieri, J. A., & Johnson, D. (2000). Effectiveness of a cognitive strategy intervention in improving arithmetic computation based on the PASS theory. *Journal of Learning Disabilities, 33,* 591–597.

Nation, K. (1999). Reading skills in hyperlexia: A developmental perspective. *Psychological Bulletin, 125,* 338–355.

Nation, K. (2005). Children's reading comprehension difficulties. In M. J. Snowling & C. Hulme (Eds.), *The science of reading: A handbook* (pp. 248–266). Oxford, UK: Blackwell.

Nation, K., Adams, J. W., Bowyer-Crane, A., & Snowling, M. J. (1999). Working memory deficits in poor comprehenders reflect underlying language impairments. *Journal of Experimental Child Psychology, 73,* 139–158.

Nation, K., Clarke, P., Marshall, C. M., & Durand, M. (2004). Hidden language impairments in children: Parallels between poor reading comprehension and specific language impairment? *Journal of Speech, Language, and Hearing Research, 47,* 199–211.

Nation, K., Clarke, P., & Snowling, M. J. (2002). General cognitive ability in children with reading comprehension difficulties. *British Journal of Educational Psychology, 72,* 549–560.

Nation, K., & Snowling, M. J. (1998). Semantic processing and the development of word-recognition skills: Evidence from children with reading comprehension difficulties. *Journal of Memory and Language, 37,* 85–101.

National Center for Educational Statistics (NCES). (2003). *National Assessment of Educational Progress: The nation's report card.* Washington, DC: U.S. Department of Education.

National Center for Student Progress Monitoring. Retrieved June 5, 2006, from http://www.studentprogress.org/.

National Joint Committee on Learning Disabilities (NJCLD). (1988). *Letter to NJCLD member organizations.* Author.

National Reading Panel (NRP). (2000). *Report of the National Reading Panel. Teaching children to read: An evidence-based assessment of the scientific research literature on reading and its implications for reading instruction* (NIH Publication No. 00-4754). Washington, DC: U.S. Government Printing Office.

Neuhaus, G., Foorman, B. R., Francis, D. J., & Carlson, C. D. (2001). Measures of information processing in rapid automatized naming (RAN) and their relation to reading. *Journal of Experimental Child Psychology, 78,* 359–373.

Nicolson, R. I., Fawcett, A. J., & Dean, P. (2001). Developmental dyslexia: The cerebellar hypothesis. *Trends in Neuroscience, 24,* 508–511.

Norman, C. A., & Zigmond, N. (1980). Characteristics of children labeled and served as learning disabled in school systems affiliated with Child Service Demonstration Centers. *Journal of Learning Disabilities, 13,* 542–547.

Nothen, M. M., Schulte-Korne, G., Grimm, T., Cichon, S., Vogt, I. R., Muller-Myhsok, B., et al. (1999). Genetic linkage analysis with dyslexia: Evidence for linkage of spelling disability to chromosome 15. *European Child and Adolescent Psychiatry, 3,* 56–59.

Oakhill, J. (1993). Children's difficulties in reading comprehension. *Educational Psychology Review, 5,* 1–15.

Oakhill, J. V., Cain, K., & Bryant, P. E. (2003). The dissociation of word reading and text comprehension: Evidence from component skills. *Language and Cognitive Processes, 18,* 443–468.

Oakhill, J., & Kyle, F. (2000). The relation between phonological awareness and working memory. *Journal of Experimental Psychology, 75,* 152–164.

Oakhill, J. V., Yuill, N., & Parkin, A. (1996). On the nature of the difference between skilled and less-skilled comprehenders, *Journal of Research in Reading, 9,* 80–91.

Oakland, T., Black, J., Stanford, G., Nussbaum, N., & Balise, R. (1998). An evaluation of the dyslexia training program: A multi-sensory method for promoting reading in students with reading disabilities. *Journal of Learning Disabilities, 31,* 140–147.

O'Connor, R. E. (2000). Increasing the intensity of intervention in kindergarten and first grade. *Learning Disabilities Research and Practice, 15,* 43–54.

O'Connor, R. E., Fulmer, D., Harty, K., & Bell, K. (2001). *Total awareness: Reducing the severity of reading disability.* Paper presented at the American Educational Research Conference, Seattle, WA.

O'Connor, R. E., Fulmer, D., Harty, K., & Bell, K. (2005). Layers of reading intervention in kindergarten through third grade: Changes in teaching and student outcomes. *Journal of Learning Disabilities, 38,* 440–455.

O'Connor, R. E., Notari-Syverson, N., & Vadasy, P. (1998). *Ladders to Literacy: A kindergarten activity book.* Baltimore: Brookes.

Ogle, J. W. (1867). Aphasia and agraphia. *Report of the Medical Research Council of Saint George's Hospital, 2,* 83–122.

O'Hare, F. (1973). *Sentence-combining: Improving student writing without formal grammar instruction.* Urbana, IL: National Council of Teachers of English.

Olson, R. K., Forsberg, H., Gayan, J., & DeFries, J. C. (1999). A behavioral–genetic analysis of reading disabilities and component processes. In R. M. Klein & P. A. McMullen (Eds.), *Converging methods for understanding reading and dyslexia* (pp. 133–153). Cambridge MA: MIT Press.

Olson, R. K., Forsberg, H., Wise, B., & Rack, J. (1994). Measurement of word recognition, orthographic, and phonological skills. In G. R. Lyon (Ed.), *Frames of reference for the assessment of learning disabilities* (pp. 243–278). Baltimore: Brookes.

Olson, R. K., & Wise, B. (2006). Computer-based remediation for reading and related phonological disabilities. In M. McKenna, L. Labbo, R. Kieffer, & D. Reinking (Eds.), *Handbook of literacy and technology* (Vol. 2, pp. 57–74). Mahwah, NJ: Erlbaum.

Olson, R. K., & Wise, B. W. (1992). Reading on the computer with orthographic and speech feedback: An overview of the Colorado Remedial Reading Project. *Reading and Writing: An Interdisciplinary Journal, 4,* 107–144.

Open Court Reading. (1995). *Collections for young scholars.* Peru, IL: Science Research Associates/McGraw-Hill.

Orton, S. (1928). Specific reading disability—strephosymbolia. *Journal of the American Medical Association, 90,* 1095–1099.

Orton, S. (1937). *Reading, writing and speech problems in children: A presentation of certain types of disorders in the development of the language faculty.* New York: Norton.

Palinscar, A., & Brown, A. (1985). Reciprocal teaching: A means to a meaningful end. In J. Osborn, P. T. Wilson, & R. C. Anderson (Eds.), *Reading education: Foundations for a literate America* (pp. 66–87). Lexington, MA: Heath.

Papanicolaou, A. C. (1998). *Fundamentals of functional brain imaging.* Lisse, the Netherlands: Swets & Zeitlinger.

Papanicolaou, A. C., Simos, P. G., Breier, J. I., Fletcher, J. M., Foorman, B. R., Francis, D. J., et al. (2003). Brain mechanisms for reading in children with and without dyslexia: a review of studies of normal development and plasticity. *Developmental Neuropsychology, 24,* 593–612.

Paulesu, E., Demonet, J. -F., McCrory, E., Chanoine, V., Brunswick, N., Cappa, S. F., et al. (2001). Dyslexia: Cultural diversity and biological unity. *Science, 291,* 2165–2167.

Pearson, P. D. (1998). Standards and assessment: Tools for crafting effective instruction? In F. Lehr & J. Osborn (Eds.), *Literacy for all: Issues in teaching and learning* (pp. 264–288). New York: Guilford Press.

Pelletier, P. M., Ahmad, S. A., & Rourke, B. P. (2001). Classification rules for basic phonological processing disabilities and nonverbal learning disabilities: Formulation and external validity. *Child Neuropsychology, 7,* 84–98.

Pennington, B. F., Filipek, P. A., Churchwell, J., Kennedy, D. N., Lefley, D., Simon, J. H., et al. (1999). Brain morphometry in reading-disabled twins. *Neurology, 53,* 723–729.

Pennington, B. F., Gilger, J. W., Olson, R. K., & DeFries, J. C. (1992). The external validity of age- versus IQ-discrepancy definitions of reading disability: Lessons from a twin study. *Journal of Learning Disability, 25,* 562–573.

Pennington, B. F., & Olson, R. K. (2005). Genetics of dyslexia. *The science of reading: A handbook* (pp. 453–472). Oxford, UK: Blackwell.

Perfetti, C. A. (1985). *Reading ability.* New York: Oxford University Press.

Perfetti, C. A., Landi, N., & Oakhill, J. (2005). The acquisition of reading comprehension skill. *The science of reading: A handbook* (pp. 227–247). Oxford, UK: Blackwell.

Peters, J. E., Davis, J. J., Goolsby, C. M., & Clements, S. D. (1973). *Physician's handbook: Screening for MBD.* New York: CIBA Medical Horizons.

Petrill, S. A., Deater-Deckard, K., Thompson, L. A., DeThorne, L. S., & Schatschneider, C. (2006a). Reading skills in early readers: Genetic and shared environmental influences. *Journal of Learning Disabilities, 39,* 48–55.

Petrill, S. A., Deater-Deckard, K., Thompson, L. A., DeThorne, L. S., & Schatschneider, C. (2006b). Genetic and shared environmental effects of serial naming and phonological awareness on early reading outcomes. *Journal of Educational Psychology, 98,* 112–121.

Petrill, S. A., Deater-Deckard, K., Thompson, L. A., Schatschneider, C., & DeThorne, L. S. (in press). Longitudinal genetic analysis of early reading: The Western Reserve Reading Project. *Reading and Writing.*

Peverly, S. T. (2006). The importance of handwriting speed in adult writing. *Developmental Neuropsychology, 29,* 197–216.

Phillips, B. M., & Lonigan, C. J. (2005). Social correlates of emergent literacy. In M. J. Snowling & C. Hulme (Eds.), *The science of reading handbook* (pp. 173–204). Oxford, UK: Blackwell.

Plomin R., & Kovas, Y. (2005). Generalist genes and learning disabilities. *Psychological Bulletin, 131,* 592–617.

Poeppel, D. (1996). A critical review of PET studies of phonological processing. *Brain and Language, 55,* 317–351.

Pokorni, J. I., Worthington, C. K., & Jamison, P. J. (2004). Phonological awareness intervention: Comparison of Fast ForWord, Earobics, and LiPS. *Journal of Educational Research, 97,* 147–157.

President's Commission on Excellence in Special Education. (2002). *A new era: Revitalizing special education for children and their families.* Washington, DC: U.S. Department of Education.

Pressley, M. (2006). *Reading instruction that works* (3rd ed.). New York: Guilford Press.

Price, C. J., & McCrory, E. (2005). *The science of reading: A handbook* (pp. 473–496). Oxford, UK: Blackwell.

Pugh, K. R., Mencl, W. E., Shaywitz, B. A., Shaywitz, S. E., Fulbright, R. K., Constable, R. T., et al. (2000). The angular gyrus in developmental dyslexia: Task-specific differences in functional connectivity within posterior cortex. *Psychological Science, 11,* 51–56.

Raberger, T., & Wimmer, H. (2003). On the automaticity/cerebellar deficit hypothesis of dyslexia: Balancing and continuous rapid naming in dyslexic and ADHD children. *Neuropsychologia, 41,* 1493–1497.

Rae, C., Harasty, J. A., Dzendrowskyj, T. E., Talcott, J. B., Simpson, J. M., Blarmire, A. M., et al. (2002). Cerebellar morphology in developmental dyslexia. *Neuropsychologia, 40,* 1285–1292.

Ralph, M. A. L., & Patterson, K. (2005). Acquired disorders of reading. In M. J. Snowling and C. Hulme (Eds.), *The science of reading: A handbook* (pp. 413–430). Oxford, UK: Blackwell.

Ramus, D. (2003). Developmental dyslexia: Specific phonological deficit or general sensorimotor dysfunction. *Current Opinion in Neurobiology, 13,* 212–218.

Ramus, F. (2001). Talk of two theories. *Nature, 412,* 393–395.

Ramus, F., Pidgeon, E., & Frith, U. (2003a). The relationship between motor control and phonology in dyslexic children. *Journal of Child Psychology and Psychiatry, 44,* 712–722.

Ramus, F., Rosen, S., Dakin, S., Day, B. L., Castellote, J. M., White, S., et al. (2003b). Theories of developmental dyslexia: Insights from a multiple case study of dyslexic adults. *Brain, 126,* 841–865.

Ransby, M. J., & Swanson, H. L. (2003). Reading comprehension skills of young adults with childhood diagnosis of dyslexia. *Journal of Learning Disabilities, 36,* 538–555.

Rashotte, C. A., MacPhee, K., & Torgesen, J. K. (2001). The effectiveness of a group reading instruction program with poor readers in multiple grades. *Learning Disability Quarterly, 24,* 119–134.

Raskind, W. H., Hsu, L., Berninger, V. W., Thomson, J. B, & Wijsman, E. M. (2000). Familial aggregation of dyslexia phenotypes. *Behavior Genetics, 30,* 385–396.

Raskind, W. H., Igo, R. P., Jr., Chapman, N. H., Berninger, V. W., Thomson, J. B., Matsushita, M., et al. (2005). A genome scan in multigenerational families with dyslexia: Identification of a novel locus on chromosome 2q that contributes to phonological decoding efficiency. *Molecular Psychiatry, 10,* 699–711.

Rayner, K., Foorman, B. R., Perfetti, C. A., Pesetsky, D., & Seidenberg, M. S. (2002). How psychological science informs the teaching of reading. *Psychological Science in the Public Interest, 2,* 31–74.

Reed, M. A. (1989). Speech perception and the discrimination of brief auditory cues in reading disabled children. *Journal of Experimental Child Psychology, 48,* 270–292.

Reschly, D. J., & Tilly, W. D. (1999). Reform trends and system design alternatives. In D. Reschly, W. Tilly, & J. Grimes (Eds.), *Special education in transition* (pp. 19–48). Longmont, CO: Sopris West.

Reynolds, C. (1984–1985). Critical measurement issues in learning disabilities. *Journal of Special Education, 18,* 451–476.

Richards, T. L., Aylward, E. H., Berninger, V. W., Field, K. M., Grimme, A. C., Richards, A. L., et al. (2006). Individual fMRI activation in orthographic mapping and morpheme mapping after orthographic or morphological spelling treatment in child dyslexics. *Journal of Neurolinguistics, 19,* 56–86.

Richards, T. L., Berninger, V., Nagy, W., Parsons, A., Field, K., & Richards, A. (2005). Brain activation during language task contrasts in children with and without dyslexia: Inferring mapping processes and assessing response to spelling instruction. *Educational and Child Psychology, 22,* 62–80.

Richards, T. L., Berninger, V., Sylward, E., Richards, A., Thomson, J., Nagy, W., et al. (2002). Reproducibility of proton MR spectroscopic imaging (PEPSI): Comparison of dyslexic and normal reading children and effects of treatment on brain lactate levels during language tasks. *American Journal of Neuroradiology, 23,* 1678–1685.

Richards, T. L., Corina, D., Serafini, S., Steury, K., Echelard, D. R., Dager, S. R., et al. (2000). The effects of a phonologically driven treatment for dyslexia on lactate levels as measured by proton MRSI. *American Journal of Neuroradiology, 21,* 916–922.

Rittle-Johnson, B., Siegler, R. S., & Alibali, M. W. (2001). Developing conceptual understanding and procedural skill in mathematics: An iterative process. *Journal of Educational Psychology, 93,* 346–362.

Rivera, D., & Smith, D. D. (1987). Influence of modeling on acquisition and maintenance of computational skills: A summary of research findings from three sites. *Learning Disability Quarterly, 10,* 69–80.

Rivera, S. M., Menon, V., White, C. D., Glaser, B., & Reiss, A. L. (2002). Functional brain activation during arithmetic processing in females with fragile X syndrome is related to FMRI protein expression. *Human Brain Mapping, 16,* 206–218.

Roberts, J. E., Schaaf, J. M., Skinner, M., Wheeler, A., Hooper, S. Hatton, D. D., et al. (2005). Academic skills of boys with fragile X syndrome: Profiles and predictors. *American Journal of Mental Retardation, 110,* 107–120.

Robinson, C. S., Menchetti, B. M., & Torgesen, J. K. (2002). Toward a two-factor theory of one type of mathematics disabilities. *Learning Disabilities Research and Practice, 17,* 81–89.

Rodgers, B. (1983). The identification and prevalence of specific reading retardation. *British Journal of Educational Psychology, 53,* 369–373.

Roeltgen, D. (2003). Agraphia. In K. M. Heilman & E. Valenstein (Eds.), *Clinical neuropsychology* (Vol. 4, pp. 75–96). New York: Oxford University Press.

Rogosa, D. (1995). Myths and methods: "Myths about longitudinal research" (plus supplemental questions). In J. M. Gottman (Ed.), *The analysis of change* (pp. 3–66). Mahwah, NJ: Erlbaum.

Romani, C., Olson, A., & Di Betta, A. M. (2005). Spelling disorders. In M. J. Snowling and C. Hulme (Eds.), *The science of reading: A handbook* (pp. 431–448). Oxford, UK: Blackwell.

Rourke, B. P. (1975). Brain–behavior relationships in children with learning disabilities: A research programme. *American Psychologist, 30,* 911–920.

Rourke, B. P. (Ed.). (1985). *Neuropsychology of learning disabilities: Essentials of subtype analysis.* New York: Guilford Press.

Rourke, B. P. (1989). *Nonverbal learning disabilities: The syndrome and the model.* New York: Guilford Press.

Rourke, B. P. (1993). Arithmetic disabilities specific and otherwise: A neuropsychological perspective. *Journal of Learning Disabilities, 26,* 214–226.

Rourke, B. P., & Finlayson, M. A. J. (1978). Neuropsychological significance of variations in patterns of academic performance: Verbal and visual–spatial abilities. *Journal of Pediatric Psychology, 3,* 62–66.

Rouse, C. E., & Krueger, A. B. (2004). Putting computerized instruction to the test: A randomized evaluation of a "scientifically based" reading program. *Economics of Education Review, 23,* 323–338.

Rovet, J., Szekely, C., & Hockenberry, M. N. (1994). Specific arithmetic calculation deficits in children with Turner syndrome. *Journal of Clinical Experimental Neuropsychology, 16,* 820–839.

Rumsey, J. M., Andreason, P., Zametkin, A. J., Aquino, T., King, A., Hamburger, S., et al. (1992). Failure to activate the left temporoparietal cortex in dyslexia. An oxygen 15 positron emission tomographic study. *Archives of Neurology, 49,* 527–534.

Rumsey, J. M., Nace, K., Donohue, B., Wise, D., Maisog, J. M., & Andreason, P. (1997). A positron emission tomographic study of impaired word recognition and phonological processing in dyslexic men. *Archives of Neurology, 54,* 562–573.

Rumsey, J. M., Zametkin, A. J., Andreason, P., Hanchan, A. P., Hamburger, S. D., Aquino, T., et al. (1994). Normal activation of frontotemporal language cortex in dyslexia, as measured with oxygen 15 positron emission tomography. *Archives of Neurology, 51,* 27–38.

Rutter, M. (1982). Syndromes attributed to "minimal brain dysfunction" in childhood. *American Journal of Psychiatry, 139,* 21–33.

Rutter, M., Caspi, A., Fergusson, D., Horwood, L. J., Goodman, R., Maughn, B., et al. (2004). Sex differences in developmental reading disability. New findings from 4 epidemiological studies. *Journal of the American Medical Association, 291,* 2007–2012.

Rutter, M., & Yule W. (1975). The concept of specific reading retardation. *Journal of Child Psychology and Psychiatry, 16,* 181–197.

Saddler, S., Moran, S., Graham, S., & Harris, K. R. (2004). Preventing writing difficulties: The effects of planning strategy instruction on the writing performance of struggling writers. *Exceptionality, 12,* 3–17.

Saenz, L., Fuchs, L. S., & Fuchs, D. (2005). Effects of peer-assisted learning strategies on English language learners: A randomized controlled study. *Exceptional Children, 71*, 231–247.

Salomon, G., & Perkins, D. N. (1989). Rocky roads to transfer: Rethinking mechanisms of a neglected phenomenon. *Educational Psychologist, 24*, 113–142.

Sandler, A. D., Watson, T. E., Footo, M., Levine, M. D., Coleman, W. L., & Hooper, S. R. (1992). Neurodevelopmental study of writing disorders in middle childhood. *Developmental and Behavioral Pediatrics, 13*, 17–23.

Sattler, J. M. (1993). *Assessment of children's intelligence and special abilities.* New York: Allyn & Bacon.

Satz, P., Buka, S., Lipsitt, L., & Seidman, L. (1998). The long-term prognosis of learning disabled children: A review of studies (1954–1993). In B. K. Shapiro, P. J. Accardo, & A. J. Capute (Eds.), *Specific reading disability: A view of the spectrum* (pp. 223–250). Parkton, MD: York Press.

Satz, P., & Fletcher, J. M. (1980). Minimal brain dysfunctions: An appraisal of research concepts and methods. In H. Rie & E. Rie (Eds.), *Handbook of minimal brain dysfunctions: A critical view* (pp. 669–715). New York: Wiley–Interscience.

Savage, R. (2004). Motor skills, automaticity and developmental dyslexia: A review of the research literature. *Reading and Writing, 17*, 301–324.

Savage, R. S., Frederickson, N., Goodwin, R., Patni, U., Smith, N., & Tuersley, L. (2005). Relationships among rapid digit naming, phonological processing, motor automaticity, and speech perception in poor, average, and good readers and spellers. *Journal of Learning Disabilities, 38*, 12–28.

Schatschneider, C., Carlson, C. D., Francis, D. J., Foorman, B. R., & Fletcher, J. M. (2002). Relationships of rapid automatized naming and phonological awareness in early reading development: Implications for the double-deficit hypothesis. *Journal of Learning Disabilities, 35*, 245– 256.

Schatschneider, C., Fletcher, J. M., Francis, D. J., Carlson, C. D., & Foorman, B. R. (2004). Kindergarten prediction of reading skills: A longitudinal comparative analysis. *Journal of Educational Psychology, 96*, 265–282.

Schulte-Korne, G. (2001). Genetics of reading and spelling disorder. *Journal of Child Psychology and Psychiatry, 42*, 985–997.

Schulte-Korne, G., Deimel, W., Muller, K., Gutenbrunner, C., & Remschmidt, H. (1996). Familial aggregation of spelling disability. *Journal of Child Psychology and Psychiatry, 37*, 817–822.

Schultz, R. T., Cho, N. K., Staib, L. H., Kier, L. E., Fletcher, J. M., Shaywitz, S. E., et al. (1994). Brain morphology in normal and dyslexic children: The influence of sex and age. *Annals of Neurology, 35*, 732–742.

Schumaker, J. B., Deshler, D. D., & McKnight, P. (2002). Ensuring success in the secondary general education curriculum through the use of teaching routines. In M. A. Shinn, H. M. Walker, & G. Stoner (Eds.), *Interventions for academic and behavior problems II: Preventive and remedial approaches* (pp. 791–823). Bethesda, MD: National Association of School Psychologists.

Scientific Learning Corporation. (1999). *Fast ForWord companion: A comprehensive guide to the training exercises.* Berkeley, CA: Author.

Seabaugh, G. O., & Schumaker, J. B. (1993). The effects of self-regulation training on the academic productivity of secondary students with learning problems. *Journal of Behavioral Education, 4*, 109–133.

Seidenberg, M. S., & McClelland, J. L. (1989). A distributed, developmental model of word recognition. *Psychological Review, 96,* 523–568.

Semrud-Clikeman, M., Guy, K., Griffin, J. D., & Hynd, G. W. (2000). Rapid naming deficits in children and adolescents with reading disabilities and attention deficit hyperactivity disorder. *Brain and Language, 74,* 70–83.

Senf, G. M. (1987). Learning disabilities as sociological sponge: Wiping up life's spills. In S. Vaughn & C. Bos (Eds.), *Research in learning disabilities: Issues and future directions* (pp. 87–101). Boston: Little, Brown.

Seymour, P. H. (2005). Early reading development in European orthographies. In M. J. Snowling and C. Hulme (Eds.), *The science of reading: A handbook* (pp. 296–315). Oxford, UK: Blackwell.

Shadish, W., Cook, T., & Campbell, D. (2002). *Experimental and quasi-experimental designs for generalized causal inference.* Boston: Houghton Mifflin.

Shalev, R. S., Auerbach, J., Manor, O., & Gross-Tsur, V. (2000). Developmental dyscalculia: Prevalence and prognosis. *European Child and Adolescent Psychiatry, 9,* 58–64.

Shalev, R. S., Manor, O., Auerbach, J., & Gross-Tsur, V. (1998). Persistence of developmental dyscalculia: What counts? Results from a 3–year prospective follow-up study. *Journal of Pediatrics, 133,* 358–362.

Shalev, R. S., Manor, O., & Gross-Tsur, V. (2005). Developmental dyscalculia: A prospective six-year follow-up. *Developmental Medicine and Child Neurology, 47,* 121–125.

Shalev, R. S., Manor, O., Kerem, B., Ayali, M., Badichi, N., Friedlander, Y., et al. (2001). Developmental dyscalculia is a familial learning disability. *Journal of Learning Disabilities, 34,* 59–65.

Shanahan, T., & Barr, R. (1995). Reading Recovery: An independent evaluation of the effects of an early instructional intervention for at-risk learners. *Reading Research Quarterly, 30,* 958–996.

Shankweiler, D., & Crain, S. (1986). Language mechanisms and reading disorder: A modular approach. *Cognition, 24,* 139–168.

Shankweiler, D., Lundquist, E., Katz, L., Stuebing, K, Fletcher, J. M, Brady, S., et al. (1999). Comprehension and decoding: Patterns of association in children with reading difficulties. *Scientific Studies of Reading, 3,* 69–94.

Shapiro, E. S., Edwards, L., & Zigmond, N. (2005). Progress monitoring of mathematics among students with learning disabilities. *Assessment for Effective Intervention, 30,* 15–32.

Share, D., & Stanovich, K. (1995). Cognitive processes in early reading development: Accommodating individual differences into a model of acquisition. *Issues in Education: Contributions to Educational Psychology, 1,* 1–57.

Share, D. J., Jorm, A. F., MacLean, R., & Matthews, R. (1984). Sources of individual differences in reading achievement. *Journal of Educational Psychology, 76,* 466–477.

Share, D. L., McGee, R., & Silva, P. D. (1989). I. Q. and reading progress: A test of the capacity notion of I. Q. *Journal of the American Academy of Child and Adolescent Psychiatry, 28,* 97–100.

Shavelson, R., & Towne, L. (2002). *Science and education.* Washington, DC: National Academy of Sciences.

Shaywitz, B. A., Shaywitz, S. E., Blachman, B., Pugh, K. R., Fulbright, R. K., Skudlarski, P., et al. (2004). Development of left occipitotemporal systems for skilled reading in children after a phonologically based intervention. *Biological Psychiatry, 55,* 926–933.

Shaywitz, B. A., Shaywitz, S. E., Pugh, K. R., Mencl, W. E., Fulbright, R. K., Constable, R. T., et al. (2002). Disruption of the neural circuitry for reading in children with developmental dyslexia. *Biological Psychiatry, 52,* 101–110.

Shaywitz, S. E. (2004). *Overcoming dyslexia.* New York: Knopf.

Shaywitz, S. E., Escobar, M. D., Shaywitz, B. A., Fletcher, J. M., & Makuch, R. (1992). Evidence that dyslexia may represent the lower tail of a normal distribution of reading ability. *New England Journal of Medicine, 326,* 145–150.

Shaywitz, S. E., Fletcher, J. M., Holahan, J. M., Schneider, A. E., Marchione, K. E., Stuebing, K. K., et al. (1999). Persistence of dyslexia: The Connecticut Longitudinal Study at adolescence. *Pediatrics, 104,* 1351–1359.

Shaywitz, S. E., Pugh, K. R., Jenner, A. R., Fulbright, R. K., Fletcher, J. M., Gore, J. C., et al. (2000). The neurobiology of reading and reading disability (dyslexia). In M. L. Kamil, P. B. Mosenthal, P. D. Pearson, & R. Barr (Eds.), *Handbook of reading research* (Vol. 3, pp. 229–249). Mahwah, NJ: Erlbaum.

Shaywitz, S. E., & Shaywitz, B. A. (2005). Dyslexia (specific reading disability). *Biological Psychiatry, 57,* 1301–1309.

Shaywitz, S. E., Shaywitz, B. A., Fletcher, J. M., & Escobar, M. D. (1990). Prevalence of reading disability in boys and girls: Results of the Connecticut Longitudinal Study. *Journal of the American Medical Association, 264,* 998–1002.

Shaywitz, S. E., Shaywitz, B. A., Pugh, K. R., Fulbright, R. K., Constable, R. T., Mencl, W. E., et al. (1998). Functional disruption in the organization of the brain for reading in dyslexia. *Proceedings of the National Academy of Sciences, 95,* 2636–2641.

Shepard, L. (1980). An evaluation of the regression discrepancy method for identifying children with learning disabilities. *Journal of Special Education, 14,* 79–91.

Siegel, L. S. (1992). An evaluation of the discrepancy definition of dyslexia. *Journal of Learning Disabilities, 25,* 618–629.

Siegel, L. S. (2003). Basic cognitive processes and reading disabilities. In H. L. Swanson, K. R. Harris, & S. Graham (Eds.), *Handbook of learning disabilities* (pp. 158–181). New York: Guilford Press.

Siegel, L. S., & Ryan, E. B. (1989). The development of working memory in normally achieving and subtypes of learning disabled. *Child Development, 60,* 973–980.

Sikora, M. D., Haley, P., Edwards, J., & Butler, R. W. (2002). Tower of London test performance in children with poor arithmetic skills. *Developmental Neuropsychology, 21,* 243–254.

Silani G., Frith, U., Demonet, J. R., Fazio, F., Perani, D., Price, C., et al. (2005). Brain abnormalities underlying altered activation in dyslexia: A voxel-based morphometry study. *Brain, 128,* 2453–2461.

Silva, P. A., McGee, R., & Williams, S. (1985). Some characteristics of 9–year-old boys with general reading backwardness or specific reading retardation. *Journal of Child Psychology and Psychiatry, 26,* 407–421.

Simmons, D. C., Kame'enui, E. J., Stoolmiller, M., Coyne, M. D., & Harn, B. (2003). Accelerating growth and maintaining proficiency: A two-year intervention study of kindergarten and first-grade children at-risk for reading difficulties. In B. R. Foorman (Ed.), *Preventing and remediating reading difficulties* (pp. 197–228). Baltimore: York Press.

Simon, T. J., Bearden, C. E., Mc-Ginn, D. M., & Zackai, E. (2005a). Visuospatial and numerical cognitive deficits in children with chromosome 22q11. 2 deletion syndrome. *Cortex, 41,* 145–155.

Simon, T. J., Bish, J. P., Bearden, C. E., Ding, L., Ferrante, S., Nguyen, V., et al. (2005b). A multilevel analysis of cognitive dysfunction and psychopathology associated with chromosome 22q11. 2 deletion syndrome in children. *Development and Psychopathology, 17,* 753–784.

Simos, P. G., Breier, J. I., Fletcher, J. M., Bergman, E., & Papanicolaou, A. C. (2000a). Cerebral mechanisms involved in word reading in dyslexia children: A magnetic source imaging approach. *Cerebral Cortex, 10,* 809–816.

Simos, P. G., Breier, J. I., Fletcher, J. M., Foorman, B. R., Bergman, E., Fishbeck, K., et al. (2000b). Brain activation profiles in dyslexic children during nonword reading: A magnetic source imaging study. *Neuroscience Reports, 29,* 61–65.

Simos, P. G., Fletcher, J. M., Bergman, E., Breier, J. I., Foorman, B. R., Castillo, E. M., et al. (2002a). Dyslexia-specific brain activation profile becomes normal following successful remedial training. *Neurology, 58,* 1–10.

Simos, P. G., Fletcher, J. M., Foorman, B. R., Francis, D. J., Castillo, E. M., Davis, R. N., et al. (2002b). Brain activation profiles during the early stages of reading acquisition. *Journal of Child Neurology, 17,* 159–163.

Simos, P. G., Fletcher, J. M., Sarkari, S., Billingsley, R. L., Francis, D. J., Castillo, E. M., et al. (2005). Early development of neurophysiological processes involved in normal reading and reading disability. *Neuropsychology, 19,* 787–798.

Simos, P. G., Fletcher, J. M., Sarkari, S., Billingsley-Marshall, R., Denton, C., & Papanicolaou, A. C. (in press). Intensive instruction affects brain magnetic activity associated with reading fluency in children with persistent reading disabilities. *Journal of Learning Disabilities.*

Simos, P. G., Papanicolaou, A. C., Breier, J. I., Fletcher, J. M., Wheless, J. W., Maggio, W. W., et al. (2000c). Insights into brain function and neural plasticity using magnetic source imaging. *Journal of Clinical Neurophysiology, 17,* 143–162.

Skinner, H. (1981). Toward the integration of classification theory and methods. *Journal of Abnormal Psychology, 90,* 68–87.

Snow, C. (2002). RAND Reading Study Group. *Reading for understanding.* Santa Monica, CA: RAND.

Snow, C., Burns, M. S., & Griffin, P. (Eds.). (1998). *Preventing reading difficulties in young children.* Washington, DC: National Academy Press.

Solan, H. A., & Richman, J. (1990). Irlen lenses: A critical appraisal. *Journal of the American Optometric Association, 61,* 789–796.

Spector, J. E. (2005). Instability of double-deficit subtypes among at-risk first grade readers. *Reading Psychology, 26,* 285–312.

Speece, D. L., & Case, L. P. (2001). Classification in context: An alternative approach to identifying early reading disability. *Journal of Educational Psychology, 93,* 735–749.

Spelke, E. A. (2005). Sex differences in intrinsic aptitude for mathematics and science? *American Psychologist, 60,* 950–958.

Spelke, E. S., & Tsivkin, S. (2001). Initial knowledge and conceptual change: Space and number. In M. Bowerman & S. Levinson (Eds.), *Language acquisition and conceptual development.* Cambridge, UK: Cambridge University Press.

Spreen, O. (1989). Learning disability, neurology, and long-term outcome: Some implications for the individual and for society. *Journal of Clinical and Experimental Neuropsychology, 11,* 389–408.

Spring, C., & French, L. (1990). Identifying reading-disabled children from listening and reading discrepancy scores. *Journal of Learning Disabilities, 23,* 53–58.

Stage, S. A., Abbott, R. D., Jenkins, J. R., & Berninger, V. W. (2003). Predicting response to early reading intervention from verbal IQ, reading-related language abilities, attention ratings, and verbal IQ-word reading discrepancy: Failure to validate the discrepancy method. *Journal of Learning Disabilities, 36,* 24–33.

Stahl, S. A. (2004). What do we know about fluency? Findings of the National Reading Panel. In P. McCardle & V. Chhabra (Eds.), *The voice of evidence in reading research* (pp. 187–212). Baltimore: Brookes.

Stahl, S. A., Heubach, K., & Cramond, B. (1997). *Fluency-oriented reading instruction.* Athens, GA/Washington, DC: National Reading Research Center/U.S. Department of Education, Office of Educational Research and Improvement, Educational Resources Information Center.

Stanovich, K. E. (1986). Matthew effects in reading: Some consequences of individual differences in the acquisition of literacy. *Reading Research Quarterly, 21,* 360–407.

Stanovich, K. E. (1988). Explaining the differences between the dyslexic and the garden-variety poor reader: The phonological–core variable-difference model. *Journal of Learning Disabilities, 21,* 590–604.

Stanovich, K. E. (1991). Discrepancy definitions of reading disability: Has intelligence led us astray? *Reading Research Quarterly, 26,* 7–29.

Stanovich, K. E. (1993). The construct validity of discrepancy definitions of reading disability. In G. R. Lyon, D. B. Gray, J. F. Kavanagh, & N. A. Krasnegor (Eds.), *Better understanding learning disabilities: New views on research and their implications for education and public policies* (pp. 273–307). Baltimore: Brookes.

Stanovich, K. E. (1994). Romance and reality. *Reading Teacher, 47,* 280–291.

Stanovich, K. E. (2000). *Progress in understanding reading.* New York: Guilford Press.

Stanovich, K. E., & Siegel, L. S. (1994). Phenotypic performance profile of children with reading disabilities: A regression-based test of the phonological–core variable-difference model. *Journal of Educational Psychology, 86,* 24–53.

Stanovich, K. E., Siegel, L. S., & Gottardo, A. (1997). Converging evidence for phonological and surface subtypes of reading disability. *Journal of Educational Psychology, 89,* 114–127.

Starkey, P., Spelke, E. S., & Gelman, R. (1991). Toward a comparative psychology of number. *Cognition, 39,* 171–172.

Stecker, P. M., Fuchs, L. S., & Fuchs, D. (2005). Using curriculum-based measurement to improve student achievement: Review of research. *Psychology in the Schools, 42,* 795–819.

Stein, J. (2001). The sensory basis of reading problems. *Developmental Neuropsychology, 20,* 509–534.

Sternberg, R. J. (1991). Are we reading too much into reading comprehension tests? *Journal of Reading, 34,* 540–545.

Sternberg, R. J., & Grigorenko, E. L. (2002). Difference scores in the identification of children with learning disabilities: It's time to use a different method. *Journal of School Psychology, 40,* 65–84.

Stevens, R., & Rosenshine, B. (1981). Advances in research on teaching. *Exceptional Education Quarterly, 2,* 1–9.

Stevenson, J., Graham, P., Fredman, G., & McLoughlin, V. (1987). A twin study of genetic influences on reading and spelling ability and disability. *Journal of Child Psychology and Psychiatry, 28,* 229–247.

Stothard, S. E., & Hulme, C. (1992). Reading comprehension difficulties in children: The role of language comprehension and working memory skills. *Reading and Writing, 4,* 245–256.

Stothard, S. E., & Hulme, C. (1996). A comparison of reading comprehension and decoding difficulties in children. In C. Cornoldi and J. Oakhill (Eds.), *Reading comprehension difficulties: Processes and intervention* (pp. 93–112). Mahwah, NJ: Erlbaum.

Strang, J. D., & Rourke, B. P. (1985). Arithmetic disability subtypes: The neuropsychological significance of specific arithmetic impairment in childhood. In B. P. Rourke (Ed.), *Neuropsychology of learning disabilities: Essentials of subtype analysis.* (pp. 167–186). New York: Guilford Press.

Strauss, A. A., & Lehtinen, L. E. (1947). *Psychopathology and education of the brain-injured child: Vol. 2. Progress in theory and clinic.* New York: Grune & Stratton.

Strauss, A. A., & Werner, H. (1943). Comparative psychopathology of the brain-injured child and the traumatic brain-injured adult. *American Journal of Psychiatry, 19,* 835–838.

Stuebing, K. K., Fletcher, J. M., LeDoux, J. M., Lyon, G. R., Shaywitz, S. E., & Shaywitz, B. A. (2002). Validity of IQ-discrepancy classifications of reading disabilities: A meta-analysis. *American Educational Research Journal, 39,* 469–518.

Swanson, H. L., & Beebe-Frankenberger, M. (2004). The relationship between working memory and mathematical problem solving in children at risk and not at risk for serious math difficulties. *Journal of Educational Psychology, 96,* 471–491.

Swanson, H. L., Harris, K., & Graham, S. (Eds.). (2003). *Handbook of learning disabilities.* New York: Guilford Press.

Swanson, H. L. (with Hoskyn, M., & Lee, C.). (1999). *Interventions for students with learning disabilities: A meta-analysis of treatment outcome.* New York: Guilford Press.

Swanson, H. L., & Sachse-Lee, C. (2001). A subgroup analysis of working memory in children with reading disabilities: Domain-general or domain-specific deficiency? *Journal of Learning Disabilities, 34,* 249–263.

Swanson, H. L., & Siegel, L. (2001). Learning disabilities as a working memory deficit. *Issues in Education, 7,* 1–48.

Tager-Flusberg, H., & Cooper, J. (1999). Present and future possibilities for defining a phenotype for specific language impairment. *Journal of Speech, Language, and Hearing Research, 42,* 1275–1278.

Talcott, J. B., Witton, C., McClean, M., Hansen, P. C., Rees, A., Green, G. G. R., et al. (2000). Visual and auditory transient sensitivity determines word decoding skills. *Proceedings of the Natural Academy of Sciences USA, 97,* 2952–2958.

Tallal, P. (1980). Auditory temporal perception, phonics, and reading disabilities in children. *Brain and Language, 9,* 182–198.

Tallal, P. (2004). Improving language and literacy is a matter of time. *Perspectives, 5,* 721–728.

Tan, L. H. Spinks, J. A., Eden, G. F., Perfetti, C. A., & Siok, W. T. (2005). Reading depends on writing, in Chinese. *Proceedings of the National Academy of Sciences USA, 102,* 8781–8785.

Tannock, R., Martinussen, R., & Frijters, J. (2000). Naming speed performance and stimulant effects indicate effortful, semantic processing deficits in attention-deficit/hyperactivity disorder. *Journal of Abnormal Child Psychology, 28*, 237–252.

Taylor, H. G., & Fletcher, J. M. (1983). Biological foundations of specific developmental disorders: Methods, findings, and future directions. *Journal of Child Clinical Psychology, 12*, 46–65.

Temple, E., Deutsch, G. K., Poldrack, R. A., Miller, S. L., Tallal, P., Merzenich, M. M., et al. (2003). Neural deficits in children with dyslexia ameliorated by behavioral remediation: Evidence from functional MRI. *Proceedings of the National Academy of Sciences, 100*, 2860–2865.

Thaler, V., Ebner, E. M., Wimmer, H., & Landerl, K. (2004). Training reading fluency in dysfluent readers with high reading accuracy: Word specific effects but low transfer to untrained words. *Annals of Dyslexia, 54*, 89–113.

Tiu, R. D., Jr., Wadsworth, S. J., Olson, R. K., & DeFries, J. C. (2004). Causal models of reading disability: A twin study. *Twin Research, 7*, 275–283.

Tomblin, J. B., & Zhang, X. (1999). Language patterns and etiology in children with specific language impairment. In H. Tager-Flusberg (Ed.), *Neurodevelopmental disorders* (pp. 361–382). Cambridge, MA: MIT Press.

Torgesen, J. K. (1991). Learning disabilities: Historical and conceptual issues. In B. Wong (Ed.), *Learning about learning disabilities* (pp. 3–39). San Diego: Academic Press.

Torgesen, J. K. (2000). Individual responses in response to early interventions in reading: The lingering problem of treatment resisters. *Learning Disabilities Research and Practice, 15*, 55–64.

Torgesen, J. K. (2002). Empirical and theoretical support for direct diagnosis of learning disabilities by assessment of intrinsic processing weaknesses. In R. Bradley, L. Danielson, & D. Hallahan (Eds.), *Identification of learning disabilities: Research to practice* (pp. 565–650). Mahwah, NJ: Erlbaum.

Torgesen, J. K. (2004). Lessons learned from research on interventions for students who have difficulty learning to read. In P. McCardle & V. Chhabra (Eds.), *The voice of evidence in reading research* (pp. 355–382). Baltimore: Brookes.

Torgesen, J. K., Alexander, A. W., Wagner, R. K., Rashotte, C. A., Voeller, K. K. S., & Conway, T. (2001). Intensive remedial instruction for children with severe reading disabilities: Immediate and long-term outcomes from two instructional approaches. *Journal of Learning Disabilities, 34*, 33–58.

Torgesen, J. K., Wagner, R. K., & Rashotte, C. (1999a). *Test of Word Reading Efficiency*. Austin, TX: PRO-ED.

Torgesen, J. K., Wagner, R. K., Rashotte, C. A., Rose, E., Lindamood, P., Conway, J., et al. (1999b). Preventing reading failure in young children with phonological processing disabilities: Group and individual responses to instruction. *Journal of Educational Psychology, 91*, 579–594.

Treiman, R., & Kessler, B. (2005). Writing systems and spelling development. *The science of reading: A handbook* (pp. 120–134). Oxford, UK: Blackwell.

Tunmer, W. E., Chapman, J. W., & Prochnow, J. E. (2003). Preventing negative Matthew effects in at-risk readers: A retrospective study. In B. R. Foorman (Ed.), *Preventing and remediating reading difficulties* (pp. 121–164). Baltimore: York Press.

U.S. Department of Education. (1999). 34 CFR Parts 300 and 303: Assistance to the states for the education of children with disabilities and the early intervention program for infants and toddlers with disabilities. Final regulations. *Federal Register, 64*, 12406–12672.

U.S. Department of Education. (2006). 34 CFR Parts 300 and 301: Assistance to states for the education of children with disabilities and preschool grants for children with disabilities. Final rules. *Federal Register, 71,* 46540–46845.

U.S. Office of Education. (1968). *First annual report of the National Advisory Committee on Handicapped Children.* Washington, DC: U.S. Department of Health, Education and Welfare.

U.S. Office of Education. (1977). Assistance to states for education for handicapped children: Procedures for evaluating specific learning disabilities. *Federal Register, 42,* G1082–G1085.

Vadasy, P. F., Sanders, E. A., Peyton, J. A., & Jenkins, J. R. (2002). Timing and intensity of tutoring: A closer look at the conditions for effective early literacy tutoring. *Learning Disabilities Research and Practice, 17,* 227–241.

Van den Broek, P., Rapp, D. N., & Kendeou, P. (2005). Integrating memory-based and constructional processes in accounts of reading comprehension. *Discourse Processes, 39,* 299–316.

VanDerHeyden, A. M., & Burns, M. K. (2005). Using curriculum-based assessment and curriculum-based measurement to guide elementary mathematics instruction: Effect on individual and group accountability scores. *Assessment for Effective Intervention, 30,* 15–31.

van der Wissell, A., & Zegers, F. E. (1985). Reading retardation revisited. *British Journal of Developmental Psychology, 3,* 3–9.

Vaughn, S., & Fuchs, L. S. (2003). Redefining learning disabilities as inadequate response to instruction: The promise and potential problems. *Learning Disabilities Research and Practice, 18,* 137–146.

Vaughn, S., & Klingner, J. K. (2004). Teaching reading comprehension to students with learning disabilities. In C. A. Stone, E. R. Silliman, B. J. Ehren, & K. Apel (Eds.), *Handbook of language and literacy: Development and disorders* (pp. 541–555). New York: Guilford Press.

Vaughn, S., Klingner, J. K., & Bryant, D. P. (2001). Collaborative strategic reading as a means to enhance peer-mediated instruction for reading comprehension and content-area learning. *Remedial and Special Education, 22,* 66–74.

Vaughn, S., Linan-Thompson, S., & Hickman, P. (2003a). Response to treatment as a means of identifying students with reading/learning disabilities. *Exceptional Children, 69,* 391–409.

Vaughn, S., Linan-Thompson, S., Kouzekanani, K., Bryant, D. P., Dickson, S., & Blozis, S. A. (2003b). Reading instruction grouping for students with reading difficulties. *Remedial and Special Education, 24,* 301–315.

Vaughn, S. R., Moody, S. W., & Schumm, J. S. (1998). Broken promises: Reading instruction in the resource room. *Exceptional Children, 64,* 211–225.

Vaughn, S. R., Wanzek, J., Woodruff, A. L., & Linan-Thompson, S. (in press). A three-tier model for preventing reading difficulties and early identification of students with reading disabilities. In D. H. Haager, S. R. Vaughn, & J. K. Klingner (Eds.), *Validated reading practices for three tiers of intervention.* Baltimore: Brookes.

Vellutino, F. R. (1979). *Dyslexia: Theory and research.* Cambridge, MA: MIT Press.

Vellutino, F. R., Fletcher, J. M., Scanlon, D. M., & Snowling, M. J. (2004). Specific reading disability (dyslexia): What have we learned in the past four decades? *Journal of Child Psychiatry and Psychology, 45,* 2–40.

Vellutino, F. R., Scanlon, D. M., & Jaccard, J. (2003). Toward distinguishing between cognitive and experiential deficits as primary sources of difficulty in learning to read: A two-year follow-up to difficult to remediate and readily remediated poor readers. In B. R. Foorman (Ed.), *Preventing and remediating reading difficulties* (pp. 73–120). Baltimore: York Press.

Vellutino, F. R., Scanlon, D. M., & Lyon, G. R. (2000). Differentiating between difficult-to-remediate and readily remediated poor readers: More evidence against the IQ–achievement discrepancy definition for reading disability. *Journal of Learning Disabilities, 33,* 223–238.

Vellutino, F. R., Scanlon, D. M., Sipay, E. R., Small, S. G., Pratt, A., Chen, R., et al. (1996). Cognitive profiles of difficult-to-remediate and readily remediated poor readers: Early intervention as a vehicle for distinguishing between cognitive and experimental deficits as basic causes of specific reading disability. *Journal of Educational Psychology, 88,* 601–638.

Vellutino, F. R., Scanlon, D. M., Small, S., & Fanuele, D. P. (2006). Response to intervention as a vehicle for distinguishing between children with and without reading disabilities: Evidence for the role of kindergarten and first-grade interventions. *Journal of Learning Disabilities, 39,* 157–169.

Vellutino, F. R., Scanlon, D. M., & Tanzman, M. S. (1994). Components of reading ability: Issues and problems in operationalizing word identification, phonological coding, and orthographic coding. In G. R. Lyon (Ed.), *Frames of reference for the assessment of learning disabilities: New views on measurement issues* (pp. 279–329). Baltimore: Brookes.

Vukovic, R. K., & Siegel, L. S. (2006). The double-deficit hypothesis: A comprehensive analysis of the evidence. *Journal of Learning Disabilities, 39,* 25–47.

Waber, D. P., Forbes, P. W., Wolff, P. H., & Weiler, M. D. (2004). Neurodevelopmental characteristics of children with learning impairments classified according to the double-deficit hypothesis. *Journal of Learning Disabilities, 37,* 451–461.

Waber, D. P., Weiler, M. D., Wolff, P. H., Bellinger, D., Marcus, D. J., Ariel, R., et al. (2001). Processing of rapid auditory stimuli in school-age children referred for evaluation of learning disorders. *Child Development, 72,* 37–49.

Waber, D. P., Wolff, P. H., Forbes, P. W., & Weiler, M. D. (2000). Rapid automatized naming in children referred for evaluation of heterogeneous learning problems: How specific are naming speed deficits to reading disability? *Child Neuropsychology, 6,* 251–261.

Wadsworth, S. J., Olson, R. K., Pennington, B. F., & DeFries, J. C. (2000). Differential genetic etiology of reading disability as a function of IQ. *Journal of Learning Disabilities, 33,* 192–199.

Wagner, R. K., Torgesen, J. K., & Rashotte, C. A. (1994). The development of reading-related phonological processing abilities: New evidence of bi-directional causality from a latent variable longitudinal study. *Developmental Psychology, 30,* 73–87.

Wagner, R. K., Torgesen, J. K., Rashotte, C. A., & Hecht, S. A. (1997). Changing relations between phonological processing abilities and word-level reading as children develop from beginning to skilled readers: A 5-year longitudinal study. *Developmental Psychology, 33,* 468–479.

Wakely, M. B., Hooper, S. R., de Kruif, R. E. L, & Swartz, C. (2006). Subtypes of written expression in elementary school children: A linguistic-based model. *Developmental Neuropsychology, 29,* 125–159.

Wechsler, D. (2001). *Wechsler Individual Achievement Test* (2nd ed.). San Antonio, TX: Psychological Corporation.

Wernicke, C. (1894). *Grundriss der psychiatrie in Klinischen vorlesungen.* Leipzig, Germany: G. Thieme.

Wesson, C. L. (1991). Curriculum-based measurement and two models of follow-up consultation. *Exceptional Children, 57,* 246–257.

Wiederholt, J. L. (1974). Historical perspectives on the education of the learning disabled. In L. Mann & D. A. Sabatino (Eds.), *The second review of special education* (pp. 103–152). Austin TX: PRO-ED.

Wiederholt, J. L., & Bryant, B. R. (2001). *Gray Oral Reading Tests* (4th ed.). Austin, TX: PRO-ED.

Wiig, E. H., Neilsen, N. P., Minthon, L., McPeek, D., Said, K., & Warkentin, S. (2002). Parietal lobe activation in rapid, automatized naming by adults. *Perceptual and Motor Skills, 94,* 1230–1244.

Wilder, A. A., & Williams, J. P. (2001). Students with severe learning disabilities can learn higher-order comprehension skills. *Journal of Educational Psychology, 93,* 268–278.

Wilkinson, G. (1993). *Wide Range Achievement Test–3.* Wilmington, DE: Wide Range.

Willcutt, E. G., & Pennington, B. F. (2000). Psychiatric comorbidity in children and adolescents with reading disability. *Journal of Child Psychology and Psychiatry, 41,* 1039–1048.

Williams, K. T., Cassidy, J., & Samuels, S. J. (2001). *Group Reading Assessment and Diagnostic Education.* Circle Pines, MN: American Guidance Services.

Williams, J. P. (2002). Using the Theme Scheme to improve story comprehension. In C. C. Block & M. Pressley (Eds.), *Comprehension instruction: Research-based best practices* (pp. 126–139). New York: Guilford Press.

Williams, J. P. (2003). Teaching text structure to improve reading comprehension. In H. L. Swanson, K. R. Harris, & S. Graham (Eds.), *Handbook of learning disabilities* (pp. 293–305). New York: Guilford Press.

Williams, J. P., Hall, K. M., Lauer, K. D., Stafford, B., DeSisto, L. A., & deCani, J. S. (2005). Expository text comprehension in the primary grade classroom. *Journal of Educational Psychology, 97,* 538–550.

Williams, J. P., Lauer, K. D., Hall, K. M., Lord, K. M., Gugga, S. S., Bak, S. J., et al. (2002). Teaching elementary students to identify story themes. *Journal of Educational Psychology, 94,* 235–248.

Wilson, K. M., & Swanson, H. L. (2001). Are mathematics disabilities due to a domain-general or a domain-specific working memory deficit? *Journal of Learning Disabilities, 34,* 237–248.

Wimmer, H., & Mayringer, H. (2002). Dysfluent reading in the absence of spelling difficulties: A specific disability in regular orthographies. *Journal of Educational Psychology, 94,* 272–277.

Wimmer, H., Mayringer, H., & Landerl, K. (2000). The double-deficit hypothesis and difficulties in learning to read a regular orthography. *Journal of Educational Psychology, 92,* 668–680.

Wimmer, H., Mayringer, H., & Raberger, T. (1999). Reading and dual-task balancing: Evidence against the automatization deficit explanation of developmental dyslexia. *Journal of Learning Disabilities, 32,* 473–478.

Wise, B., Ring, J., & Olson, R. K. (1999). Training phonological awareness with and without attention to articulation. *Journal of Experimental Child Psychology, 72,* 271–304.

Wise, B., Ring, J., & Olson, R. K. (2000). Individual differences in gains from computer-assisted remedial reading with more emphasis on phonological analysis or accurate reading in context. *Journal of Experimental Child Psychology, 77,* 197–235.

Wolf, M., & Bowers, P. G. (1999). The double-deficit hypothesis for the developmental dyslexias. *Journal of Educational Psychology, 91,* 415–438.

Wolf, M., Miller, L., & Donnelly, K. (2002). Retrieval, Automaticity, Vocabulary Elaboration, Orthography (RAVE-O): A comprehensive, fluency-based reading intervention program. *Journal of Learning Disabilities, 33,* 375–386.

Wolf, M., & Obregon, M. (1992). Early naming deficits, developmental dyslexia, and a specific deficit hypothesis. *Brain and Language, 42,* 19–47.

Wolf, M., O'Brien, B., Adams, K. D., Joffe, T., Jeffrey, J., Lovett, M., et al. (2003). Working for time: Reflections on naming speed, reading fluency, and intervention. In B. R. Foorman (Ed.), *Preventing and remediating reading difficulties* (pp. 355–380). Baltimore: York Press.

Wolff, P. (1993). Impaired temporal resolution in developmental dyslexia: Temporal information processing in the nervous system. In P. Tallal, A. Galaburda, R. Llinas, & C. von Euler (Eds.), *Annals of the New York Academy of Sciences, 682,* 87–103.

Wong, B. Y. L. (1991). The relevance of metacognition to learning disabilities. In B. Y. L. Wong (Ed.), *Learning about learning disabilities* (pp. 231–258). San Diego: Academic Press.

Wood, F. B., & Felton, R. H. (1994). Separate linguistic and attentional factors in the development of reading. *Topics in Language Disorders, 14,* 42–57.

Wood, F. B., Felton, R. H., Flowers, L., & Naylor, C. (1991). Neurobehavioral definition of dyslexia. In D. D. Duane & D. B. Gray (Eds.), *The reading brain: The biological basis of dyslexia* (pp. 1–26). Parkton, MD: York Press.

Wood, F. B., & Grigorenko, E. L. (2001). Emerging issues in the genetics of dyslexia: A methodological preview. *Journal of Learning Disabilities, 34,* 503–512.

Woodcock, R., McGrew, K., & Mather, N. (2001). *Woodcock–Johnson III Tests of Achievement.* Itasca, IL: Riverside.

World Health Organization. (1992). *The ICD-10 classification of mental and behavioral disorders: Clinical descriptions and diagnostic guidelines.* Geneva: Author.

Wristers, K. J., Francis, D. J., Foorman, B. R., Fletcher, J. M., & Swank, P. R. (2002). Growth in precursor reading skills: Do low-achieving and IQ-discrepant readers develop differently? *Learning Disability Research and Practice, 17,* 19–34.

Wynn, K. (1992). Addition and subtraction by human infants. *Nature, 358,* 749–750.

Wynn, K. (2002). Do infants have numerical expectations or just perceptual preferences? *Developmental Science, 5,* 207–209.

Ysseldyke, J. E., & Marston, D. (1999). Origins of categorical special education services in schools and a rationale for changing them. In D. Reschly, W. Tilly, & J. Grimes (Eds.), *Special education in transition* (pp. 1–18). Longmont, CO: Sopris West.

Zabell, C., & Everatt, J. (2002). Surface and phonological subtypes of adult developmental dyslexia. *Dyslexia, 8,* 160–177.

Zeleke, S. (2004). Self-concepts of students with learning disabilities and their normally achieving peers: A review. *European Journal of Special Needs Education, 19,* 145–170.

Ziegler, J. C., & Goswami, U. (2005). Reading acquisition, developmental dyslexia, and skilled reading across languages: A psycholinguistic grain size theory. *Psychological Bulletin, 131,* 3–29.

Ziegler, J. C., Perry, C., Ma-Wyatt, A., Ladner, D., & Schulte-Korne, G. (2003). Developmental dyslexia in different languages: Language-specific or universal? *Journal of Experimental Child Psychology, 86,* 169–193.

Zigmond, N. (1993). Learning disabilities from an educational perspective. In G. R. Lyon, D. B. Gray, J. F. Kavanagh, & N. A. Krasnegor (Eds.), *Better understanding learning disabilities: New views from research and their implications for education and public policies* (pp. 27–56). Baltimore: Brookes.

Zigmond, N. (2003). Searching for the most effective service delivery model for students with learning disabilities. In H. L. Swanson, K. R. Harris, & S. Graham (Eds.), *Handbook of learning disabilities* (pp. 110–124). New York: Guilford Press.

Zinkstok, J., & van Amelsvoort, T. (2005). Neuropsychological profile and neuroimaging in patients with 22Q11. 2 deletion syndrome: A review. *Child Neuropsychology, 11,* 21–37.

Index